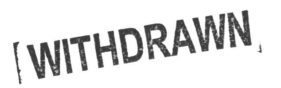

Delirium

Delirium
Acute confusional states in palliative medicine

SECOND EDITION

Augusto Caraceni

Chief Palliative Care, Pain Therapy and Rehabilitation,
Fondazione IRCCS Istituto Nazionale dei Tumori, Milan, Italy

Professor of Palliative Medicine,
Department of Cancer and molecular biology,
Norwegian University of Science and Tecnology NTNU,
Trondheim, Norway

and

Luigi Grassi

Professor and Chair of Psychiatry, Section of Psychiatry,
Chair Department of Medical and Surgical Disciplines of
Communication and Behaviour, University of Ferrara, Italy;

Chief Clinical and Emergency Psychiatry Unit, Integrated
Department of Mental Health and Drug Abuse, Ferrara, Italy

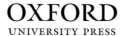

OXFORD
UNIVERSITY PRESS

OXFORD

UNIVERSITY PRESS

Great Clarendon Street, Oxford OX2 6DP

Oxford University Press is a department of the University of Oxford.
It furthers the University's objective of excellence in research, scholarship,
and education by publishing worldwide in

Oxford New York

Auckland Cape Town Dar es Salaam Hong Kong Karachi
Kuala Lumpur Madrid Melbourne Mexico City Nairobi
New Delhi Shanghai Taipei Toronto

With offices in

Argentina Austria Brazil Chile Czech Republic France Greece
Guatemala Hungary Italy Japan Poland Portugal Singapore
South Korea Switzerland Thailand Turkey Ukraine Vietnam

Oxford is a registered trade mark of Oxford University Press
in the UK and in certain other countries

Published in the United States
by Oxford University Press Inc., New York

First published 2003
Second edition published 2011

British Library Cataloguing in Publication Data
Data available

Library of Congress Cataloging-in-Publication Data
Caraceni, Augusto.
    Delirium : acute confusional states in palliative medicine /
Augusto Caraceni and Luigi Grassi. — 2nd ed.
        p. ; cm.
    Includes bibliographical references and index.
    ISBN 978-0-19-957205-2
 1. Delirium. 2. Palliative treatment. I. Grassi, Luigi. II. Title.
 [DNLM: 1. Delirium. 2. Palliative Care—methods. WL 340]
    RC520.7.C37 2011
    616.8'4—dc22
                                                2010040668

Typeset in Minion by Glyph International Bangalore, India
Printed in Great Britain
on acid-free paper by
CPI Antony Rowe, Chippenham, Wiltshire

ISBN 978–0–19–957205–2

10 9 8 7 6 5 4 3 2 1

This book is dedicated to
Giannina Rita and Valeria,
Giuseppe and Tommaso,
Cinzia and Francesca,
Eleonora, Davide, and Marco

Foreword to the first edition

Delirium is among the most prevalent and challenging clinical problems. Its assessment and management must be individualized based on both a biomedical understanding of the disease and its comorbidities, and a more nuanced understanding of the prognosis, risks, and benefits of treatment. Every intervention must be informed by a critical understanding of the changing goals of care. These complexities are critically explored in this volume.

Given the diversity of clinical presentations associated with neurological and psychiatric disorders in the medically ill, considerable efforts have been made during the past decade to derive meaningful diagnostic criteria for delirium. Consensus on diagnostic criteria is needed as a foundation for future investigations focused on the epidemiology, aetiologies, and treatments of this disorder. Even distinctions that appear simple in some populations, such as the difference between delirium and dementia, can become clouded when an underlying disease is progressing and the patient is exposed to complex therapies for the disease itself and for its consequences. If an acute confusional state that is expected to be transitory never clears, should it still be called a delirium? If one or two of the elements that together characterize delirium—for example, changes in alertness, psychomotor activity, cognition, perception, mood, or sleep–wake cycle—occur in isolation, is this delirium?

One of the most important barriers to the adequate treatment and management of delirium is the fact that it is so commonly under-recognized or misdiagnosed. Its protean manifestations make it a syndrome that is often misdiagnosed.

The development of validated measures to identify delirium, and grade its severity, has been an important advance. These developments highlight the need for additional studies that will clarify the phenomenology of delirium, establish evidence-based criteria for diagnosis, and rationalize the type of clinical assessment that is needed to define a treatment strategy. Studies that separately assess consciousness, cognition, perception, and mood potentially could define subpopulations that may benefit from more targeted interventions. Ultimately, treatable pathophysiologies linked to a particular phenomenology might be elucidated.

Even the most sophisticated research, however, will never obviate the clinical challenge in managing delirium in populations with advanced illness. Death is commonly preceded by a period of somnolence or confusion, which may be as brief as hours or as long as months. Although the decline might be attributable to specific biomedical causes, it is not considered pathological if it is perceived to be part of the normal dying process. If this is the case, interventions are limited to those necessary to ensure comfort and reassure the family. Efforts to assess and reverse the underlying causes, which are essential in other clinical settings, would be inappropriate here.

Thus, the clinical problem of delirium resonates with a broad range of profound challenges in palliative care. Clinicians are notoriously poor prognosticators; yet some understanding of the time left is needed to inform judgements about the evaluation and management of delirium. If there is a chance for meaningful survival, and the goals of care are consistent with this, the delirious patient may undergo a very aggressive evaluation and complex interventions designed to reduce contributing causes and reverse the disorder. If the patient is perceived to be imminently dying, however, the overriding concern may be the control of agitation or fear. No effort is then made to identify or treat potential causes.

Ethical considerations are prominent in this decision-making and are under intense discussion among specialists in palliative care. Should the delirious patient at the end of life empirically receive hydration, a simple intervention that would reverse one potential contributing factor? Or does the belief that death is imminent preclude this intervention? If the delirious patient is agitated, what are the ethical considerations in using sedative doses of drugs until death occurs? These are complex issues, and require case-by-case reasoning.

Delirium is not a disorder whose impact is confined to the patient alone, particularly in the palliative care setting. Recent studies (Breitbart, et al. 2002a; 43: 183–94) suggest that delirium in the palliative care setting is distressing for patients, family members, and health care providers. While patients experience high levels of delirium-related distress, particularly when delirium is accompanied by delusions and paranoia, family members score even higher than their loved ones who are delirious, on measures of distress. Many family members become distraught at the thought that in addition to a terminal physical illness, their loved one now has a 'psychiatric' illness and has 'lost his/her mind'; an emotional or cognitive death where they have lost the patient as a 'human being'. Then they experience a 'second death' when the patient physically dies. Nurses are highly distressed as well when caring for dying delirious patients. Caring for these patients is very emotionally difficult work for all concerned. These data suggest that educational interventions for families and care-givers on the true medical nature of delirium and what can be expected in the dying process regarding delirium may be beneficial. They also make the case, as is made in this text, that delirium can be expected to occur as part of the dying process and that not only should families and caregivers be prepared for this event they should also be aware of it as a harbinger of decline and impending death. Important discussions regarding treatment preferences and advanced directives, rituals of reconciliation and forgiveness, and other practical issues should take place in advance of the inevitable delirium. The events of delirium, given their potential for causing distress in families, inevitably influence the bereavement process, and must be considered in the aftercare of family members.

In conclusion the scientific and clinical characterization of delirium is as yet rudimentary, but clinicians must do the best they can. The need for mutual and comprehensive cooperation by a variety of disciplines (i.e. medicine, palliative care practitioners, neurologists, and psychiatrists) emerges as an important message from this book in which Caraceni and Grassi offer a critical evaluation of the existing literature and recommendations for a holistic approach to this complex syndrome.

The authors' personal experiences, as shown by a number of clinical examples, provide a good foundation for the challenges faced at the bedside. The addition of appendices with many of the most utilized delirium tools is a great advantage of this textbook.

February 2003

Russell K. Portenoy MD
Chairman, Department of Pain
Medicine and Palliative Care,
Beth Israel Medical Center,
New York, NY Professor of Neurology,
Albert Einstein College of Medicine,
Bronx, New York

William Breitbart, MD,
Chief, Psychiatry Service, Department of
Psychiatry and Behavioral Sciences,
Attending Psychiatrist, Pain and
Palliative Care Service, Department of
Neurology, Memorial Sloan-Kettering
Cancer Center, New York, NY and
Professor of Psychiatry, Department of
Psychiatry, Weill Medical College of
Cornell University, New York

Foreword to the second edition

When I was asked to write a foreword to the second edition of this book by Caraceni and Grassi on delirium in palliative medicine, I looked back at my copy of the first edition, which I discovered was well-worn, heavily underlined, and marked with innumerable tabs. I then read the manuscript of this edition and found it to be equally valuable.

Delirium is a common, serious, and often unrecognized complication of medical and surgical illness in hospitalized patients, particularly in the elderly and in the palliative care setting. When delirium complicates the patient's illness, it prolongs hospitalization, increases mortality, and distresses both the patient and the patient's loved ones. Delirium has many symptoms and a myriad of underlying causes making diagnosis and treatment challenging. Even the criteria for diagnosis, as this book points out, differ somewhat in different classification systems. However, all agree that delirium is a disorder of attention and alertness.

At Memorial Sloan-Kettering Cancer Center, delirium is among the most common reason for physicians and surgeons to request a neurologic or psychiatric consultation. Unfortunately, the number of consultations underestimates the problem as delirium is frequently unrecognized by caregivers, although more likely to be recognized by family and nurses than by physicians.

Delirium presents in two major but not mutually exclusive forms: quiet and withdrawn (hypoactive) or hyperactive and agitated. In as many as one-half of patients suffering from the hypoactive form, the abnormality is unrecognized or, if recognized, is mistaken for depression associated with the medical illness. However, even brief daily bedside mental status examinations by the patient's physicians using some of the instruments tabulated in this book will usually establish the diagnosis. Moreover, examination of the mental status of all patients on admission to the hospital may reveal risk factors, such as mild to moderate dementia, that may predict the subsequent appearance of delirium.

Establishing the cause of delirium is often more difficult than making the diagnosis and may require careful physical examination, laboratory evaluation, and diagnostic imaging. All too frequently, more than one cause is found, particularly in critically ill patients. However, successfully treating one of the several causes often ameliorates the delirium. Even if one cannot identify and treat the underlying cause, supportive care is often helpful. Frequent visits by family members, repeated attempts to orient the patient, and removal of distractions are all helpful interventions. In some patients, methylphenidate is beneficial.

The hyperactive form of delirium characterized by agitation, tremulousness, and hallucinations is easy to diagnose but often difficult to treat. Patients may do themselves considerable harm, particularly in the postoperative period, by removing dressings and catheters. Drugs such as haloperidol are mandatory and some patients require restraints.

Physicians and other caregivers must learn to recognize delirium in all of its forms and prescribe appropriate treatment, whether that be medication or supportive care. This excellent updating of delirium and its treatment by Caraceni and Grassi will substantially assist physicians in delivering appropriate care.

Jerome B. Posner M.D.
Attending Neurologist
Memorial Sloan-Kettering Cancer Center
New York
USA

Preface to the first edition

Delirium is a complex syndrome with a multifactorial aetiology and is characterized by marked disturbances of consciousness, attention, memory, perception, thought, and the sleep–wake cycle, and by fluctuation of symptoms. Over the last few years, clinicians, especially in geriatric and intensive care settings, have concentrated on delirium. However, since delirium is also very frequent in palliative care settings, attention to this topic has progressively increased among palliative care physicians. In fact, patients who are affected by serious and incurable diseases, have multiple organ failures, receive multiple pharmacological treatments, and are often advanced in age and are at an increased risk for the development of the disorder.

A good description of what could correspond to prodromal symptoms of delirium, and to a pre-delirium state in a patient with a rapidly disseminating disease, is given by Alessandro Manzoni (1840; English translation 1972) in the last part of the famous novel *I promessi sposi* (*The Betrothed*). At the height of the pestilence, which affected Milan in the second decade of 1600, Don Rodrigo, one of the co-protagonists, who is already affected by plague, is returning home at night: 'as he walked along', Manzoni writes, 'he began to feel a discomfort, a fatigue, a weakness in the legs, a difficulty in drawing breath, and a feeling of internal burning which he would have been only happy to attribute to the wine he had drunk... .' Then, when Don Rodrigo is going to bed,

> the blankets seemed to weigh a ton. He threw them back, curled up and tried to doze off, for he was half dead with the need for sleep. But his eyes had only been shut for a moment when he woke up again with a jerk, as if someone had spitefully given him a shake... . After much tossing and turning, he finally got to sleep, and began to dream the ugliest and most tangled dreams in the world. As they went on, he seemed to find himself in a great church, right in the middle of it, among a huge crowd. He stood there, without any idea of how he had got there, especially at that time; and this infuriated him. He looked at those who were around him. All of them had yellowish emaciated faces, with dazed, unseeing eyes and hanging lips. The rags in which they were clad were falling off them, and through the gaps he could see the bubonic swellings and discoloured patches that were the symptoms of the plague. 'Out of my way, you swine!' he cried in his dream, looking at the door, which was a great way off. Though he accompanied the words with a threatening scowl, he did not raise his hand, but rather shrank into himself, to avoid further contact with those filthy bodies, which already pressed upon him all too closely from every side. But none of those crazy figures showed any sign of wanting to get out of his way, or even of having heard him. In fact they crowded in upon him more tightly than ever, and one of them in particular seemed to be jabbing him with something, perhaps an elbow, in the left side, between heart and armpit. Don Rodrigo felt a painful pricking sensation there, a feeling of heaviness. And as he twisted away to try and free himself from it, something else, at once, seemed to prick him in the same spot. Angered by this, he felt for his sword; but it seemed to have been jostled half out of its scabbard by the crowd, so that it was its hilt that had been pressing against his side. But he put his hand there, there was no sign of the sword, and he felt a yet sharper stab. He shouted; he was all out of breath; he was trying to shout

louder still; and then it seemed as if all those faces suddenly turned to look in one direction. He glanced that way too, and saw a pulpit, over the edge of which appeared something round and smooth and shining. Then a bald cranium rose clearly to view, followed by a pair of eyes, the rest of a face, and the long white beard. A friar stood there, visible from the waist upwards above the edge of the pulpit. It was Father Cristoforo. His threatening gaze passed all round the whole audience, and finally seemed to fix itself on Don Rodrigo. The friar's hand was raised in the same attitude as when he had denounced Don Rodrigo in one of the great rooms of his palace. Then Don Rodrigo raised his own hand quickly and made a violent effort trying to leap forward and grab that outstretched arm. Words which had been choking in his gullet burst forth in a terrible scream and he woke up... he had some difficulty in regaining consciousness.

Manzoni continues:

he felt violent stifling palpitations of the heart, a constant buzzing or whistling in his ears, a burning in his body and a heaviness in his limbs, worse than when he had gone to bed... . he was aware that his mental processes were growing darker and more confused, and felt the approach of a moment when he would have no thought left in his head except the thought of abandoning himself to utter despair.

That Don Rodrigo is severely ill and his physical and mental status is rapidly deteriorating is apparent, since, as the novel continues, we find Don Rodrigo dying in the lazzareto, where he has been cast by *monatti*: 'The unhappy man was stretched out motionless. His eyes were wide open, but unseeing, his face pale and covered with dark blotches. His lips were black and swollen. It might have been the face of a corpse, except for a violent contraction of the features which bore witness to a tenacious will to live. His chest heaved from time to time in a painful struggle for breath.'

In spite of its prevalence and the relevance and the distressing nature of its symptoms for the patient (and his/her family), and the high mortality, delirium goes often unrecognized and is not properly treated in palliative care settings.

In starting to write this book, we had some considerations in mind and some challenges to address. First, as neurologists and psychiatrists, we are often involved in palliative care programmes on a consultation basis, while the integration of these disciplines in palliative care might greatly contribute to the field, as far as delirium is concerned. Second, regarding the assessment of delirium, most of the available instruments were elaborated by psychiatrists and geriatricians and tested on specific populations other than patients in an advanced phase of illness, including terminally ill patients. Therefore, testing these instruments on the more heterogeneous palliative care population and training palliative care teams on the use of the assessment methods are important aims for both clinical and research reasons. Third, in considering the dying population, the actual prevalence of delirium is unknown. If brain failure is part of the process of dying and the dying process is not an acute event, it is likely that delirium could be considered as part of the dying process itself. This condition has not been fully described. Fourth, often delirium cannot be promptly reversed both in the terminal cases and in patients with potential for recovery. It is distressing for the patient and the family and palliative treatment is required. Palliative care professionals have therefore more than one responsibility in mastering the diagnosis, management, and treatment of this disorder. Fifth, the development of home-care assistance for terminally ill patients in many countries, including Italy, run by primary care physicians and/or primary care teams coordinated by general practitioners, makes evident the need for specific training in this underrecognized clinical area.

This book is designed to address these problems and to provide palliative care professionals with what our experience and the most recent literature can offer in terms of theory and clinical practice with regard to the classification, aetiology, phenomenology, and management of delirium. We hope this book will also provide a stimulus to further exploration of this area and to a more integrated approach in daily assistance to terminally ill patients and their families.

In Chapter 1, we focus attention on the definition and conceptualization of delirium over time, starting with the historical roots of Hippocratic medicine, through the first attempt of classification during the nineteenth and early twentieth centuries, to the most recent classifications of the World Health Organization (1992; *International Classification of Disease*—ICD-10) and the American Psychiatric Association (2000; *Diagnostic and Statistical Manual of Mental Disorders*—DSM-IV-TR).

Chapter 2 addresses the neuropathophysiology of delirium, including the anatomical, neurotransmitter, metabolic, and molecular levels of dysfunction, which are considered to be involved in the pathogenesis of the disorder.

Chapter 3 deals with the problem of incidence and prevalence of delirium in clinical settings, while, in Chapter 4, the core clinical symptoms and signs of the prodromal phases of delirium (pre-delirium) and full-blown delirium are presented and discussed in detail.

Chapter 5 discusses the relevant problem of differential diagnosis between delirium and other significant neurological and psychiatric disorders, such as dementia and psychiatric disorders with psychotic features.

The different clinical subtypes of delirium and the populations at risk of delirium are the themes of Chapters 6 and 7. Chapter 6 examines the most common forms of delirium, such as alcohol withdrawal delirium (delirium tremens) and other withdrawal deliria, delirium due to metabolic causes, and delirium due to structural brain lesions. Chapter 7 looks at the populations that are particularly exposed to the development of delirium, such as advanced cancer patients, HIV-infected subjects, the elderly, and patients who have undergone surgery. The problem of terminal delirium is also discussed here.

In Chapter 8, we examine the main diagnostic examinations, including laboratory (e.g. blood chemistry, urine analysis, drug level screening) and instrumental diagnostic tests (e.g. electroencephalogram, computed tomography, magnetic resonance imaging). We also review the most used delirium assessment tools to be applied in clinical practice (e.g. diagnostic algorithms, rating scales, and other tests).

Chapter 9 considers the management of delirium and presents the most useful strategies, examining the characteristics of psychotropic drugs, especially antipsychotics, and their correct use. The application of educational and environmental strategies by health staff professionals is also discussed.

The final chapter is dedicated to the often neglected area of the family of terminally ill patients. It provides a synthesis of the struggle of family members to adjust and respond to the multiple demands both in the terminal phase of illness of their loved one and bereavement, including the problems that can emerge during this phase, such as complicated grief.

Finally, a consideration that supports the comprehensive character of the book. While we are more than aware of the relevance that terminal care has within the frame of palliative care, we strongly support the view that palliative medicine and palliative care are not to be considered equivalent to 'end-of-life care', because, on the contrary, they cover a much wider span of the evolution of progressive incurable illnesses crossing the fields of oncology, neurology, anaesthesiology, and internal medicine at least and building an autonomous and specific area of cultural and practical development in medicine.

We are indebted to all the patients and families we have encountered in our clinical activity for what they have taught us. We would like to thank all the clinical units of the National Cancer Institute of Milan and of the S. Anne University Hospital in Fenase for their continuous trust in referring their patients to us. A special thank you goes to the Diagnostic Radiology Unit A and its director Professor Renato Musumeci (National Cancer Institute, Milan) for their friendly collaboration in reproducing many of the radiological images presented. We are also grateful to Paul Packer for his valuable contribution in editing the manuscript and to Lea Baider for her thoughtful comments and suggestions on Chapter 10.

Augusto Caraceni
Luigi Grassi
February 2003

Preface to the second edition

When Ludovico Ariosto, one of the most important and influential poets of the Italian Renaissance at the Court of the Este family and their dukedom in Ferrara, first published his romantic epic *Orlando Furioso* (*The Frenzy of Orlando*)[1] in 1516, he could have never imagined that the description of an acute psychotic and confusional state would be used, five hundred years later, in the preface of a book on delirium. The catatonic motoric behaviour of the hero of the poem, Orlando, the possible metabolic alterations due to his forced refusal of food and water, then the onset of a hyperactive agitated state are fully described by Ariosto in Canto XXIII (132-4):

> Soaked with his sweat, he falls upon the grass
> And gazes at the sky without a word.
> He neither sleeps nor eats; though three days pass,
> Three times the dark descends, he has not stirred.
> His grief so swells, his sorrow so amass
> The madness clouds him, in which long he erred.
> On the fourth day, by fury roused once more
>
> .   .   .   .   .
>
> His rage and fury mount to such a pitch
> They obfuscate and darken all his senses.

Then, in Canto XXXIX (57-60), the intervention of the English knight Astolfo, who is able to reconquer Orlando's wit on a journey to the Moon and to restoring him to a normal state of consciousness and sanity, is also described by Ariosto in terms of what, today, could be described as a sort of pharmacological and supportive treatment:

> Astolfo had prepared the precious phial
> In which Orlando's wits preserved had been,
> And placed it to his nose in such a style
> That with one breath he drew the contents in
> And straightaway emptied it. O miracle!
> His intellect returned to its pristine
> Lucidity as brilliant as before,
> As his fair discourse later witness bore.
> As one who wakes from a distressful dream
> Of gruesome monsters which could never be,
> However grim and menacing they seem,
> Or of committing some enormity,
> And though his senses have returned to him,
> From his amazement cannot yet shake free,
> So now Orlando, wakened from illusion,

---

[1] Ariosto L. *Orlando Furioso (1516-1532): translated into English Heroical Verse by Sir John Harington (1591)*. New edition *The Frenzy of Orlando. A Romantic Epic by Ludovico Ariosto*, ed. Barbara Reynolds, vols I and II (Penguin, London, 1977).

Remained in stupefaction and confusion.

.   .   .   .   .

Then like Silenus when he was secured
By captors in a cave, 'Solvit me',
Orlando said; and they, being reassured
By his expression of serenity
Released him, and [...]
They consoled him, for bitter grief
Which overwhelmed him then was past belief.

Acute confusional states are extremely common in medical settings and their feature, without careful assessment, can easily be confused with many different psychiatric syndromes, such as acute psychotic episodes, dementia, and depression. If correctly diagnosed it can be a treatable syndrome, by both examining the underlying causes and using symptomatic treatments to comfort patients and to allow better management in medical units.

In palliative care the assessment and management of delirium are of extreme importance. Since the first edition of this book, several steps have been made in the understanding of this syndrome in terms of etiopathogenesis, clinical characteristics, assessment, and treatment, including the important aspect relative to the effect of delirium in caregivers and family members. Particular emphasis has also been given to the need for a regular evaluation of confusional states and its differentiation from other disorders, with many new studies published with the aim of favouring physicians and health care professionals involved in palliative care.

In Chapter 1, we discuss the conceptualization of delirium by starting form the historical roots of Hyppocratic medicine and the first classification during the nineteenth and early twentieth centuries, through the criteria of the World Health Organization's *International Classification of Disease*, 10th edition (ICD-10), and the American Psychiatric Association's *Diagnostic and Statistical Manual of Mental Disorders*, 4th edition (DSM-IV-TR), with some details about what the upcoming nosographic systems (ICD-11 and DSM-V) are proposing in the classification of delirium.

In Chapter 2 the most recent data regarding the neuropathophysiology of delirium, the anatomical, neurotransmitter, metabolic, and molecular levels of dysfunction, are described for a comprehension of the syndrome.

Chapter 3 discusses the problem of incidence, prevalence, and prognosis of delirium, with particular reference to delirium in the elderly, post-operative delirium, delirium tremens, and delirium in cancer. In Chapter 4, the core clinical symptoms and signs of delirium are presented and discussed in detail, including the most recent data on consciousness and motoric behaviour.

Chapter 5 presents the problem of differential diagnosis between delirium and other neurological and psychiatric disorders, such as dementia and psychiatric disorders with psychotic features. In Chapter 6 we examine the most common forms of delirium, such as alcohol and other withdrawal deliria, delirium due to metabolic causes, and delirium due to structural brain lesions, with an update of the recent literature regarding these issues. The segments of the population particularly exposed to the development of delirium is the object of Chapter 7, in which the most recent details about delirium in advanced cancer patients, HIV-infected subjects, the elderly, and patients who have undergone surgery are presented. The specific issues of terminal delirium and the new area of delirium in children are also discussed in this chapter.

Chapter 8 deals with the diagnostic assessment for delirium, including laboratory and instrumental tests, the most used and newest tests and rating scales, and diagnostic algorithms.

The management of delirium from a psychopharmacological point of view is given in Chapter 9, where the most recent drugs, especially antipsychotics, and their use are detailed. Educational and environmental strategies for both the patient and the family are also presented.

In Chapter 10 the family issues are examined in detail for a more complete vision of delirium in palliative care. The role of the family as a unit in dealing with delirium and the terminal illness of their loved one, the assessment of family functioning and the possible psychosocial disorders in the family, and the important area of anticipatory grief, bereavement, complicated grief, and different possible intervention are described and updated.

We hope that this new edition can provide further insight into the often-underevaluated problem of delirium and can help clinicians in both medical settings and specifically in palliative care to deal with this syndrome and the vast implications it has on the patients, their families, and health care professionals.

We deeply acknowledge all the patients and families we have encountered in our clinical activity, all the clinical units of the National Cancer Institute in Milan and the University Hospital and Health Agency in Ferrara for their trust in us and in our work, and all those who supported us with suggestions and encouragement, in our journey on book-revising.

Augusto Caraceni
Luigi Grassi
May 2010

Contents

List of Abbreviations

5-HT	5-hydroxytryptamine (serotonin)		ESRS	Extrapyramidal Symptom Rating Scale
ACh	acetylcholine		GABA	c-aminobutyric acid
AChE	acetylcholinesterase		GBL	gamma-butyrolactone
ADS	Agitation Distress Scale		GHB	gamma-hydroxybutyric acid
APA	American Psychiatric Association		ICD	*International classification of disease* (WHO)
ARAS	ascending reticular activating system		ICD-10-DCR	*ICD-10 Classification of Mental and Behavioural Disorders—Diagnostic Criteria for Research* (WHO)
b.i.d.	twice a day			
BZD	benzodiazepine			
CABG	coronary artery bypass graft		ICDSC	Intensive Care Delirium Screening Checklist
CAM	Confusion Assessment Method			
CAM-ICU	CAM for use in intensive care units		ICIDH-2	*International Classification of Functioning and Disability* (WHO)
CDCG	clinical descriptions and diagnostic guidelines (ICD-10)			
			ICU	intensive care units
			IL-2	interleukin 2
CI	confidence interval		IM	intramuscular
C–L	Consultation–Liaison (psychiatry)		IV	intravenous
			LOS	length of stay (in hospital)
COPD	chronic obstructive pulmonary disease		LSD	lysergic acid diethylamide
			MAO	monoamine oxidase
CS	Communication Capacity Scale		MCS	minimally conscious state
CSE	Confusional State Evaluation		MDAS	Memorial Delirium Assessment Scale
CTD	Cognitive Test for Delirium			
DA	dopamine		MMSE	Mini-Mental State Examination
DI	Delirium Index		NA	noradrenaline
DIC	disseminated intravascular coagulation		NCSE	non-convulsive status epilepticus
			NMS	neuroleptic malignant syndrome
DSI	Delirium Symptom Interview		NuDESC	Nursing Delirium Screening
DSM	*Diagnostic and Statistical Manual (of Mental Disorders)* (American Psychiatric Association)		OR	odds ratio
			OSAS	obstructive sleep apnoea syndrome
DRS	Delirium Rating Scale		PaP	palliative prognostic (score)
DT	delirium tremens		PCA	patient-controlled anaesthesia (pump)
DWT	Delirium Writing Test			
ECT	electroconvulsive therapy		PCP	phencyclidine
EEG	electroencephalography		PEG	polyethylene glycol

PET	positron emission tomography	SIADH	syndrome of inappropriate antidiuretic hormone secretion
pMHPG	plasma-free 3-methoxy-4-hydroxyphenyl (ethylene) glycol	SPECT	single-photon emission computerized tomography
p.r.n.	*pro re nata* ('as circumstances may require'; of dosage)	SSRIs	selective serotonin re-uptake inhibitors
q.h.s.	*quaque hora somni*, before going to sleep	TCAs	tricyclic antidepressants
		TdP	torsades de pointes
q.i.d.	four times a day	TICS	telephone interview for cognitive status
REM	rapid eye movement		
SAA	serum anticholinergic activity	t.i.d.	three times a day
SAS	Specific Activity Scale	TRP	tryptophan
SC	subcutaneous	VS	vegetative state
SCLC	small-cell lung cancer	WHO	World Health Organization

Chapter 1

From history to present definitions

1.1 **Historical note**

The first chapter of Lipowski's seminal book on delirium is a magnificent source on the history of the definition, taxonomy, and fluctuating denominations of this syndrome throughout the centuries (Lipowski 1990b).

Celsus (first century AD) was the first to use the term 'delirium' to describe a mental condition developing in different contexts, but often in association with fever, and to unify the conditions already known as *frenitis* and *lethargus* by observing the frequent transition between the two. The detection of mental or psychic changes due to medical illnesses was already established by Hippocrates, who described the occurrence of delirium due to fever, meningitis, trauma, and pneumonia. Hippocratic medicine is based on observation and its merit can be well appreciated today given that 2500 years ago clinical findings were clearly described and their association with disease and prognosis correctly interpreted. Hippocrates uses different words (παραφροσύνη, παράνοιαν, ἔκπληξισ, παραλήροι, φρενίτισ) for describing an altered mental status with incoherence of thought, altered sleep–wakefulness pattern, inability to recognize known people, and psychomotor agitation. Most of these words have been translated into English using the word *delirium* (1931). He distinguishes this condition from cases characterized by sleepiness and immobility often evolving in coma, pointing out also that agitated states can often evolve in lethargic conditions and vice versa. It is likely that the most commonly used word, παραφροσύνη, corresponds to delirium secondary to fever, while φρενίτισ is a primary brain affection such as meningitis.

It is interesting to quote a few original statements from Hippocrates.

'When in continued fevers occur difficulty of breathing and delirium (παραφποσύνη), it is a fatal sign' (*Aphorisms*, IV, L).

'As to the motion of the arms I observe the following facts. In acute fevers, pneumonia, phrenitis and headache, if they move before the face, hunt in the empty air, pluck nap (κροκύδασ) from the bedclothes, pick up bits (καρφολογεούσασ), and snatch chaff from the walls—all these signs are bad, in fact deadly' (*Prognostic*, IV).

'Acute pain of the ear with continuous high fever is dangerous for the patient is likely to become delirious and die' (*Prognostic*, XXII).

These and other examples and the clinical descriptions found in the *Books of epidemics* shows that Hippocrates put the aetiology of delirium in the brain, described most of the relevant clinical findings with words used until today (such as crocysdismos, = 'picking at the bed clothes', and carphologia = 'picking at the walls') and associated its onset with the presence of unresolving fevers of several aetiologies. He observed that often agitated deliria evolved in lethargic states and that the resolution of delirium was a favourable prognostic sign. It is also likely that his interpretation included cases of primary brain origin (phrenitis), and others originating secondarily from other affections such as pneumonia and fever (paraphrosine). Galenus (Galeno 1978) clearly distinguishes cases due to noncerebral causes, giving rise, by 'sympathetic' effect on the brain, to 'a certain type of delirium', from those due to primary brain affections, causing lethargus or frenitis. Galenus' understanding of medicine reflected mainly Hippocratic theories and his own fascinating clinical observations and intuitions.

The dualism between the word phrenitis–which is increasingly used to describe acute mental insanity—and lethargy hold validity in the medical literature until the 18th century (Fredreriks 2000).

Many good clinical descriptions of the phenomena that characterize delirium can be found throughout medical literature from Roman times until the eighteenth century, including Areteus from Cappadocia who distinguished chronic conditions (dementias) from acute deliria and recommended boiled poppy and rest as therapy (Adams 1861; Azorin et al. 1992; Ey et al. 1989; Lipowski 1990b).

The main topics which made the genesis of a unitary concept of delirium so difficult were clearly delineated: primary cerebral affection versus secondary, differential diagnosis with psychoses, constant association with fever, acute onset versus chronic conditions such as dementia and mania, during which time and more recently, core concepts were elaborated that lead to the modern understanding of delirium.

In the nineteenth century, the terminology describing delirium exhibited significant ambiguity. In France, a number of authors used different terms to describe similar syndromes, such as Pinel's *idiotisme acquis* (1809), Esquriol's *démence aiguë* (1814), Georget' *stupidité* (1820). In Germany, Wille (1888) described the *Verwirrtheit* as a functional disorder of the brain, usually with acute or, more rarely, chronic features, characterized by confusion, hallucinations, delusions, disturbances of the consciousness, and stupor (see Lipowski 1990). Later on, Meynert (1890) described a similar syndrome by introducing the term 'amentia'. In England, Norman (1890) described 'acute confusional insanity' as a syndrome with a rapid evolution characterized by hallucinations and disturbances of the consciousness.

Greiner (1817) pioneered the concept of the clouding of consciousness (*Verdunkelung des Bewusstseins*) as the main pathogenetic feature of delirium in a treatise that gave a very comprehensive picture of the psychopathology of the syndrome. Chaslin's (1895) account of *la confusion mentale* (mental confusion is a French definition) identified the inability to think coherently, reduced perceptual discrimination, and memory failure as the unifying features of the syndrome with the possibility that oniric aspects were superimposed as in delirium tremens. This definition has remained constant in French literature since the term *délire* was restricted to describing thought pathology (delusion), and confusion has come to occupy the conceptual space of delirium up to the present time (Berrios 1981; Gil 1989).

Bonhoeffer (1908–12, cited in Neumarker 2001) described acute organic brain disorders as acute exogenous reactions (symptomatic psychoses), which included a group of different syndromes, such as epileptic excitement, crepuscular states, hallucinosis, amentia, and catatonic psychosis. Bonhoeffer's contribution was very important in suggesting that the brain could react in a similar way to very many exog-enous noxae due to physical illnesses in what he called 'acute exogenous reaction types', which were all characterized by a clouding of consciousness. From his work came the concept of the disergastic reaction (Wolf and Curran 1935). The contribu-tion of Hughling Jackson, and of his theory of a hierarchic organization of the central nervous system (CNS), should also be acknowledged as he defined consciousness as one function of the CNS that could be deranged by different agents leading to positive and negative signs (Jackson 1932).

It is only in the twentieth century that Engel and Romano (1959) made one of the most important observations to date on the pathogenesis of delirium by showing that delirious patients were affected by a reduction of consciousness that corresponded to a slowing of electroencephalographic (EEG) activity and, in their interpretation, to a general cerebral metabolic insufficiency. In their unitary interpretation the disturbance of consciousness could result in failure at different cognitive tasks, fluctuating levels of awareness, psychomotor hyper- or hypoactivity, agitation, or lethargy.

Lipowski classified all the psychic manifestations due to a direct, specific, demon-strable aetiology residing in brain dysfunction under the taxonomy of organic brain syndromes. Delirium in his view is a 'transient, global disorder of cognition, consciousness and attention regardless of the level of consciousness (awareness) or psychomotor activity that a given patient exhibits which may often change from one extreme to another in the course of a single day' (Lipowski 1990b, p. 44) or 'a transient organic mental syndrome of acute onset, characterized by global impairment of cog-nitive functions, a reduced level of consciousness, attentional abnormalities, increased or decreased psychomotor activity and disordered sleep-wake cycle' (Lipowski 1990b, p. 41). His ideas proved to be in accordance with the definition of 'delirium' estab-lished in English medical literature by the end of the nineteenth century. In *Tuke's Dictionary of Psychological Medicine* (1892) delirium is defined as a condition compli-cating a wide range of non-mental diseases manifesting with intellectual and cognitive impairment (Lipowski 1990b). Lipowski's definition has been very influential on the most recent psychiatric nosological systems, such as the *Diagnostic and Statistical Manual of Mental Disorders* (DSM), developed by the American Psychiatric Association (APA; see next paragraph). However, this definition is broad and deserves further research to prove how well it identifies various clinical conditions from a pathophysi-ological point of view. Still open to discussion is the question whether delirium tre-mens has peculiar clinical and pathophysiological features, deserving a specific taxonomy. In our opinion, the definition should be judged from an empirical point of view by evaluating its ability to identify a homogeneous group of patients in terms of psychopathology whilst more research is conducted to identify the exact or more precise aetio-pathogenetic subgroups (Camus et al. 2000).

1.2 International terminology—differences and similarities

Medical and lay terminology should be viewed differently from diagnostic concepts. We are not able to review here how the word delirium translates in all languages but a few examples will explain where semantic diversity is only at a linguistic level and where it could reflect more profound changes in meaning (Table 1.1). In the Italian editions of DSM-III and DSM-IV the word delirium is not translated and is endorsed as it is. The medical term in Italian corresponds to Lipowski's definition of 'acute confusional state' (*Stato confusionale acuto*) (Caltagirone and Carlesino 1990), even though the closest medical term to delirium in Italian is *delirio*. However, *delirio*, like the French term *délire*, corresponds to the English term 'delusion' and the German *Wahn*, as a specific thought disorder, which can be found in many different psychiatric disorders, including schizophrenia, acute psychotic states, mood disorders with psychotic features, and delirium. To add to the confusion, the Italian *delirio* in the lay vocabulary can be considered a translation of the Latin 'delirium'—and has a non-medical meaning very close to the English 'delirium'.

In one Italian neurology textbook 'confusional state' is described under the chapter on consciousness alterations as: 'a condition where the patient suffers a generalized alteration of the content of consciousness, time and often space disorientation, memory impairment, perceptual errors (mainly visual); it is fluctuating, with the possibility of lucid phases. Sleep-wakefulness cycle impairment is possible, agitation or reduced level of consciousness with sensory obtundation and somnolence' (Capitani 1985). A well-known French psychiatry short textbook (Lemperiere and Feline 1977) reports

Table 1.1 International terminology related to the specificity of delirium vocabulary

Delirium	English word for acute mental change secondary to exogenous noxae affecting the brain
Delirio	Italian word for delusion
Delire	French word for delusion
Acute confusional state	Term synonymous of delirium accepted also by Anglophone authors, used mainly in non-Anglophone textbooks (French, Italian)
Encephalopathy	Neurological term that identifies brain syndromes not due to focal lesions or to specific neurological diseases, characterized by generalized suffering of brain structure often manifesting with delirium
Oneirism	Term from the French literature that describes those clinical aspects of delirium-acute confusional state that resemble dreaming such as hallucinations, complex hallucinatory, and delusional behaviours
Clouding of consciousness	Term from the German literature that proved useful when coined since it pointed to an important pathophysiological aspect of delirium, but it soon became a source of confusion and is now of limited clinical usefulness
Toxic psychosis	Acute mental syndrome caused by drug or poison, obsolete
Exogenous, organic, or symptomatic psychosis	Acute mental syndromes due to systemic illnesses, term often used in German neurology (*Hirnorganisches Psychosyndrom*)

all the clinical characteristics of delirium under the chapter on confusional states. Main clinical features are disturbances of vigilance, memory, and orientation to space and time. Additional findings include oneirisim (alteration of perception and behaviour resembling that of dreams), which French tradition prefers to keep as a separate concept (Sellal and Collard 2001). These conditions have organic causes and are acute and generally transient.

We think that authors from many different linguistic and cultural background recognize that the DSM-IV definition of delirium can be used to describe acute confusional states well. The history of the words used to define the syndrome is intertwined with the origins of many psychopathological concepts and in its complexity is beyond the scope of this chapter Table 1.2 summarizes some of the important conceptual steps made by different authors and shows how, across the different languages, the present clinical definition was borne through contribution, during the nineteenth and twentieth centuries, from at least three cultural areas: anglophone, French, and German. Recently Morandi et al. (2008) pointed out that the different terms related to delirium (e.g. Intensive Care Unit syndrome, acute brain dysfunction, acute brain failure, psychosis, confusion, encephalopathy) internationally are hindering cross-talk and collaborative research and has led to scientific 'confusion' regarding published data and methodology within studies, which is further exacerbated by organizational, cultural,

Table 1.2 Important steps in the evolution of the modern concept of delirium in the nineteenth century

---

◆ Acute versus chronic

Delirium was separated from the concept of psychoses before these latter were nosologically identified as such, by distinguishing the acute insanity associated with fever, i.e. delirium (délire aigue in French), from chronic insanity, i.e. madness (délire chronique).

◆ Fever

Acute onset and fever have often been required as necessary adjuncts of delirium; the absence of fever was a differential diagnostic criterion to separate madness from delirium, although already in the nineteenth century it was clear that fever was not a condition *sine qua non* for delirium (Berrios 1981).

◆ Consciousness and confusion

The concepts of a consciousness and of its disturbances expressed by 'clouding of consciousness' resulted in the nineteenth century in differentiating another important concept from other forms of insanities. Complimentary to the new definition of clouded consciousness, oneiric consciousness, or narrowing of consciousness, French psychiatry coined the term *confusion mentale*, while *délire* came to be defined specifically as 'delusion'. Similarly German authors used *Verwirrtheit*, amentia, or *dysnoia*. Chaslin (1895) gave unitary form to the concept and linked it to organic causes.

◆ Exogenous cause

By the beginning of the twentieth century an exogenous cause was finally considered essential for the diagnosis of delirium or acute confusion as systematized by Bonhoeffer (see Neumarker 2001).

and language barriers. The authors studied the different ways in which various countries define delirium and found, among thirteen languages utilizing Romanic characters. delirium, *delirio*, delirium tremens, *délire, confusion mentale, delir, delier, Durchgangs-Syndrom, acute verwardheid, intensiv-psykose, IVA-psykos, IVA-syndrom,* and *akutt konfusion/forvirring*. While 100% use delirium tremens to define delirium due to alcohol withdrawal, conversely, only 54% use the term delirium to indicate the disorder as defined by the DSM-IV as an acute change in mental status, inattention, disorganized thinking, and altered level of consciousness.

Homogenity must be reached on substance not by accident.

1.3 **Recent classification systems**

The most remarkable change in the concept of delirium occurred with the significant revolution in psychiatry in the early 1970s and again in the early 1980s with the introduction of diagnostic criteria and the development of psychiatric nosologic systems, particularly thanks to the American Psychiatric Association (APA) and the World Health Organization (WHO). There are several reasons for introducing diagnostic criteria and implementing psychiatric diagnostic classification (Dilling 2000; Lindesay 1999; Tucker 1999; Williams 1999). First, it reflects the need to bring some order to the chaotic psychiatric terminology created decades ago, secondary to the different theoretical models and existing schools. As we have already pointed out, this problem involved delirium for many years. Second, it indicates the need for creating a common language and a better communication between clinicians when describing psychiatric disorders. Lastly, it has the advantage of allowing psychiatrists to approach mental disorders in a more constructive way, in terms of epidemiology (e.g. incidence and prevalence), comprehension of underlying mechanisms, clinical differences, course, and response to treatment.

During the past two decades, the diagnostic criteria and consequent classification of delirium have changed according to the new data that research and clinical experience have accumulated. Thus, the most recent classification of delirium and relative criteria are the result of efforts to create a nomenclature sharing a common conceptual and clinical construct within the entity of the former confusional states. A review of the two nosological systems currently used in psychiatry, the *Diagnostic and Statistical Manual of Mental Disorders* (DSM) of the APA and the *International Classification of Disease* (ICD) of the WHO, is introduced here.

1.3.1 **DSM classification**

DSM-III and DSM-III-R

The third edition of the DSM (DSM-III) (American Psychiatric Association 1980) had a significant impact on psychiatric classification in many respects. It explicitly introduced diagnostic criteria for each mental disorder and it provided a multiaxial system for evaluating patients (axis I for main psychiatric disorders, axis II for personality disorders and mental retardation, axis III for medical disorders, axis IV for coding stressful events, and axis V for coding individual psychosocial functioning on a 0–100 scale).

In DSM-III delirium entered for the first time as a specific diagnostic entity, under the rubric of 'Organic Mental Disorders'. The chapter included, along with delirium, dementia, amnestic syndrome, organic delusional syndrome, organic hallucinosis, organic mood syndrome, organic personality syndrome, intoxication of and withdrawal from substances, and mixed or atypical organic mental syndrome. It was conceived that (i) delirium could be determined by a specific aetiology or physiopathological process (e.g. a medical disorder classified on axis III according to the ICD) or by an unknown cause; (ii) it could be superimposed onto a diagnosis of dementia (primary degenerative dementia, pre-senile onset or senile onset, and multi-infarct dementia); (iii) it could be secondary to intoxication from substances (amphetamine or similarly acting sympathomimetic, phencyclidine or similarly acting arylcyclohexylamine) or to withdrawal from substances (alcohol, barbiturates, or similarly acting sedative, and hypnotics); (iv) it could be secondary to other or unspecified substances.

Clouding of consciousness (reduced clarity of awareness of environment), with reduced capacity to shift, focus and maintain attention to environmental stimuli was considered the first important symptom with the presence of at least two more symptoms, including perceptual disturbance (e.g., misinterpretations, illusions, hallucinations), incoherent speech, disturbance of sleep-wake cycle, increased or decreased psychomotor activity. Also disorientation and memory impairment, rapid onset (usually hours to days) and fluctuation of the symptoms during the day and were indicated as main criteria. There would have been evidence of an etiologic factor though the history, physical examination, and laboratory tests.

In the revised version of the DSM-III (DSM-III-R) (American Psychiatric Association 1987), delirium still remained under the rubric of 'Organic Mental Syndromes and Disorders', which was similar to the DSM-III classification—apart from the introduction of the new diagnosis of organic anxiety syndrome and the modification of mixed or atypical organic mental syndrome into organic mental syndrome not otherwise specified (Table 1.3). The classification of delirium also remained quite similar, although the criteria for delirium changed in comparison with the DSM-III, in particular the replacement of clouding of consciousness with reduced ability to maintain and to shift attention to external stimuli. Among the symptoms to be present (at least two), the DSM-III-R added, in comparison to the DSM-III, reduced level of consciousness while memory impairment and disorientation were indicated as different dimensions, and incoherent speech was deleted from the list (see Table 1.4 for a comparison between the DSM systems).

DSM-IV and DSM-IV-TR

The development of the fourth edition of the DSM (DSM-IV; American Psychiatric Association 1994) was complementary to the work of the WHO on the new edition of the ICD, the ICD-10. Major changes occurred throughout the DSM-IV in comparison with the DSM-III-R, as far as the conceptualization, classification, and diagnostic criteria of mental disorders, including delirium. With regard to classification, the term 'Organic Mental Syndrome and Disorder' has been left out in DSM-IV on the basis that it incorrectly implied the existence of 'non-organic' mental disorders which do not have a biological basis (Table 1.3). Thus, in DSM-IV, the disorders formerly called

Table 1.3 DSM-III-R disorders in which a diagnosis of delirium is possible and relative Codes

Code	Disorder
Dementias	
290.30	Primary degenerative dementia of the Alzheimer type, senile onset, with delirium
290.11	Primary degenerative dementia of the Alzheimer type, presenile onset, with delirium
290.41	Multi-infarct dementia, with delirium
Psychoactive substance-induced organic mental disorders	
Withdrawal	
291.00	Alcohol withdrawal delirium
292.00	Sedative, hypnotic, or anxiolytic withdrawal delirium
Intoxication	
292.81	Amphetamine or similarly acting sympathomimetic delirium
	Cocaine delirium
	Phencyclidine (PCP) or similarly acting arylcyclohexylamine delirium
	Other or unspecified psychoactive substance delirium
Axis III disorders (or aetilogy is unknown)	
293.00	Delirium secondary to physical disorder and conditions to be registered on axis III)

'Organic Mental Syndromes and Disorders' were grouped into three distinct sections: (1) delirium, dementia, and amnestic and other cognitive disorders; (2) mental disorders due to a general medical condition; and (3) substance-related disorders. In the first category the predominant element is given by a clinically significant deficit in cognition or memory, implying a significant change from a previous level of functioning. For each disorder, the aetiology is considered either a general medical condition (although the specific general medical condition may not be identifiable) or a substance (i.e. a drug of abuse, medication, or toxin), or a combination of these factors. Thus, delirium is classified according to presumed aetiology in the following categories: delirium due to a general medical condition, substance-induced delirium (in the variants of substance intoxication delirium and substance withdrawal delirium), delirium due to multiple aetiologies, and delirium not otherwise specified (if the clinician is unable to determine a specific aetiology for the delirium) (Table 1.5).

With regard to the diagnostic criteria, the essential characteristic of delirium is considered the disturbance of consciousness with impairment in the ability to focus, sustain, or shift attention (criterion A), accompanied by a change in cognition (e.g. memory deficit, disorientation, language disturbance) or the development of a perceptual disturbance that cannot be better accounted for by a pre-existing or evolving

Table 1.4 Differences in the diagnosis of delirium between the DSM systems

DSM-III (1983)	DSM-III-R (1987)	DSM-IV (1994) and DSM-IV-TR (2000)
Delirium in the rubric Organic Mental Disorders	Delirium in the rubric Organic Mental Syndromes and Disorders	Delirium in a specific rubric Delirium, Dementia, and Amnestic and Other Cognitive Disorders; the rubric Organic Mental Syndrome and Disorders is eliminated
The main criterion is reduced clarity of awareness of environment, with reduced capacity to shift, focus and maintain attention to environmental stimuli	The main criterion is reduced ability to maintain attention to external stimuli and to appropriately shift attention to new external stimuli	The main criterion is a reduced clarity of awareness of the environment (i.e. disturbance of consciousness) with reduced ability to focus, sustain, or shift attention.
Disorientation and memory impairment as a specific criterion	Disorganized thinking as a specific criterion	Change in cognition (e.g. memory deficit, disorientation, language disturbance) or the development of a perceptual disturbance not better accounted for by dementia (preexisting, established, evolving), as a specific criterion.
At least 2 symptoms present among a series of 4 (perceptual disturbance, incoherent speech, sleep-wake cycle disturbance, increase or decreased psychomotor activity	At least 2 symptoms present among a series of 6 (reduced level of consciousness, perceptual disturbance, sleep-wake cycle disturbance, increased or decreased psychomotor activity, disorientation to time, place, or person, memory impairment)	——
Acute onset and fluctuation of symptoms as a specific criterion	Acute onset and fluctuation of symptoms as a specific criterion	Acute onset and fluctuation of symptoms as a specific criterion
Organic etiologic nature as a specific criterion with evidence from the history, physical examination, or laboratory tests of a specific organic factor judged to be etiologically related to the disturbance	Organic etiologic nature as a specific criterion with either evidence from the history, physical examination, or laboratory findings of a specific organic factor (or factors) judged to be etiologically related to the disturbance, or in the absence of such evidence, an etiologic organic factor can be presumed if the disturbance cannot be accounted for by any non organic mental disorder	A specific criterion regarding etiology indicated by evidence from the history, physical examination, or laboratory findings that a) the disturbance is caused by the direct physiological consequences of a general medical condition, or b) the symptoms developed either during Substance Intoxication or medication use is etiologically related to the disturbance, or c) the symptoms developed during, or shortly after, a withdrawal syndrome or d) the disturbance is related to more than one factor (e.g., more than one etiological general medical condition, a general medical condition plus Substance Intoxication or medication side effect)

Table 1.5 DSM-IV (and DSM-IV-TR) Classification of Delirium (and Relative Codes)

Delirium	Code
Delirium due to a general medical condition	293.0 (indicate the general medical condition and code it on axis III)
	290.41 Vascular dementia, with delirium
Substance-induced delirium	
Substance intoxication delirium	291.0 Alcohol
	292.81 Amphetamine (or amphetamine-like substance), cannabis, hallucinogen, inhalant, opioid, phencyclidine (or phencyclidine-like substance), sedative, hypnotic, or anxiolytic; other (or unknown substance) (e.g. cimetidine, digitalis, benztropine)
Substance withdrawal delirium	291.0 Alcohol
	292.81 Sedative, hypnotic, or anxiolytic; other [or unknown] substance)
Delirium due to multiple aetiologies	Multiple codes reflecting specific delirium and specific aetiologies, e.g.
	293.0 Delirium due to viral encephalitis
	291.0 Alcohol withdrawal delirium
Delirium not otherwise specified	780.09

dementia (criterion B). It is stated that the disturbance develops over a short period of time, usually hours to days, and tends to fluctuate during the course of the day (criterion C). As for the DSM-III and DSM-III-R, there should also be evidence from the history and physical examination of the patient, or from laboratory tests that the delirium is a direct physiological consequence of a general medical condition, substance intoxication or withdrawal, use of a medication, or toxin exposure, or a combination of these factors (criterion D).

Both the classification and the diagnostic criteria are retained in the text revision of the DSM-IV (DSM-IV-TR) (American Psychiatric Association 2000), in which new information has been introduced according to the research data accumulated over the past ten years. In particular data concerning the prevalence of delirium, the course of the disturbance, and its consequences in terms of medical complications and mortality have been updated.

As far as the differential diagnosis, the DSM-IV-TR indicates the need to ascertain whether the person has a dementia rather than a delirium, has a delirium alone, or has a delirium superimposed on a pre-existing dementia. From a clinical point of view, although memory impairment is common to both delirium and dementia, the disturbance in consciousness is characteristic of a delirium.

Other psychiatric disorders that should be distinguished from delirium, especially if vivid hallucinations, delusions, language disturbances, and agitation are present, are brief psychotic disorder, schizophrenia, schizophreniform disorder, other psychotic disorders, and mood disorders with psychotic features. Usually, fragmentation and poor systematization of psychotic symptoms are more typical of delirium. When anxiety and mood changes are significant, differential diagnosis with anxiety and mood disorders should also be made, while, when delirium is associated with fear, anxiety, and dissociative symptoms (e.g. depersonalization), a diagnosis of acute stress reaction (secondary to traumatic event) should be ruled out. In delirium, psychotic, anxiety, mood, and dissociative symptoms tend to fluctuate, occur in the context of a reduced ability to appropriately maintain and shift attention, and are usually associated with EEG abnormalities. Other differential symptoms are represented by memory impairment and disorientation, which are more typical of delirium, and the evidence of an underlying general medical condition, substance intoxication or withdrawal, or medication use. Delirium must be distinguished also from malingering and from factitious disorder, given the often atypical presentation in malingering and factitious disorder and the absence of a general medical condition or substance aetiologically related to the apparent cognitive disturbance. Individuals may present with some but not all symptoms of delirium. Subsyndromal presentations need to be carefully assessed because they may be harbingers of a full-blown delirium or may signal an as yet undiagnosed underlying general medical condition. Such presentations should be coded as cognitive disorder not otherwise specified.

1.3.2 **ICD-10**

A few years before the publication of the DSM-IV, the WHO published the tenth revision of the *International Classification of Diseases* (ICD-10), with substantial changes with respect to the former ICD-9, published in 1979 (World Health Organization 1992). The number of categories available for the classification was higher, ICD-9 numeric codes (001-999) were replaced by an alphanumeric coding scheme (codes with a single letter followed by two numbers at the three-character level (A00-Z99).

With regard to the 'Classification of Mental and Behavioural Disorders' (Chapter V-F) the ICD-9 categories were replaced by 100 categories in the ICD-10. There are many similarities between the ICD-10 (Chapter V) and the DSM.IV, especially when one considers the mutual contributions between the two task forces which worked on the systems. However, unlike the DSM-IV, (i) the multiaxial system is conceptualized in a different way, with one axis for psychiatric and medical diagnosis, one axis for disability (similar to DSM axis V),[1] and one axis covering psychosocial and environmental stressors (similar to the DSM axis IV); (ii) the terms neurosis and psychosis are maintained in a number of syndromes; (iii) the terms 'organic mental syndrome' and 'organic mental disorder' are retained, and (iv) the diagnostic criteria are more flexible (Dilling 2000).

---

[1] The WHO has published the draft full version of the *International Classification of Functioning and Disability* (ICIDH-2; World Health Organization, *International Classification of Functioning and Disability (ICDH-2)*, full draft version, World Health Organization, Geneva, 2001), which groups functional states associated with health conditions (i.e. a disease, disorder, injury or trauma, or other health-related state) with the aim to provide a unified and standard language and framework for the description of human functioning and disability as an important component of health, including mental health.

However, as a general rule, the codes and terms provided by the ICD-10 are compatible with the DSM-IV and DSM-IV-TR, as a result of co-joint consultations between the WHO and APA and the mutual coordination in the development of the two systems. Revisions of the ICD-10 are regularly implemented (World Health Organization, 2007), but without modification of Chapter V, 'Classification of Mental and Behavioural Disorders: Clinical Descriptions and Diagnostic Guidelines'. A clinical modification of the ICD-10 (ICD-10-CM) is currently available in the United States, where it is expected to replace use of the ICD-9-CM by October 2013.[2] Its 2010 edition makes it easier for clinicians to use both systems; as well it contains conversion tables for clinical and administrative purposes.

Clinical description and diagnostic guidelines for delirium

In the ICD-10 classification, delirium is in part subsumed under the rubric of 'organic, including symptomatic, mental disorders' (categories F00-09), and in part under the rubric of 'mental and behavioural disorders due to psychoactive and other non-prescribed substance use' (categories F10-19) (Table 1.6).

The rubric of 'organic, including symptomatic, mental disorders' (categories F00-09), consists of dementia in Alzheimer's disease (F00), vascular dementia (F01), dementia in other diseases classified elsewhere (F02), unspecified dementia (F03), organic amnesic syndrome, not induced by alcohol and other psychoactive substances (F04), and delirium, not induced by alcohol and other psychoactive substances (F05). According to the ICD-10, 'the term "organic" used in this section does not mean that the other psychiatric disturbances are "non-organic", in the sense of not having a cerebral substrate.', but 'organic means simply that the syndrome so classified can be attributed to an independently diagnosable cerebral or systemic disease or disorder' (World Health Organization 1992).

As far as the rubric of 'mental and behavioural disorders due to psychoactive substance use' is concerned, it is stated that delirium can be also a complication of all the *acute intoxication* states of the substances (specification of the code F1x.03), or *withdrawal* from the substance (F1x.40 without convulsions, F1x.41 with convulsions). The latter category includes also alcohol withdrawal syndrome or *delirium tremens,* described as a toxic confusional state, which is short in its length, can be life-threatening, and is characterized by the classical triad of reduced level of consciousness, intense hallucinations or illusions, and marked tremor.

----

[2] As indicated the National Center for Health Statistics' (NCHS) website, the federal agency responsible for use of the *International Statistical Classification of Diseases and Related Health Problems*, 10th revision (ICD-10) in the United States, the clinical modification represents a significant improvement over ICD-9-CM and ICD-10. Specific improvements include the addition of information relevant to ambulatory and managed care encounters; expanded injury codes; the creation of combination diagnosis/symptom codes to reduce the number of codes needed to fully describe a condition; the addition of sixth and seventh characters; incorporation of common fourth and fifth digit subclassifications; laterality; and greater specificity in code assignment. The new structure will allow further expansion than was possible previously with ICD-9-CM.

Table. 1.6 ICD-10 Classification of delirium

F00–F09 Organic, including symptomatic, mental disorders

F05 Delirium, not induced by alcohol and other psychoactive substances

F05.0 Delirium, not superimposed on dementia, so described

F05.1 Delirium, superimposed on dementia

F05.8 Other delirium

F05.9 Delirium, unspecified

F10–F19 Mental and behavioural disorders due to psychoactive substance use[a]

F1x.03 Acute intoxication, with delirium

F1x.4 Withdrawal state with delirium;

F1x.40 Without convulsions

F1x.41 With convulsions

[a] 'x' in the entries stands for the psychoactive substances as follows. Mental and behavioural disorders due to: use of alcohol (F10); opioids (F11); cannabinoids (F12); sedatives or hypnotics (F13); cocaine (F14); other stimulants, including caffeine (F15); hallucinogens (F16); tobacco (F17); volatile solvents (F18); other psychoactive substances (F19).
Data from World Health Organization, *The ICD-10 Classification of Mental and Behavioral Disorders: Clinical Descriptions and Diagnostic Guidelines*, WHO Publications, Geneva, 1992.

The general clinical descriptions and diagnostic guidelines for delirium are quite similar to those proposed by the DSM-IV and DSM-IV-TR, as indicated in Table 1.7. The ICD-10-CDCG defines delirium as

an etiologically non specific syndrome characterized by concurrent disturbances of consciousness, and attention, perception, thinking, memory, psychomotor behaviour, and the sleep–wake cycle. It is stated that the syndrome can develop at any age, even if it is more common in after the age of 60. The delirious state is transient and of fluctuating intensity; most cases recover within four weeks or less. Delirium lasting, with fluctuations, for up to six month is not uncommon, however, especially when arising in the course of chronic liver disease, carcinoma, or subacute bacterial endocarditis. The distinction that is sometimes made between acute and subacute is of little clinical relevance; the condition should be seen as a unitary syndrome of variable duration and severity ranging from mild to very severe. A delirious state may be superimposed on, or progress into, dementia. The onset is usually rapid and the course fluctuating during the day. The total length of the syndrome is less than six months.

If delirium is superimposed to dementia, this should be registered (F05.1). Delirium with multiple aetiologies and subacute confusional states include 'other delirium' (F05.8), while a diagnosis of 'unspecified delirium' (F05.9) is given when it is not possible to specify clinical or aetiological aspects of delirium. In the differential diagnosis approach delirium should be distinguished by other organic syndromes, specifically dementia (F00–F03), acute transient psychosis (F23), acute states of schizophrenia (F20), and confusional states possibly present in affective syndromes (F30–39).

Table 1.7 ICD-10 clinical guidelines for the diagnosis of delirium

To meet the diagnosis symptoms (mild or severe) must be present in each of the following areas:

1 Impairment of consciousness or attention on a continuum from clouding to coma; reduced ability to direct, focus, sustain, and shift attention

2 Global disturbance of cognition (perceptual distortions, illusions, hallucinations, most often visual; impairment of abstract thinking and comprehension with or without transient delusions, but typically with some degree of incoherence; impairment of immediate recall and recent memory but with relatively intact remote memory; disorientation for time as well as, in more cases, for place and person)

3 Psychomotor disturbances (hypo- or hyperactivity or unpredictable shifts from one to the other; increased reaction time; increased or decreased flow speech; enhanced startle reactions)

4 Disturbances of the sleep–wake cycle (insomnia or, in severe cases, total sleep loss or reversal of the sleep–wake cycle; daytime drowsiness; nocturnal worsening of symptoms; disturbing dreams or nightmares, which may continue as hallucinations after awakening)

5 Emotional disturbances, for example, depression, anxiety or fear, irritability, euphoria, apathy, or wondering perplexity

Data from World Health Organization, *The ICD-10 Classification of Mental and Behavioral Disorders: Clinical Descriptions and Diagnostic Guidelines,* WHO Publications, Geneva, 1992.

Diagnostic criteria for research

In 1993, the *ICD-10 Classification of Mental and Behavioural Disorders—Diagnostic Criteria for Research* (ICD-10-DCR) was published (World Health Organization 1993). This had the obvious aim to help clinicians in research settings, but also to increase the congruence and reduce the differences between the DSM and WHO systems. The criteria of the ICD-10-DCR are more restrictive, although they are completely compatible with the ICD-10-CDDG. Regarding delirium, the ICD-10-DCR indicates six criteria:

◆ Impairment of consciousness, i.e., reduced awareness of the environment, with reduced ability to focus, sustain, and shift attention;

Global disturbance of cognitive functions consisting bothimpairment of immediate recall and recent memory but with relatively intact remote memory, anddisorientation for time, place, or person;

◆ At least one of the following psychomotor disturbances:

(1) Rapid and unpredictable shifts from hypoactivity to hyperactivity;

(2) Increased reaction time;

(3) Increased or decreased flow speech;

(4) Enhanced startle reactions

◆ Disturbances of the sleep or the sleep–wake cycle, as indicated by the presence of at least one of the following:

(1) Insomnia which, in severe cases, can cause total sleep loss, with or without daytime drowsiness, or reversal of the sleep–wake cycle;

(2) Nocturnal worsening of symptoms;

(3) Disturbing dreams or nightmares, which may continue as hallucinations or illusions after awakening

♦ Rapid onset and fluctuations of symptoms during the day

♦ Evidence (from the history, physical and neurological examination, or instrumental and laboratory findings) of an underlying cerebral or systemic disease or disorder (not due to psychoactive substances) that can be responsible for the clinical symptoms described in criteria A–D.

The ICD-10-DRC note also that emotional disturbances (e.g. for example, depression, anxiety or fear, irritability, euphoria, apathy, or wondering perplexity), perceptual distortions (illusions, hallucinations, most often visual), and transient delusions are typical but are not specific criteria for the diagnosis.

1.4 Emerging problems for future classifications of delirium and conclusions

According to several authors (Gupta et al. 2008; Liptzin 1999; Meagher et al. 2008) some caveats should be taken into account in the discussion of delirium classification and the criteria currently used.

First, delirium is recognized and systematized as a nosological entity, even if the classification of the disorder and its diagnostic criteria have changed over recent decades.

Second, despite the tendency to make explicit the criteria according to the specificity of the symptoms of delirium, it must be remembered that certain clinical situations can be a source of confusion in the diagnosis. For example, hospitalization and diagnostic procedures, as well as physical symptoms, such as pain or breathing difficulties, can determine pseudo-delirium symptoms such as sleep disorders and psychomotor disturbances in hospitalized elderly and physically ill patients (Liptzin 1999).

Third, subsyndromal delirium should be considered as an entity to recognize in clinical practice when dealing with confused patients (Levkoff et al. 1996; Ouimet et al. 2007). Subsyndromal delirium is described as a disorder which has some symptoms of delirium (e.g. clouding of consciousness, disorientation), but does not meet the full diagnosis. It also falls on a continuum between delirium and 'normality', and its risk factors are identical to those for delirium.

Fourth, the balance between different nosological systems is necessary to avoid the risk of false-positive or false-negative cases when making the diagnosis of delirium. With respect to this, several authors have shown the poor correlation between the different systems, such as DSM-III, DSM-III-R, DSM-IV, and ICD-10, with the highest rate of delirium being reported through use of the DSM-III (about 35%) and the lowest through use of the ICD-10 (about 10%) (Liptzin et al. 1991; Monette et al. 2001). Similar data were recently reported in a study carried out by Laurila et al. (2003; 2004) on more than 400 elderly subjects admitted to hospitals or nursing homes, of whom

24.9% met the criteria for delirium according to the DSM-IV and only 10.1% accord-ing to the ICD-10. These results indicate, obviously, that too inclusive or to restrictive criteria can cause marked differences in prevalence rates of delirium.

A final aspect is the fact that knowledge about the diagnosis and treatment of delirium is still limited to certain medical fields, such as psychiatry, neurology, geriat-rics, and palliative medicine. As stated by Francis 1999), there is a strong need to expand the level of awareness of the problem of delirium to all health professionals who care for patient that can develop this disorder (e.g. intensivists, anaesthesiolo-gists, surgeons, internal medicine physicians, oncologists, and general practitioners working in the home setting). With regard to this, the involvement of medical disci-plines, other than psychiatry, specifically primary care, has been the aim of recent publications of both the APA, with the *DSM-IV-Primary Care Version* (American Psychiatric Association 1995) and the WHO, with the *ICD-10-DMCG Primary Care Version* (World Health Organization 1996). However, it has been repeatedly stated that current psychiatric taxonomies require major revision in order to provide a useful basis for communication and research about the most frequent presentations in the community, physical/psychiatric co-morbidity (Strain, 2005). This applies also to delirium, and future editions of both the DSM and the ICD should recognize prob-lems that emerged in the past 10 years in research carried out on delirious patients in different clinical contexts.

Regarding the next fifth edition of the DSM (DSM-V), some proposals have been raised by Meagher and Trzepacz (2007), who suggested that the differing courses of delirium symptoms (acute transient versus recurring versus persistent improving/not improving) should be categorized in the DSM-V and that the new classification should include phenomenological details about syndromal and subsyndromal delirium, including the relative frequency of all core and associated symptoms. The authors also pointed out that the DSM-V should more strongly encourage differential diagnosis of delirium and subsyndromal delirium in the dementia sections as possible reasons for the clinical presentation during the course of illness or responsiveness to treatments, including the need that dementia research should more carefully examine any deliri-um component by utilizing specific instruments (e.g. the Delirium Rating Scale-Revised).

More problems have been reported for the ICD-10 classification, and future devel-opment of the eleventh edition of the ICD (ICD-11) should recognize these problems. According to Meagher et al. (2008), ICD-10 criteria for delirium in fact have not been extensively used by researchers, partly because ICD-10 requires the presence of too many features that often cause lack of sensitivity of the nosological system in correctly identifying true cases of delirium.

For this reason, Meagher et al. (2008) underlined that the ICD-11 can change the criteria for delirium by taking into account the available research and include better account of non-cognitive features, more guidance for rating contextual diagnostic items, clearer definition regarding the interface with dementia, and accountability for illness severity, clinical subtypes, and course (Table 1.8).

Sachdev et al. (2009) have indicated that some modifications are currently part of the revision of the taxonomy in DSM-V and ICD-11 by using the DSM-V Task Force

Table 1.8 Problems and suggestions for the classification of delirium in upcoming
DSM-V and ICD-11 nosological systems

Sources of information in determining delirium caseness: it needs to be made explicit (e.g.
timeframes over which delirium can be diagnosed, extent to which third-party information
contributes to the diagnosis, status of information derived from patient interviews)

Attention as the core sign of delirium: it needs to be examined in more detail
(e.g. disproportionate disturbance of attention but with high correlation with other
cognitive elements of delirium, assessment of attention complicated by the frequent
presence of low arousal, need for clarification of the assessment method for inattention)

Cognitive deficits in delirium: problems in the area of cognitive deficits (e.g, disturbances of
both memory and orientation not always evident, with orientation prone to great
fluctuation; the extent to which deficits in elements of attention and other cognitive
domains occur separately is unknown; comprehension, visuospatial function, vigilance, and
executive abilities less studied)

Arousal and motor activity in delirium: DSM-IV disturbance of consciousness demonstrable
via attentional deficits (DSM-IV), an 'impairment of consciousness and attention (ranging
from clouding and coma; reduced ability to direct, focus, sustain and shift attention).'
(ICD-10). Possible remedy by substituting 'conscious level or attention' even at the risk of
losing some specificity.

Other neuropsychiatric features: More detailed study of the character and frequency of
disturbances in other domains (e.g. disturbances of motor activity and sleep–wake cycle,
affective changes, thought process abnormalities, thought content, and perceptual
disturbances) is needed

Context of delirium symptoms: emphasis on short time frames for onset and fluctuation
can bias definitions (e.g. many cases are more gradual in onset and the degree of symptom
fluctuation within 24 h may be less for hypoactive delirium, prodromal phase of 2–4 days
and/or subsyndromal delirium are clinically relevant phenomena)

Aetiological attribution: it needs to be studied)e.g. evidence that aetiology impacts
upon phenomenological presentation and/or treatment is lacking.; role of genetic factors
identified in studies of alcohol-related delirium not considered in non–alcohol-related cases)

Duration, course, and severity of delirium: all these issues should be more extensively
taken into account in classification

Clinical subtypes: Motor variants of delirium (hyperactive, hypoactive, and mixed) need
to be re-examined according to recent data emphasising motor disturbances that are
relatively specific to delirium (rather than associated psychomotoric symptoms)

Syndromal vs. subsyndromal delirium: further clarification of the significance of
individual features is required with need for formal recognition of subsyndromal illness.

(From Meagher et al., 2008, modified with permission from Elsevier)

Study Group criteria for re-defining in clusters the range of mental disorders for
DSM-V and ICD-10 (Andrews et al. 2009). This can be reached by taking into account
the data of research and some general criteria, including shared genetic risk factors,
familiarity, shared specific environmental risk factors, shared neural substrates, shared
biomarkers, shared temperamental antecedents, shared abnormalities in cognitive or

emotional processing, symptom similarity, high rates of co-morbidity among disorders, course of illness, and treatment response. On these bases, a new cluster, the 'neurocognitive cluster', has been indicated as a better way, in comparison with the classification of 'delirium, dementia and amnestic and other cognitive disorders' (DSM-IV) and 'organic, including symptomatic mental disorders' (ICD-10), to capture, as far as delirium is concerned, the concepts of cognitive disturbance as well as its neural substrate.

Chapter 2

Pathophysiology

2.1 **General considerations**

The pathophysiology of delirium is not fully understood but several anatomical, neurophysiological, and neurotransmitter mechanism have proved helpful in interpreting clinical findings and can be discussed in some detail.

According to the DSM-IV and previous definitions, delirium is an affection of cognition, arousal, and attention. The usefulness of this definition is to correctly classify patients and to allow communication among professionals minimizing taxonomic ambiguity. In this respect the DSM IV definition has the advantage of covering a broad clinical spectrum, but it also implies a great complexity. The areas of neurological function identified are indeed wide and can hardly be attributed to the activity of discrete cerebral structures. Also controversial is the interpretation that the syndrome is caused by the ability of different aetiological factors to impact on a final common pathway producing stereotyped clinical consequences.

2.2 **Delirium as a disorder of consciousness**

A discussion on the definition of consciousness is beyond the scope of this book, but it is certainly relevant to the DSM-IV definition of delirium (Giacino 1997; Zeman 2001). Consciousness can be defined as the brain function that allows the awareness of oneself and of the environment and is characterized by two main aspects: the level of consciousness and the content of consciousness (Plum and Posner 1980b). The level of consciousness reflects arousal and vigilance: being awake, asleep, or comatose. The content of consciousness, or part of it, is experienced by the subject as awareness of him- or herself and of the environment when awake and normally alert. Delirium can be interpreted as an abnormality of the level of consciousness. The level of consciousness is behaviourally equivalent to the degree of wakefulness, often also designated in neurological language as the level of brain arousal (Posner et al. 2007). The normal degree of wakefulness varies from asleep to awake, and it has been described as the degree of sensory stimulation required to keep the patient awake and vigilant. The content of consciousness and cognition can be examined only if at least a certain degree of wakefulness and alertness are preserved. Patients with delirium can be defined as hypoalert or hyperalert (often hypo- or hypervigilant are used synonymously) (Posner et al. 2007)

One fundamental aspect of the pathophysiology of delirium is the recognition of the functional dissociation of cognition and awareness from arousal on clinical and neuroanatomical grounds. In simplistic terms arousal is a general activation of the cortical and subcortical functions, which is a prerequisite for cognition and awareness, and is also related with sleep–wakefulness cycle regulation. Arousal and the sleep–wake cycle can be intact in patients with profound cognitive failure, such as in the demented, and even more dramatically in patients without any sign of active cognition including awareness, such as in a vegetative state (Plum and Posner 1980b).

In delirium both level of consciousness and awareness are abnormal. In coma awareness is absent and the patient cannot be awakened.

Another compelling clinical observation points out that in most of the cases presenting with delirium, if the cause cannot be removed, the condition evolves into stupor and then a coma: hence the interpretation that the cerebral structures involved in the modulation of alertness and arousal must be affected in delirium (Young 1998). In this case, delirium, as the condition characterized by selective altered arousal, is the trigger of all or most of the other disordered brain functions.

This concept requires the possibility of distinguishing between brain structures or functions responsible for a basic form of brain activation (crude consciousness, wakefulness, arousal; i.e. the level of consciousness) and structures responsible for higher cognitive processes, emotion, memory (i.e. the content of consciousness). Arousal is the prerequisite for the content of consciousness to be experienced and expressed.

Any type of lesion diffusely affecting the brain will impact on the level of consciousness. It has been shown that integrative brain functions are lost proportionally to the amount of brain matter lost but also to the rapidity of the onset of the pathological insult (Plum and Posner 1980b, Posner et al. 2007). This observation agrees with current evidence on the relevance of brainstem and medial thalamic structures together with cortical brain areas (especially associational areas) for the development of delirium.

2.3 Delirium as a disorder of attention

Attention is the ability to focus, sustain, and switch mental activity on environmental or internal stimuli. Arousal and attention are linked. Arousal is necessary for vigilance and alertness, which have been defined as the tonic and phasic components of attention (Seltzer and Mesulam 1990). Vigilance is the tonic component of attention and is characterized by circadian physiological fluctuations including the sleep–wake cycle—which can overlap with the level of consciousness. Alertness is the phasic component that can be enhanced or diminished by physiological activation for the performance of cognitive or praxic activities or by pathological conditions in the hyper- or hypoalert states typical of delirium (see also Chapter 4). One meaningful synthetic definition suggests that attention can be viewed as 'the sentry at the gate of consciousness' (Bath and Rockwood 2007).

If level of consciousness and attention are abnormal, changes in perception of internal and external stimuli can occur, thereby compromising awareness.

A failure of selective attention, which is the ability to select in the environment significant stimuli and to focus attention on them for a protracted time, is found in all cases of delirium and has also been suggested as the essential feature of the syndrome (Mesulam 1985). This is easier to demonstrate in the early stages and in mild cases allowing detailed neuropsychological examination (Osmon 1984). Selective lesion of cortical association areas in the right (non-dominant) cerebral hemisphere (posterior parietal, inner temporo-occipital, and prefrontal) can produce attention failure and acute confusional states (Mesulam et al. 1976). Other symptoms that charaterize delirium—such as language and memory alterations, writing and constructional apraxia, disruption of the sleep–wakefulness cycle, or hallucinations—can be early findings in the course of the syndrome and also isolated findings of partial syndromes. These symptoms suggest focal origins. This emphasis on the phasic component of attention is not completely accepted. In fact the more general definition now accepted in DSM-IV includes attention and level of consciousness, which, in other terms, correspond better to alertness (= phasic component of attention) and vigilance (= tonic component of attention) (Sellal and Collard 2001).

The observations that focal lesion of cortical association areas important for attentional process can produce delirium as the diffused metabolic states are not contradictory. Diffuse metabolic causes can affect first the most sensitive cerebral structures and give rise to symptoms that will subsequently combine in the full delirium syndrome or evolve into more severe states of impaired consciousness.

Arousal and attention are the product of the integrative function of different cerebral structures that can be affected by acute events both diffuse and focal. In particular the primary impairment of attention could be due to the dysfunction of the association cortical areas of the right hemisphere, but also a lesion of the reticular activating system can impact on both arousal and attention. The combination of diffuse cause with focal sensitivity and with the ability of cerebral structures to vicariate the function of the affected regions will result in the final clinical picture. Clarifying the complexity of the previous two examples can be helpful. For example, in the case quoted earlier (Mesulam et al. 1976) a focal vascular lesion of a cortical area crucial for the higher integration of attention abilities can manifest with delirium. In contrast thiamine deficiency will affect diffusely all the brain neurons and produce early dysfunction of sensitive structures in the medial thalamus, hypothamic mammillary bodies, and oculomotor nuclei, with subsequent memory deficit and ocular palsy. The full clinical effects will result in the Wernicke–Korsakoff syndrome, which is a form of dementia, but in earlier phases delirium may be the only clinical manifestation (Barbato and Rodriguez 1994; O'Keeffe et al. 1994).

In the delirium syndrome which follows electroconvulsive therapy for depression an electroencephalographic (EEG) study on 12 patients showed the prevalence of EEG-slowing frequencies (in the theta rhythm) in the anterior cyngulate cortex as the main finding in correlation with disorientation, and attention, recall, and awareness failure (Reischies et al. 2005).

One synthetic concept tried to define the neurological dysfunctions associated with delirium as the impairment in mechanisms underlying arousal time perception and attention (Bath and Rockwood 2007). This view is consistent with findings of the Mini-Mental Status Examination of a large population of delirious patients, which demonstrated that four items used to evaluate temporal orientation (orientation to year and date) and attention skills (backwards spelling and copy design) were sufficient to screen patients for delirium (Fayers et al. 2005).

2.4 **Cerebral structures implied in the pathogenesis of delirium**

2.4.1. **Arousal**

The central nervous system (CNS) structures responsible for arousal, attention, and regulating the sleep–wake cycles are partially known and their functions overlap. Several brainstem neural groups are important for these functions and some neurostransmitters are linked to the functions of these cells.

The ascending reticular activating system (ARAS) was described more than 50 years ago by Moruzzi and Magoun (1949) (Figure 2.1). These authors demonstrated that the dorsal mesencephalic reticular formation with its rostral projection system is necessary for sustaining arousal, that its lesion is associated with coma, and that its stimulation produces behavioural and electroencephlographic arousal. The same authors demonstrated that the dorsal hypothalamus and the subthalamic region could also modulate (increase) the arousal level (Magoun 1952). Other relevant brainstem structures with different functions are the locus coeruleus and the raphe nuclei. The ARAS projects to the intralaminar and the reticular nuclei of the thalamus, which in turn regulate the thalamic-specific nuclei outflow to the cortical mantle and also project to the cortex itself (Brodal 1981). These areas overlap with neurons relevant to the regulation of the sleep–wakefulness cycle. Cases of persistent vegetative state confirm that the preservation of brainstem and hypothamic structures can be sufficient to sustain

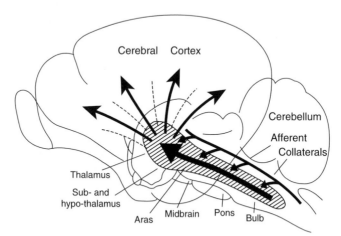

Fig 2.1 One of the first representations of the ascending reticular activating system (ARAS). The schematic drawing shows how the brainstem and thalamic reticular formation should influence, by means of its cortical projections, the maintenance and regulation of the level of consciousness. The connections named 'afferent collaterals' would serve to explain how peripheral inputs can modulate the activity of the ARAS and be carried to the conscious level in the cortex after being filtered by the ARAS itself and the thalamus. Reproduced from Starzl et al. (1951). Copyright 1951 by American Physiological Society. Reproduced with permission of the American Physiological Society.

arousal and the sleep–wake cycles while cognition is lost (Kinney et al. 1994). The importance of brainstem structure for the regulation of normal wakefulness is supported also by cases of delirium, autoptically proven to be associated with degeneration of the reticular formation, raphe nuclei, and locus coeruleus (Fukutani et al. 1993). The anatomical model by Moruzzi and Magoun (Figure 2.1) integrated with modern understanding of neurochemistry and neurophysiology is still valid today.

2.4.2. **Attention**

Attention is closely related to arousal. Lesions in the same brainstem areas affecting arousal will also affect attention. As mostly implicated in the selection of relevant stimuli, attention must rely on the ability of the brainstem and thalamic structures to distinguish between relevant from irrelevant external stimuli, in letting them influence the higher cortical area. At the cerebral cortical level the right parietal lobe, the cyngulate gyrus, and the dorsolateral prefrontal cortex are all important areas to direct and sustain attention. Ischaemic lesions of some of these areas and reduced metabolism in the same structures have been associated with cases of delirium (Mesulam et al. 1976; Trzepacz 1994a). Two studies have shown that visual-spatial attention and visual memory tests could discriminate delirious patients from demented patients (Hart et al. 1997; Mach et al. 1996). These types of visual cognitive abilities are associated with right hemisphere functions.

2.5 **Neurophysiological and functional studies in humans**

Electroencephalography is viewed as a method of assessing the activity of a great number of neurons to reflect the function of the mass of cortical neurons in their interconnections. This activity is modulated as already shown by subcortical structures. Engels and Romano (1959) in their unmatched pioneering work described the EEG findings typical of delirium. They demonstrated that independent of the aetiology of delirium the EEG showed a diffuse slowing of its frequency, which paralleled the severity of the disease. In mild cases the EEG could be slowed in comparison with the patient baseline, albeit being within normality ranges, and at recovery the EEG rhythm could be restored.

An increase of fast EEG rhythms in the beta frequency range (13–35 c/sec) can be found as a typical sign of delirium tremens and other drug withdrawal deliria.[1] This inhomogeneity is the basis for the major criticism of the unifying theory of delirium as a syndrome of cerebral insufficiency.

Similar findings were reproduced experimentally by injecting anticholinergic drugs into normal volunteers (Itil and Fink 1968). Depending on the dose, the subjects experienced delirium with reduced arousal, hallucinations, and agitated behaviour or stupor, and their EEG showed typical changes (alpha rhythm disruption, delta and theta rhythms, and superimposed fast activity). When the same subjects experiencing

---

[1] EEG recording is conventionally classified according to the frequency of the electrical signal as follows: alpha (α) = 8–13 Hz; beta (β) = 13–35 Hz; delta (δ) < 4 Hz; theta (θ) = 4–8 Hz.

anticholinergic toxicity were challenged with other drugs, some cholinergics could reverse both the clinical and EEG findings, amphetamines improved alertness, whilst lysergic acid diethylamide (LSD) aggravated the agitated and hallucinated clinical picture when the EEG showed increased fast activity. Chlorpromazine abolished psychomotor agitation and hallucinations and produced stupor with slow EEG frequencies (Itil and Fink 1968). This experiment was considered an example of anticholinergic delirium and is a useful model for suggesting the presence of EEG excitatory phenomena associated with hyperactive delirium, while a dominant slow EEG rhythm is the hallmark of reduced alertness and psychomotor activity.

A few studies (Trzepacz 1994a) suggest that evoked potentials are affected in delirious patients at a subcortical level (Trzepacz et al. 1989b). A study using the bispectral analysis technique to monitor EEG frequencies showed that the reduction of arousal quantified by the reduction of EEG frequencies documented by bispectral analysis could occur independently of the presence of delirium. This finding could be interpreted to conclude that a reduction of arousal alone is not enough or not invariably associated with the complete delirium syndrome (Ely et al. 2004).

SPECT studies (Trzepacz et al. 1994) showed reduced global cerebral metabolism in some cases and in others selective areas of reduced energy consumption, in the orbitofrontal and prefrontal cortical areas, while enhanced cerebral metabolisms characterized delirium tremens. It is important, however, to remember that the techniques still employed today are still not yet sensitive enough to document with precision the brainstem and the thalamic physiological activity.

2.6 **Neurotransmitters**

The neurochemical characterization of the arousal and sleep–wake cycle regulation points to the importance of several neurotransmitters, namely acetylcholine, cathecolamines, serotonin, and histamine (Flacker and Lipsitz 1999a; Trzepacz 1994a, 1999). Table 2.1 gives a simplified synthetic summary of the neurotransmitter implications of delirium.

2.6.1 **Acetylcholine (ACh)**

Cholinergic transmission from the basal forebrain and from the brainstem-activating system to cortical areas is one relevant biochemical substrate of some aspects of arousal and sleep, attention and memory (Perry et al. 1999; Robbins and Everitt 1995) (Figure 2.2). The importance of the cholinergic system as the potential final common pathway of many deliriogenic conditions is suggested by its impairment in dementia and in aging of the brain, both of which are conditions that lead to a higher risk of delirium.

Anticholinergic drugs are indeed among the most frequent causes of delirium. The use of drugs with anticholinergic effects is associated with delirium especially in the elderly (Han et al. 2001) and in the postoperative period (Tune et al. 1993). One animal model of delirium has been produced in rats by the administration of an anticholinergic agent, biperidene (Tamura et al. 2006), and one recent hypothesis linked anticholirgic activities in the brain with neuroinflammatory mechanisms (van Gool et al. 2010).

Table 2.1 Brain centres and neurotransmitters active in maintaining and modulating normal wakefulness and level of consciousness

Neurotransmitters	Pathophysiology role in delirium, possible pharmacological interventions and toxicity
Acetylcholine	Promotes wakefulness and cognition
	Inhibition by drugs produces sedation, cognitive impairment, and delirium (e.g. atropine, opioids, tricyclic antidepressants)
	A major role in cholinergic pathways dysfunction is likely in many cases of delirium
Dopamine	Promotes wakefulness
	Hyperactivation can be responsible for delusion, hallucinations, and psychomotor agitation in delirium
	Neuroleptics (haloperidol) are used in delirium mainly for their inhibitory activity on these receptors in order to obtain tranquillization without sedation
Noradrenaline (norepinephrine)	Promotes wakefulness
	Hyperactivation can be important for agitated deliria, particularly in alcohol and other substance withdrawal
	Alpha 2 adrenergic agents (e.g. clonidine) can inhibit this pathway, are useful in sedation, and can be used in hyperactive delirium such as delirium tremens due to alcohol withdrawal
Serotonin	Modulates sleep–wakefulness cycle
	Excessive serotonergic activity is associated with delirium (serotonergic syndrome)
	Can be caused by serotonergic drugs such as many antidepressants, some antiemetics and analgesics
	New generation neuroleptics have setotonin inhibitory effects on subsets of serotonin receptors
Histamine	Promotes wakefulness, inhibition causes sedation
	Antihistamine drugs are sedative (e.g. promethazine)
Orexin (hypocretin)	Promotes wakefulness and attention in cooperation with the histaminergic and cholinergic systems
	In cases of excessive sedation due to drug toxicity or other factors, drugs acting on orexin receptors (modafinil) can improve arousal and vigilance
Gamma-aminobutyric acid (GABA)	The final common pathway of all sleep-promoting neurotransmitters
	Benzodiazepines, barbiturates, and general anaesthetics sedative effects are all mediated by GABA receptors
	Level of consciousness is reduced and risk of developing delirium is increased electively by benzodiazepines

Their potential role in the pathophysiology of delirium is highlighted together with the pharmacological interventions that can be useful for treating delirium and potential toxic causal agents for the development of delirium.
Reproduced from Caraceni and Simonetti (2009) with permission from Elsevier.

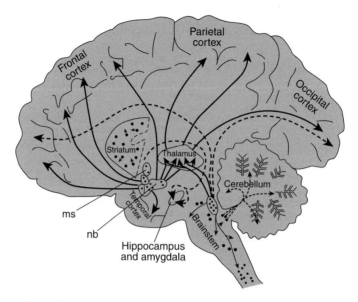

Fig. 2.2 Major cholinergic systems in the human brain with diffused cortical projections from the basal forebrain and hypothalamic areas (nb, ms, and adjacents), from the thalamus, and from the brainstem to the thalamus. The role of acetylcholine in cognition, dementia, and delirium is discussed in the text. This picture represents the evolution from anatomy (Fig. 2.1) to neuropharmacology in interpreting the regulation of consciousness.
Reproduced from Perrry et al. (1999) with permission from Elsevier.

2.6.1.1 Serum anticholinergic activity

Several studies tried to demonstrate a link between the level of serum anticholinerigic activity (SAA) (Tune et al. 1992) with the risk of developing delirium and gave ambiguous results. SAA should be hypothetically absent in humans and has been considered to reflect the effect of drugs or other substances (Flacker and Lipsitz 1999a; Tune et al. 1992). Some studies showed that SAA is associated with an increased risk of delirium (see Flacker and Lipsitz 1999a for a review). Acute changes in SAA status were seen during febrile illnesses but could not be related to the development of delirium (Flacker and Lipsitz 1999b). Another study recently found that SAA use of neuroleptics and benzodiazepines was independently associated with the occurrence of delirium in a group of 61 elderly patients (Mussi et al. 1999). Anticholinergic activity due to endogenous substances, independent of any drug effect, has been demonstrated in elderly patients with acute illness (Flacker and Wei 2001). Changes in blood SAA is associated with CSF anticholinerigic activity (Plaschke et al. 2007a), but the evidence that increased serum SAA is a marker of delirium has also been also recently challenged (Plaschke et al. 2007b, Thomas et al. 2008). Differences in study results can depend on essay methods for determining SAA, but it is more likely that they reflect the complex interaction of external factors with the individual patient response, and it is probable that SAA reflects an aspecific stress response of elderly subjects to illness or inflammation (Flacker and Lipsitz 1999b).

2.6.2 Dopamine (DA)

The role of dopaminergic and noradrenergic pathways is closely linked to the cholinergic system in regulating sleep–wakefulness states (Zeman 2001). An imbalance between the activities of these systems is likely to contribute to delirium symptoms with a relative overactivity of the dopaminergic system and hypoactivity of cholinergic transmission. Agents that block DA activity and in particular DA2 receptors are used to control delirium symptoms, whereas certain substances (such as cocaine) or conditions (such as electroconvulsive therapy, ECT) that enhance DA levels can cause delirium. Interestingly ECT often causes hyperactive deliria and has also been used to resolve untreatable delirium (Fink 1993; Levin et al. 2002; Liston and Sones 1990; Rao and Lyketsos 2000). On the other hand the central activating system pharmacology involves at least ACh, DA, noradrenaline (NA; norepinephrine), serotonin (5-hydroxytryptamine, 5-HT), and histamine in a complex and integrated network. For instance, ACh and NA seem to serve different aspects of attention functions (Robbins and Everitt 1995). The role of dopamine transmission changes in the development of delirium has been recently underlined by genetic studies (see below).

2.6.3 Serotonin (5-HT)

The raphe nuclei in the brainstem also have a cortical projection and contain serotonin. Serotoninergic neurons in the raphe nuclei and in the hypothalamus are considered important for sleep regulation, in particular for those phases of sleep characterized by dreams (rapid eye movement (REM) sleep), and perhaps in the genesis of hallucinations as supported by the observation that LSD-like drugs exert their hallucinogenic activity probably acting as 5HT-2 agonists (Ross 1991). The serotonergic syndrome is a recognized complication of drugs which selectively enhance 5-HT transmission and is characterized by delirium (Gillman 1999).

A number of studies tried to link 5-HT or 5-HT metabolites to delirium in the postoperative, septic, and hepatic deliria and in the elderly populations. Both high and low levels of 5-HT have been associated with delirium. The balance of 5-HT CNS availability can be compromised by the reduced uptake by the brain of triptophan, which is the precursor of 5-HT, due to an altered metabolism of amino acids. In particular the increase of phenilalanine and large-chain neutral amino acids under certain pathological conditions, such as liver failure, postoperative stress, and poor general conditions, could be the initial cause of 5-HT reduction and simultaneously of increased noradrenergic and dopaminergic function and finally predispose to delirium (van der Mast and Fekkes 2000; van der Mast et al. 1991). On this basis branched amino acid infusions have been tried with some success in septic and hepatic failure deliria (Flacker and Lipsitz 1999a). The stress response and immune activation may also influence the levels of plasma amino acids. This mechanism may be involved in the development of postoperative delirium in the elderly, more vulnerable patients (van der Mast and Fekkes 2000).

2.6.4 **Gamma-aminobutyric acid (GABA)**

GABAergic thalamic interneurons have an inhibitory effect on the thalamocortical projection, and GABA is in general the major inhibitory transmitter within the CNS. The anxiolitic and hypnotic effects of benzodiazepines and barbiturates are mediated by GABAergic effects. In patients with hepatic encephalopathy circulating benzodiazepine-like substances that could act on the GABA inhibitory system at the cortical level to produce EEG and behavioural signs of reduced arousal and delirium are found. While a role of the GABAergic system in producing hepatic encephalopathy (HE) is confirmed (Meyer et al. 1998) the role of benzodiazepine-like substances is uncertain (Macdonald et al. 1997). In fact the benzodiazepine antagonist flumazenil is effective in improving clinical and EEG findings in only a minority of patients with HE (Annese et al. 1998; Barbaro et al. 1998; Gyr et al. 1996; Laccetti et al. 2000).

2.6.5 **Histamine, other neurotransmitters, and recent findings**

Histamine-containing neurons are also present in the hypothalamus, and H2 histamine receptors in the cortex and hippocampus mediate sedative effects; in particular, the activity of histaminergic neurons in the anterior hypothalamus promotes vigilance, while the posterior hypothalamic areas promote sleep.

Some years ago a new peptide was identified in the hypothalamus and was named hypocretin 1 (Silber and Rye 2001). This peptide, or better to say its receptors (known also as orexin system) (Mieda and Sakurai 2009), is present in all areas that are important for regulating arousal and the sleep–wake cycle, including cholinergic neurons of the basal forebrain and in the brainstem, histaminergic neurons in the hypothalamus, dopaminergic neurons of the ventral tegmental area, serotonergic neurons of the raphe nuclei, and noradrenergic neurons of the locus coeruleus Siegel 2009). Hypocretin 1 is thought to play an important role in activating the ascending reticular activating system and its deficiency seems to be a cause of daytime somnolence and abnormalities of REM sleep found in narcolepsy (Kroeger and de Lecea 2009; Silber and Rye 2001). The role of this peptide in many other disorders of arousal, including some forms of delirium, should be investigated. The activity of a relatively new drug, modafinil, which has been used to improve vigilance in hypersomnic and sedated states due to different neurological diseases (e.g. narcolepsy, Parkinson's disease, depression) (Holder et al. 2002; Nieves and Lang 2002; Rammonah et al. 2002) has been linked to the histaminergic neurons function within the anterior hypothalamus (Scammell et al. 2000).

2.7 **Metabolic and molecular levels of dysfunction**

The cholinergic hypothesis on the pathogenesis of delirium tends to demonstrate that both predisposing factors (age, dementia) and exogenous insults (thiamine deficiency, exogenous toxic substances, hypoxia, ion disturbances) act on a final common pathway at the cellular and molecular level, which has one unifying step, namely the failure of cholinergic transmission (Gibson et al. 1991). Altered cerebral metabolism due to different causes such as hypoxia, ageing, and nutritional deficiency would impact the cholinergic system, causing the symptoms of delirium (Blass and Gibson 1999). Changes in other neurotransmitters, such as dopamine and glutamate, may also occur and the second messenger systems are implicated in fundamental damaging mechanisms at cellular level. And finally the neurotransmitter imbalance, inflammatory, and stress responses may be players of a game we still poorly understand, leading to functional and in some cases structural failure of definite cell groups and activities serving our higher attentional, vigilance, and cognitive functions.

2.7.1 The role of thiamine deficiency

The main neurological disease due to thiamine (vitamin B1) deficiency, Wernike-Korsakoff encephalopathy, characterized by memory loss, ocular movement disturbances, and dementia, is often associated with peripheral neuropathy and occurs more often in patients with alcohol abuse. Recently partial syndromes have been thought to occur more often than the classic full-blown encephalopathy. Elderly institutionalized patients with poor general health are considered at risk of malnutrition. Therefore thiamine deficiency should be frequently suspected in cases presenting with a change in cognition and reduced food intake or absorption. In the hospitalized elderly a definite thiamine deficiency has been found in 5% (Papersack et al. 1999) to 17% (O'Keeffe et al. 1994) of patients. In a group of 50 subjects admitted to a palliative care unit, 28% had significant thiamine deficiency defined with the same level of essay sensitivity (Barbato and Rodriguez 1994). Cognitive performance correlated with thiamine levels in the palliative care setting and was associated with delirium in one geriatric study (O'Keeffe et al. 1994), but not in a subsequent, in-depth study (Papersack et al. 1999).

2.8 Stress, inflammatory, and immune response

2.8.1 Endogenous steroids

A relationship between delirium and cortisol is suggested by the potential development of delirium, sometimes also called steroid psychosis, during the therapeutic administration of glucocorticoids and by observation of psychoses and delirium occurring in the course of Cushing's syndrome. An impaired regulation of the hypothalamo-pituitary-adrenal axis, resulting in increased cortisol levels or activity, has been observed in delirious patients (Robertsson et al. 2001), and to be a risk factor for the development of delirium in the elderly according to O'Keeffe and Devlin (1994). The theory that delirum can be caused by endogenous cortisol and favoured by a low threshold to stress is hypothetical (Flacker and Lipsitz 1999a). A recent study linked the preoperative plasma levels of cortisol with the onset of postoperative delirium and cerebrospinal fluid (CSF) cortisol levels in a group of 20 patients, of whom 7 developed delirium (Pearson et al. 2010).

2.8.2 Cytokines and inflammation

The therapeutic administration of interleukins (IL-2) can cause delirium (Denikoff et al. 1987) and subclinical cognitive changes (Caraceni et al. 1992). IL-1 and prostaglandin D2 play a role in sleep regulation. The role of cytokines as potential direct or indirect toxic factors in the development of post-surgical or infectious delirium is unknown (Flacker and Lipsitz 1999a). Studies on the relationships, if any, between neuroendocrine and dysfunction of the immune system in the course of delirium are lacking (Broadhurst and Wilson 2001; Stefano et al. 1994). One article on a limited series of 20 cases demonstrated an association between the level of proinflammatory chemokines and the onset of delirium after cardiac surgery (Rudolph et al. 2008b). Interleukin-6 and interleukin-8 were increased in patients with medical and post-surgical deliria (de Rooij et al. 2007, Van Munster et al. 2008). A recent theory has suggested that anticholinergic control of neuroinflammatory mechanisms at the microglia level could account for the presence of chemokines in delirium and for the link between delirium and chronic cognitive deterioration (van Gool et al. 2010).

2.9 Genetic factors

The application of genetic factor analysis is recent in delirium research and can be a useful tool for explaining part of the multifactorial pathophysiological cascade implied in individual cases of delirium. In fact individual sensitivity to similar external or physiological conditions could be modified by genetic characteristics affecting the main pathophysiological pathways, such as the neurotransmitter systems. Patients with cognitive impairment and advanced age share a common risk for delirium; genetic variability could add to that by facilitating or, on the other hand, providing resilience to delirium onset. Candidate genes regulating dopamine cerebral function and inflammatory reactions have been associated with delirium, but results, although interesting, are still preliminary (Smit et al. 2010; van Munster et al. 2009a, 2010a, b). Similar results pointing at the relevance of dopamine transmission control to delirium tremens have also emerged (van Munster et al. 2007a). New genetic approaches and careful classification of patients according to delirium predisposing and precipitating factors in large population studies will be needed to address and quantify the role of genetic variability in explaining different clinical courses.

2.10 Conclusions

The pathogenesis of delirium is still controversial and largely unknown. However, the DSM-IV definition requires altered state of arousal and attention to be present. Physiological and anatomical knowledge suggests a main role for brainstem-thalamo-cortical connections for the regulation of arousal and the sleep–wakefulness cycle. A useful model can identify in this system the main target for most, if not all, the noxae which can cause delirium. Discussion on the role of different neurotransmitters in the pathogenesis of delirium has been thus far mainly academic and supported with almost no good animal model research (Flacker and Lipsitz 1999a; Gibson et al. 1991; Ross 1991; Tamura et al. 2006; Trzepacz 1994a, 1999).The identification of a specific pathway or system which could be responsible for delirium seems unlikely, and reasonably delirium could be conceived as 'the failure of a high-order function in a complex system that is close to system failure' (Bath and Rockwood 2007). The relative role played by several associated aetiological and pathophysiological mechanisms may be difficult to interpret as they may reflect different aspects of a final common pathway modifying, for instance, neurotransmitter regulation.

In definite risk categories, such as the elderly or the severely ill, it would seem sensible to reducing anticholinergic effects, supplementing thiamine, and introducing stress and inflammation modifying interventions as a means of reducing the risk of developing delirium (Ancelin et al. 2006).

Chapter 3

Epidemiology

3.1 **Incidence—prevalence**

The difficulties encountered in defining diagnostic criteria, the fluctuating clinical course, and uneven methods of assessment explain the late development of valid epidemiological research on delirium. While it has been clearly demonstrated that, as expected, retrospective chart studies are totally unreliable (Johnson et al. 1992), it is important to realize that the population of interest is a crucial epidemiological factor. In fact the risk of developing delirium varies enormously across different patients and contexts of care. This chapter will review studies that used prospective methods and specific criteria for diagnosis and will distinguish as much as possible the population at risk. Table 3.1 compares some of the evidences and gives a broad overview of the magnitude of the problem in different clinical settings (Caraceni and Simonetti 2009).

3.1.1 **Elderly**

Over the past years, the epidemiology of delirium in the elderly population has received more attention, due to the high frequency of the syndrome, its impact on hospital care and costs (Britton and Russell 2007; Inouye et al. 1999b), and its evident link with senile dementias. In fact, delirium may affect 60% of frail elderly people in hospital and, among the cognitively impaired, 45% have been found to develop delirium. In one of the first studies on this topic, of 2000 consecutive admissions of patients aged 55 or older, 9% were demented—41% of which were delirious at admission (Erkinjutti et al. 1986). Other studies have described the prevalence of delirium at the time of hospital admission, and the incident cases developing during the hospital stay in elderly patients admitted to general medical and surgical wards over significant periods of time. Table 3.1 summarizes these data (Brauer et al. 2000; Francis et al. 1990; Inouye and Charpentier 1996; Inouye et al. 1993, 1999a; Levkoff et al. 1992; Pompei et al. 1994). It must be pointed out that all of the above-mentioned studies excluded terminal patients. Although not identical, the design of these studies was homogeneous also in respect to the diagnostic criteria employed. In fact all studies used DSM-III or DSM-III-R criteria for diagnosis (the Confusion Assessment Method is based on DSM-III-R criteria). Therefore the variability in prevalence, greater still in the number of incident cases observed after admission, is very interesting.

In more heterogeneous populations of elderly with chronic debilities, prevalent cases can increase. For instance, in a cross-sectional survey of patients aged 75 or more admitted to emergency hospital, nursing homes, or long-term geriatric facilities or receiving home-care, the prevalence of delirium reached 43.9% (Sandberg et al. 1999).

Table 3.1 Prevalence and incidence of delirium: comparison of the elderly, medically ill population with palliative care and oncology patients

Authors	Prevalence (%) at admission	Incidence (%) during admission	Population (age if elderly)
Francis et al. (1990)	16.0	06.0	≥ 70
Levkoff et al. (1992)	10.5	31.3	≥ 65
Inouye et al. (1993)		25.0	≥ 70
Inouye and Charpentier (1996)		18.0	≥ 70
Ljubisavljevic and Kelly (2003)		18.0	Medical oncology
Gaudreau et al. (2005a)		16.5	Medical oncology
Minagawa et al. (1996)	28.0		Hospice
Lawlor et al. (2000b)	42.0	45.0	Hospital palliative care unit
Caraceni et al. (2000)	28.0	—	Palliative care program including homecare
Massie et al. (1983)		85	Dying cancer patient (on a group of only 13)

Reproduced from Caraceni and Simonetti (2009) with permission from Elsevier.

The number and the complexity of risk factors, individual vulnerability, and environmental factors identified by these authors and in other studies can explain this variability. In the series of studies performed at Yale University the number of incident cases decreased over time, and has been lower still in the most recent reports. However, it must be remembered that this study selected a population at intermediate or high risk for developing delirium according to previously identified risk factors. Time-related changes of environmental factors may have contributed to this variability (Inouye et al. 1999a; McCusker et al. 2001a). Risk factors identified by several authors are summarized in Table 3.2.

One model identified the role of predisposing vulnerability factors, combined with the role of precipitating factors. In independent groups of elderly patients (≥ 70 years old), vision impairment, pre-existing cognitive impairment, severity of illness, and high blood urea nitrogen/creatinine ratio were defined as vulnerability factors (Inouye et al. 1993) and were used to assign patients to different risk groups (Inouye and Charpentier 1996). The effect of precipitating factors on these risk groups was then assessed (Inouye and Charpentier 1996). Precipitating factors were represented by the patients' need for physical restraints, their malnutrition, the use of more than three medications, the use of a bladder catheter, and any iatrogenic event (Inouye and Charpentier 1996). The model demonstrates the interaction of vulnerability factors (the soil) with precipitatig factors (potentially aetiological) in contributing to the final individual risk of developing delirium (Inouye and Charpentier 1996), therefore confirming an early intuition by Lipowski (1990a).

Table 3.2 Risk factors for the development of delirium in the elderly hospitalized patients at multivariate analyses

Variable	Francis et al. (1990)	Levkoff et al. (1992)	Schor et al. (1992)	Inouye et al. (1993)	Pompei et al. (1994)	McCusker et al. (2002)
Age (years)		* (>80)	* (>80)			
Previous cognitive failure	*	*	*	*	*	
Fracture Illness severity	*	*	*	*	*	
Psychoative drugs, neuroleptics, opioids	*	*	*			
Fever, infection	*					
Renal function	*			*		
Abnormal sodium	*					
Institutionalization, vision impairment environmental factors		*				*
Male sex			*			
Depression					*	
Alcoholism					*	

* Indicates that the study found variable to be a risk factor.

The role of environmental factors, for long time considered relevant in the onset of delirium episodes in the elderly, has been recently confirmed in an article that identified number of room changes, absence of a clock or watch, and absence of reading glasses as potentially modifiable risk factors (McCusker et al. 2001a).

It is worth saying that statistical associations leading to the definition of risk factors or precipitating factors are not a substitute for the recognition of aetiological factors or true biological causes, but they can suggest the role of potential causes or of conditions associated with such causes. The same authors demonstrated indeed that by acting on some of the environmental/physiological factors identified it was possible to reduce the incidence of delirium (Inouye et al. 1999a).

Despite all these data, delirium in the elderly seems still to be an underreported phenomenon in certain settings. In a retrospective study examining delirium and related confusional diagnoses recorded in patients older than age 60 discharged from Veterans Affairs (VA) acute inpatient units nationally in 1996 ($n = 267,947$), only 4% of patients had delirium or related confusional diagnoses recorded (Kales et al. 2003).

3.1.2 Postoperative delirium

The frequency of postoperative delirium is highly variable depending on preoperative vulnerability factors, type of surgery, and intraoperative and postoperative factors.

For elective non-cardiac surgery the incidence of delirium in the first five postoperative days is 9% (Marcantonio et al. 1994a). A clinical prediction score showing that preoperative factors and type of surgery will affect enormously the number of incident cases has been developed and validated (see Chapter 7 for more detailed description; Marcantonio et al. 1994a; Williams-Russo et al. 1992). This model was also valid in a consecutive series of 138 patients operated on for head-and-neck cancer (Weed et al. 1995). A new predictive model has been specifically validated for cardiac surgery, which bears per se an increased risk of delirium (Rudolph et al. 2009), and is discussed in Chapter 7.

Very high incidences have been observed in emergency surgery for higher risk elderly (42.5% after hip fracture, 42.3% after bypass surgery for lower limb ischaemia; Sasajima et al. 2000), after open heart surgery (14 to 59%; van der Mast et al. 1999), lung trasplant (73%; Bitondo Dyer et al. 1995).

Intra- and perioperative factors contributing to the risk of postoperative delirium are the use of psychoactive drugs, especially benzodiazepine, meperidine, and drugs with anticholinergic activity (Berggren et al. 1987; Marcantonio et al. 1994b); low postoperative oxygen saturation (Berggren et al. 1987); and blood loss with hematocrit reduction during and immediately after surgery (Marcantonio et al. 1998).

The presence of more severe postoperative pain has also been associated with the occurrence of delirium while opioids type and dose were not (Lynch et al. 1998). This finding combines with other observations documenting higher incidence of delirium in patients with poorly controlled pain (Schor et al. 1992), no difference in delirium incidence in patients randomized to IV opioids versus epidural analgesia (Williams-Russo et al. 1992), and higher pain score with more postoperative confusion in patients treated with intramuscular (IM) morphine injection rather than those using patient-controlled analgesia (Egbert et al. 1990). At the same time both higher pain and higher opiod dose used were associated with the occurrence of delirium (Leung et al. 2009, Vaurio et al. 2006). It can be concluded that pain, or factors associated with more severe pain, and the careful use of opioid medication contribute to the risk of delirium in the postopeative period.

New risk associations were demonstrated with early postoperative cognitive dysfunction (Rudolph et al. 2008a) and atherosclerosis (Rudolph et al. 2005). The specific role of these conditions is unknown; early postoperative cognitive dysfunction can be detected only by detailed neuropsychological testing and therefore can reflect a preexisting individual predisposition to cognitive failure. The same can be true for atherosclerosis as a specific role of cardiac embolisms has been ruled out by studies in cardiac surgery.

3.1.3 Delirium tremens

The frequency of delirium tremens (DT) reflects the specificity of this withdrawal syndrome but also its continuity with other general factors implied by the mechanisms underlying acute confusional reactions. Among 200 alcoholics hospitalized for alcohol withdrawal or detoxification, 24% developed DT (Ferguson et al. 1996). At multivariate analysis, the amount of days since last drink was a risk factor for DT (Odds ratio (OR) = 1.3, 95% confidence interval (CI) = 1.09–1.61), but a significantly higher risk was associated by co-morbidity with an acute medical illness (OR = 5.1, CI = 2.07–12.55). Patients with no risk factors had 9% probability of developing DT, those with one or two risk factors had 25 and 54%, respectively, chance of developing DT during hospitalization. In a recent study on patients admitted for alcohol withdrawal (334 cases), 6.9% developed alcohol withdrawal delirium after admission. The patients at risk of developing delirium were those diagnosed as having concurrent infections, tachycardia (above 120 bpm), a history of seizures and delirium, or serum alcohol levels of more than 1 g/L (Palmstierna 2001). In a more recent study of 147 patients diagnosed as having alcohol dependence (Lee JH et al. 2005), DT developed in 59 cases (33%) during hospitalization. Previous history of DT and high pulse rate (above 100 bpm) were significant predictors for developing DT. DT developed in just 20.4% of cases without any predictors, in 45.6% when one predictor was present, and in all cases (100%) when two predictors were present. Thrombocytopenia was also found as a significant predictor of DT and/or seizures among patients fulfilling the diagnoses of alcohol dependence and alcohol withdrawal syndrome according to DSM-IV (Berggren et al. 2009).

3.1.4 Cancer

The most quoted statistics on the epidemiology of delirium in cancer settings come from the work done by Derogatis and his collegues (1983) on the prevalence on psychiatric disorders among cancer patients. This study was a prospective cohort assessment of all new admissions of patients with a Karnofsky performance status of 50 or more, engaged in active treatment at in- or outpatient facilities at three major US cancer centres. In this sample, based on DSM-III definitions, 32% of patients had a diagnosis of adjustment disorder and 4% of organic brain syndrome, the latter representing 8% of all psychiatric diagnoses. From the article it is impossible to say how many of these patients would have fulfilled the criteria for delirium. Indirect data show that change in mental status is a common reason for neurological and psychiatric (Levine et al. 1978) consultations in oncology (17% of neurological consultations) and toxic/metabolic encephalopathy the most frequent final diagnosis (Caraceni et al. 1999; Clouston et al. 1992; Tuma and DeAngelis 2000), which often corresponds to the clinical features of delirium. More recently data referring to 7- to 10-day hospital admission periods estimate the prevalence of delirium in hospitalized cancer patients at around 15% (95% CI 9–18%) (Ljubisajevic and Kelly 2003; Gaudreau et al. 2005a).

Patients with advanced cancer admitted to palliative care (PC) units or hospices are nowadays assessed more carefully in the area of cognitive function and more recent data confirm earlier anecdotal observation about the high prevalence of delirium in this population (Massie et al. 1983). Cognitive failure developed in 83% of patients before death in one PC unit (Bruera et al. 1992b). Using specific clinical criteria for delirium, prevalence was found to be 28% at hospice admission (DSM-III-R) (Minagawa et al. 1996; Morita et al. 1999), and 27.7% at referral to PC units in an Italian multicentre study (CAM criteria) (Caraceni et al. 2000). In this study the diagnosis of delirium at referral was associated with brain metastases, lower performance status, male gender, and poorer clinical prediction of survival. Two prospective studies found the prevalence of delirium to be 42% at admission to a tertiary PC unit (Lawlor et al. 2000b) and 20% in a hospice (Gagnon et al. 2000), with incident cases thereafter rising to 45% (Lawlor et al. 2000b) and 33% (Gagnon et al. 2000), respectively, among patients monitored until death.

Table 3.3 compares the risks of developing delirium as evidenced in some relevant clinical populations by statistical association with multifactor analysis.

3.2 Prognosis

Three main issues relate to the prognosis of a delirium episode: its reversibility, the potentially increased mortality, and the risk of developing dementia.

3.2.1 Reversibility and outcome

It can be obvious that acute confusional states related to readily identifiable causes or conditions, such as drug intoxication or acute febrile illnesses, are to be counteracted

Table 3.3 Factors associated with the risk of developing delirium resulting from multivariate analysis in at least one study

Factor	Cancer patients	General elderly medical population	Postsurgical patients
Advanced age	+	+	+
Previously impaired cognition	+	+	+
Severity of illness	+	+	
Benzodiazepines	+	+	+
Functional impairment		+	+
Metabolic abnormalities		+	+
Low albumin	+		
Bone metastases	+		
Liver metastases	+		
Haematological malignancies	+		
History of delirium	+		
Metastases to brain or meninges	+		
Opioids (dose-related)	+		+
Corticosteroids (dose-related)	+		
Visual/hearing impairment		+	
Infection		+	
Alcohol abuse			+
Atherosclerosis			+
Type of surgery (cardiac thoracic surgery bears a higher risk)			+

Modified from Caraceni and Simonetti (2009) with permission from Elsevier.

by reverting or withdrawing the cause. It is less obvious in more complex situations in the elderly and the severely ill, where the cause can be more difficult to identify and the explanation of the course of delirium is not easy to be found. In these cases the precipitating cause is likely to be combined with a number of co-morbidities or predisposing factors. In one study only 4% of elderly patients with delirium had complete recovery from the syndrome at discharge and about 30% still fulfilled the DSM-III criteria for delirium (Levkoff et al. 1992).

Patients diagnosed with delirium had a greater probability of a longer stay in the hospital or to be placed in an institution after discharge (Francis and Kapoor 1992; Levkoff et al. 1992) and of more severe cognitive and functional decline at follow-up independently from other risk factors or morbid conditions (Francis and Kapoor 1992; McCusker et al. 2001b). Furthermore, higher scores on the delirium rating scales, reflecting more severe cases, are associated with poorer clinical outcome (Wada and Yamaguchi 1993; Marcantonio et al. 2000, 2002). In patients with dementia delirium episodes are associated with further progression of the cognitive decline (Fong et al. 2009).

In advanced cancer patients delirium was reversible in a minority of cases and often preceded death by about 2 weeks (Bruera et al. 1992b). More systematic clinical observation showed that 49% of delirium episodes were evaluated as reversible in an acute PC unit setting with very high prevalence of delirious patients on admission, and 27% in hospice (Lawlor et al. 2000b; Leonard et al 2008). The most frequent aetiological factor associated with reversible cases was opioid toxicity, whereas factors more often associated with irreversibility were lung disease and infection-causing hypoxia (Lawlor et al. 2000b). In the second study only organ failure was more common in irreversible delirium (Leonard et al. 2008).

3.2.2 Mortality

As reported in Chapter 1, the earliest medical observation had indicated that delirium was a sign of impending death. When and how this prediction is borne out is a more difficult question. Hildegard of Bingen (1098–1179; Ildegarda di Bingen 1997) observed that cases of delirium secondary to different diseases can evolve to death; at the same time she stated that if delirium resolves, the disease is also likely to recover. She anticipated one of the most recent, maybe non-surprising, research findings in palliative care, showing that reversible delirium is associated with longer survival than irreversible delirium (Leonard et al. 2008).

Several observations have indicated that mortality is more likely in patients with delirium (Curyto et al. 2001; van Hemert et al. 1994). Some good studies (Francis and Kapoor 1992; Levkoff et al. 1992; Pompei et al. 1994) have suggested that early mortality was increased in delirious patients irrespective of the medical condition, whereas long-term mortality (90 days, 6 months, 1 year) was increased in patients who developed delirium secondarily to the severity of their medical illness. Mortality was not increased, instead, in the year following the delirium episode. More sophisticated analyses, however, could demonstrate that, in the elderly, delirium was an independent predictor of mortality for patients without dementia and that this association was stronger depending on delirium severity (McCusker et al. 2002). However, preoperative delirium was not correlated with long-term survival in liver transplant candidates (Trzepacz and DiMartini 1992), while number of days with delirium has been reported to be associated with higher 1-year mortality in elderly patients after intensive care units (ICU) admission (Pisani et al. 2009).

When looking at more selected acutely ill populations, such as patients with advanced cancer under palliative care, the occurrence of delirium is independently associated with a worse prognosis (Metitieri et al. 2000). The diagnosis of delirium in this population has been used successfully to design a prognostic model (Bruera et al. 1992b; Caraceni et al. 2000; Morita et al. 1999). Also in a case series of patients with cancer, delirium was associated with more advanced disease and had a poor prognostic impact for overall outcome. Thirty-day mortality was 25%, and 44% of patients died within 6 months. Younger patients and those with hypoxemia or kidney or liver dysfunction were more likely to die (Tuma and DeAngelis 2000).

The mortality rate in septic patients who had been admitted to ICU and developed encephalopathy and delirium was found to be higher (33–9%) than among septic patients who did not develop encephalopathy (16–27%) (Eidelman et al. 1996).

The prediction of an accurate prognosis is very important in palliative care. Research has focused on a number of clinical variables in helping to formulate accurate intermediate- and short-term prognosis. A systematic analysis of the literature includes cognitive failure among the factors that are definitely associated with survival in terminal cancer patients (Viganò et al. 2001). On the other hand, the onset of delirium is, per se, an occasion during which an accurate prognostic assessment is of immediate value, for care planning and family counselling.

Two prognostic scores have been published so far to be used in patients with advanced cancer. The palliative prognostic index by Morita is based on the presence of

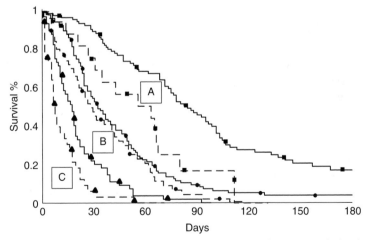

Fig. 3.1 Survival curves of three different prognostic groups of patients, admitted to a palliative care program, according to the PaP score (Table 3.4). A (squares) best prognosis, B (circles, intermediate prognosis), C (triangles, worst prognosis). The survival of delirious patients at referral is represented by the dotted lines and that of non-delirious patients by continuous lines. The impact of delirium on survival is evident in all groups and particularly in the best prognostic group.
Reproduced from Caraceni et al. (2000) with permission.

Table 3.4 The Palliative Prognostic (PaP) score

Variable		Score
Dyspnea	No	0
	Yes	1
Anorexia	No	0
	Yes	1
Karnofsky performance status	≥ 50	0
	30–40	0
	10–20	2.5
Clinical prediction of survival		
Weeks	>12	0
	11–12	2.0
	9–10	2.5
	7–8	2.5
	5–6	4.5
	3–4	6.0
	1–2	8.5
Total white blood cells (cell/mm³)	4,800–8,500	0
	8,501–11,000	0.5
	>11,000	1.5
Lymphocyte rate (%)	20.0–40.0	0
	12.0–19.9	1.0
	0–11.9	2.5
Risk group	30-day survival probability (%)	PaP score
A, best prognosis	> 70	0.0–5.5
B, intermediate prognosis	30–70	5.6–11.0
C, worst prognosis	< 30	11.1–17.5

Adapted from Caraceni et al. (2000) with permission.

dysphagia, dyspnoea, oedema, and delirium. This score showed an 80% sensitivity and 85% specificity in predicting 3-week survival (Morita et al. 1999).

The palliative prognostic score (PaP score) by Maltoni et al. (1999) (Table 3.4) is particularly interesting for evaluating the effects of delirium on survival because it has been designed without the contribution of cognitive function assessment. This score is based on the presence of some symptoms (anorexia and dyspnoea), performance status, lymphocytes and granulocytes count, and the clinical prediction of survival expressed by a PC physician (Pirovano et al. 1999). When the diagnosis of delirium was combined with the PaP score it proved to an independent factor in predicting patients' survival (Caraceni et al. 2000) (Figure 3.1). The PaP score can therefore be used in delirious patients to try to improve prognostication. In addition, as shown by Lawlor et al. (2000b) a better understanding of irreversible delirium will certainly help in defining true terminal cases. This has been recently emphasized in a very detailed observational study on 121 consecutive cases of delirium seen in a hospice PC unit, demonstrating that the survival of patients with reversible delirium was 37 ± 70 days while patients with irreversible delirium died after 15 ± 9 days after its onset (Leonard et al. 2008).

3.3 **Conclusions**

The functional and survival outcomes of different populations affected by delirium are intertwined with the underlying neuropathological and general condition. Often delirium will be a sign of the underlying impaired brain reserve due to either primary or secondary causes, therefore justifying different outcomes such as chronic cognitive decline in the elderly (dementia) or death in the acutely ill.

Chapter 4

Clinical phenomenology

Delirium, as already observed, is a syndrome and not a disease, and is therefore defined by a cluster of symptoms and signs. Chapter 8 on diagnostic criteria will further elaborate the way to use clinical findings in a consistent classification system useful to distinguishing the clinical conditions of a single patient. Clinical presentation of subjective and objective findings are the aim of this chapter. The study of the phenomenology of delirium has received little attention, in recent times, in comparison with other areas of clinical interest. Invaluable information on phenomenology is available in old accounts (Farber 1959; Wolf and Curran 1935), but accurate clinical observations with modern methodology should help in clarifying pathophysiology, and clinical course and outcome (Gupta et al. 2008; Meagher et al. 1998; Meagher and Trzepacz 1998, Stagno et al. 2004).

4.1 Disordered level of consciousness

According to Plum and Posner (1980b), consciousness is the 'state of awareness of the self and environment'. Others defined it as the capacity for subjective experience while awareness is the ability to react to or manifest that experience.

Arousal, alertness, or wakefulness can be used somehow interchangeably and define one aspect of consciousness, also called the level as opposed to the content of consciousness. In the absence of wakefulness it is impossible to explore the content, if any, of consciousness and especially the patient's awareness of such content (Giacino 1997). It is difficult to separate the concept of level of consciousness from that of arousal. The relevance of the reticular formation, hypothalamus, and other structures in modulating arousal and therefore the level of consciousness has already been discussed in Chapter 2.

As a clinical concept, arousal has been operationally defined as the intensity of sensory stimulation needed to arouse a subject from sleep, or to keep him awake, and the duration of this state following stimulation. 'Easily arousable' or 'arousable only with intense stimulation' are common clinical expressions reflecting the need to quantify the arousal level. Arousal has been distinguished into 'tonic arousal', which explains the spontaneous fluctuations in the level of wakefulness occurring during the daylight hours, independent of sensory stimulation (equivalent to vigilance according to some authors; Sellal and Collard 2001), and 'phasic arousal' (equivalent to alertness; Sellal and Collard 2001), which can be understood as the orienting reaction that enhances arousal in response to new or sudden stimuli (Giacino 1997). Phasic arousal induces an attentional reaction. The ability to sustain attention has been linked to the concept of alertness, and the brain structures involved in phasic arousal largely overlap with those implied in attentional processes. The lesion of the structures responsible for tonic arousal will produce a reduced level of consciousness while a lesion of the phasic arousal system will cause distractibility or reduced ability to direct and maintain attention.

The appreciation of the theoretical boundaries between these concepts also underlines the substantial degree of clinical overlap reflected in the DSM-IV first criterion that combines the need of a disordered level of consciousness with attention failure. It is therefore necessary to assess the level of consciousness if delirium is to be differentiated from dementia, mania, or inattention.

The level of consciousness or arousal that can be found in delirious patients is, on the other hand, difficult to define. By definition, symptoms in delirium are fluctuating. An oscillating level of arousal identifies patients who are at times stuporous or even in coma and may be delirious when arousal improves. The arousal can be enhanced or diminished either way, pathologically, to the extent that it interferes with attention and cognition. Therefore the patient with delirium can be hypo- or hyperalert, which is typical of delirium tremens and other excited states. This should happen while maintaining a sufficient level of arousal or vigilance to allow the assessment of attention and cognitive functions. Drawing the line of this clinical boundary may be difficult, because severely delirious patients may be unable to perform most cognitive tasks. However, delirium is certainly found in patients with a disorder of arousal on the continuum between hyperalertness, normal wakefulness, stupor, and coma or that can be classified on this continuum (Ross 1991). Folstein et al. (1975), in proposing the Mini-mental State Examination (MMSE) for assessing acute or chronic changes in cognition, inserted after the questionnaire a visual analogue scale to quantify the level of arousal exactly on this continuum.

The correct diagnosis of an abnormal level of arousal requires some familiarity with the differential diagnosis of the main syndromes of impaired consciousness (Giacino 1997; Plum and Posner 1980b; Young 1998), which are briefly summarized in Table 4.1. Table 4.1 can also be useful for underlining how content (cognition) and level of consciousness are linked but also differentially affected under different clinical conditions.

The assessment of arousal in cases of delirium will disclose that patients can be hyperaroused and agitated, display a reduced level of arousal and be somnolent, or have mixed features at different assessment times. Lipowski (1990b), in forming a unitary concept of the syndrome, proposed the adoption of the definitions of hypoactive, hyperactive, and mixed delirium. One study used factor analysis to confirm the existence of two types of clinical presentations characterized by the clustering of different symptoms: the hyperactive form associated with agitation, aggressiveness, hallucinations, delusions, and the hypoactive variant with decreased reactivity, motor and speech retardation, and facial inexpressiveness (Camus et al. 2000).

In one study, 58 delirious patients were assessed in terms of their arousal level as somnolent or activated: 39 were found to be hypoactive and 19 were activated (Ross et al. 1991). The activated group was more likely to display an agitated behaviour and to have delusions, hallucinations, and illusions. In another study on 125 elderly patients with delirium 15% were rated as only hyperactive while 19% were only

Table 4.1 Syndromes of impaired consciousness and states of unresponsiveness

Syndrome	Arousal—level of consciousness	Cognition—content of consciousness
Delirium—acute confusional state	Impaired, diminished, or increased interfering with attention and cognition, often fluctuating. The patient is awake or easily arousable.	Impaired
Stupor	Impaired. The patient is arousable only with vigorous stimuli. If the stimulus is withdrawn the patient lapse back into the unresponsive state. The patient lays with closed eyes, unresponsive.	Not assessable
Minimally conscious state (MCS)	Preserved or slightly impaired	Impaired. Inconsistent but reproducible behavioural evidence of awareness of self and environment. Inconsistent but reproducible ability to perform easy tasks: follow command, gestural, verbal yes/no responses
Akinetic mutism	Preserved or slightly impaired	Impaired with mainly elective failure of volitional drive. The patient is totally apathetic, shows occasional, infrequent speech or movement to command. Has been described as subcategory of MCS.
Vegetative state (VS)	Preserved eye can be opened and sleep–wakefulness cycle documented on EEG	Absent. No evidence of self environment awareness
Coma	Absent, non-sleep–wakefulness cycle on EEG recording. The patient lays, unresponsive with eye closed.	Absent. No evidence of self environment awareness
Locked-in syndrome	Preserved	Preserved. The patient is unresponsive due to supranuclear palsy or spinal and cranial nerves, but can usually respond by blinking.
Dementia	Preserved	Impaired. At extreme extent of progression the condition can mimic VS.
Psychogenic unresponsiveness Catatonia	Preserved	Difficult to assess; preserved.

hypoactive, 52% had a mixed clinical picture, and 14% had neither hyper- or hypoactivity (Liptzin and Levkoff 1992). Although this study a priori codified specific symptoms or behaviours as belonging to the hyper- or hypoactive series and did not specify a way of assessing the arousal state specifically, its results are useful in showing the high prevalence of mixed clinical presentations.

A study using an activity scale to rate psychomotor behaviour found that of the 94 elderly delirious patients analysed, 21% had an hyperactive form, 29% were hypoactive, and 43% presented mixed features (O'Keeffe 1999). Patients with hypoactive deliria were more frequently affected by more severe illness and had longer hospital stay than hyperactive cases, but the mortality rate did not differ. In the same study patients with withdrawal syndromes and with drug toxicity had more hyperactive deliria while metabolic disturbances were more often hypoactive (O'Keeffe 1999). In another study deliria due to anticholinergic toxicity were more often hypoactive (Meagher et al. 1998, 2000).

However, it has been repeatedly shown by both clinical observation and research studies that normal psychomotor activity and hyperactive deliria have a more favourable outcome as far as time of recovery and prognosis are concerned (Kiely et al. 2007; Kobayashi et al. 1992; Olofson et al. 1996). Similar results were reported in a recent study of 441 patients aged 65 years and older with delirium (Yang et al. 2009), in which the hypoactive/mild class was associated with a higher risk of mortality among those with dementia ($N = 166$), whereas greater severity was associated with mortality, regardless of psychomotor features, among those without dementia ($N = 275$).

4.2 **Attention**

As mentioned earlier, the clinical assessment of attention and arousal often overlap to a significant extent. Indeed, changes in arousal level will affect performances used to assess or measure attention abilities. Some authors consider attention deficit the core of the neurological dysfunction characterizing delirium (Geschwind 1982; Mesulam 1985). According to the phenomenological definition adopted by the DSM-IV, we should distinguish attention failure that can be found due to several central nervous system (CNS) lesions affecting the cerebral cortex and especially the frontal lobes, from attention failure associated with disordered arousal, as characteristic of delirium. Attention is the process that enables one to select relevant stimuli from the environment, to focus and to sustain behavioural responses to such stimuli, and to switch mental activity towards a new stimulus, reorienting the individual behaviour according to the relevance of the stimulus. Although attention, consciousness, and cognition can be variably explained, consciousness is in general considered the prerequisite for experiencing and expressing a cognitive content, cognition would derive from the ability to elaborate and respond to the content of consciousness, while attention is conceptualized as the processing ability related to this content and the consequent behavioural responses. The simplest clinical assessment of attention is limited to the recognition of clear-cut symptoms such as the following:

◆ Distractability is reported when the subject is unable to sustain a task for a more or less prolonged time, a very common sign of delirium, considered among its essential characteristics by the DSM-IV.

◆ Neglect is the selective failure of attention for a given sensory modality usually due to focal brain lesion, though true neglect is seldom found in delirium.

◆ Perseveration is due to the failure of redirecting behaviour towards new stimuli while perseverating in the present task. Perseverating behaviours can often be seen in severely delirious patients.

The quantitative assessment of attention capacity can rely on different test and neurophysiological measures (Deutsche Lezak 1995; Whyte 1992; Zacny 1995). It is worthwhile recalling that many of the tasks commonly included in many bedside neuropsychological tests are better explained as tests of attention. This is the case for short-term memories for numbers, objects, and easy calculations as required in the popular serial sevens. Several specific assessment tools include operationalized items for addressing attentional failures (e.g. see the Delirium Rating Scale, the Memorial Delirium Assessment Scale, and the Cognitive test for delirium). By applying modern criteria and using these types of tools, inattention has been described in 97% of cases of delirium.

By using computerized assessments of attention, Lowery et al. (2007, 2008; 2010) found that differences in reaction time, global cognition, accuracy, and variability of reaction time could distinguish between 'no delirium' and 'sub-syndrome delirium' patients after surgery, stressing the role of accurate and prospective examination of attention as an early marker and predictor of delirium.

4.3 Sleep–wakefulness cycle alteration

The inversion of the sleep–wakefulness cycle in confused patients, with drowsiness during waking hours and insomnia during the night, is a very old clinical observation (Lipowski 1990b) and often an early sign of a developing delirium. Studies on both the structure of sleep during the course of delirium and the circadian wakefulness state are limited to one old observation of a change in the organization of the electroencephalograph (EEG) during the day and night-time sleep (Lipowski 1990b). Delirium as a disorder of arousal implies the notion that sleep–wakefulness mechanisms are likely to be involved, since the structures responsible for these functions overlap in the brainstem, thalamus, and hypothalamus. This theory combines well with the clinical observation that sleep is practically always abnormal in delirious patients and that symptoms tend to worsen during the night. In a recent study of the pattern of wakefulness in delirium, Jacobson et al. (2008) found that delirious patients had fewer night-time minutes resting, fewer minutes resting over 24 hours, greater mean activity at night, and a smaller amplitude of change in activity from day to night, confirming a state of pathologic wakefulness in delirium.

The terms sundowning and sundowner have been used to designate the night-time deterioration of cognitive functions and even the onset of full-blown delirium, especially in the elderly and in patients with overt or masked dementia (Duckett and Scotto 1992; Vitiello et al. 1992).

Palliative care patients, using breakthrough analgesia and adjusting doses as needed, who developed delirium, were using more analgesic doses in the evening and at night, while non-delirious patients tended to use analgesia more often in the morning. The authors speculate that this may be related to an effect of delirium on the normal circadian rhythm (Gagnon et al. 2001).

4.4 Cognition

The definition and assessment of cognitive functions is a wide chapter of neurology and neuropsychology, which cannot be developed within the scope of the present book. More detail has been given to attention because of its potential specific implication in the clinical phenomenology of delirium. One useful interpretation key is that all aspects of cognition, higher cerebral functions in Jacksonian terms, will be affected if the arousal mechanisms in the lower more primitive part of the brain are impaired. Depending on the severity of the delirious state, cognitive tasks will be affected proportionally to the attention demand implied by the task. Calculation ability will be affected before immediate memories and in serial sevens the more difficult subtractions (usually crossing decades) will prompt more confused responses than the easiest ones. One of our patients was oriented to time, space, and person, and able to subtract 7 from 100 and from 79, but when asked to subtract 7 from 93, he was not only unable to do it, but made easily avoidable mistakes such as giving a number higher then 93. Memory for recent events will be affected when past history can be recalled precisely. This hierarchy of mental function derangement can be used with benefit in examining patients. The same observations could be used to argue that the tests with gradually more attention demand are more easily failed.

4.4.1 Orientation

Orientation to person, space, and time is the most common and first-line clinical assessment of cognition traditionally performed by physicians and nurses at the bedside, often considered an hallmark of confusion. In fact, 66% of patients presented defects in orientation in an old study (Farber 1959). Orientation does not explore a specific cognitive function, whereas it represents a synthetic evaluation of attention, arousal, and memory. Although delirious patients very rarely forget who they are, they often become disoriented with regards to space and almost always to time. This hierarchic structure of the construct of orientation can be verified easily in clinical practice and is confirmed from the experience with electroshock showing a reverse order (person, space, time) in the recovery from the confusional state that follows the procedure. Patients may forget where they are and often locate themselves in a known, familiar place, and if delusion occurs, they may also act out their usual occupation, according to the 'rule' of mistaking the unfamiliar for the familiar (Lipowski 1990b). One of our patients, who sustained a long-lasting post-liver transplant delirium and was a farmer from the Po River valley, was convinced of being near his barn and urged that it was time for milking his cow. Commonly the hospital is mistaken for another hospital more familiar to the patient or for a hotel. One patient who had just recovered from a severe delirious episode due to a sudden increase in the plasma level of an immunosuppressive agent (tacrine) went on for at least 24 hours professing that the waitress (a nurse) had brought him a pill that morning.

Hospitalized elderly patients who loose their familiar environmental context may experience disorienting episodes especially at night, either unmasking previously compensated cognitive deficits or precipitating true delirious episodes in the situation often described as sundowning.

The concept of orientation has no known normative data as such, but it is included in the Mini-mental State Examination, which has been accurately studied and which, with some limitations, is still a very useful tool for assessing the mental status of potentially delirious patients (see Chapter 8). Within the MMSE orientation items proved to be among the most useful for screening patients for delirum (Fayers et al. 2005).

4.4.2 **Language**

Language is impoverished in delirium. Delirious subjects can appear silent and inhibited or they may persevere on odd or irrelevant subjects, with difficulties in finding words or concepts that can lead to the inadvertent use of 'passe-par-tout' words or expressions to fill in gaps ('you know what I mean'). Paranomias, i.e. the use of a different, but well-recalled word in place of one not coming explicitly to mind, are frequent. Language difficulties are probably due more to the disordered arousal and attention levels than to a specific cause, or, alternatively, they can disclose an altered thought process. In severe cases of global impairment, frank confabulation can dominate, leaving little opportunity to assess language, memory, and thought content. Often language and speech, including reading, are less affected than writing, especially in mild or early cases.

Few specific observations on language disturbances found in the course of delirium are available. In one study misnamings were very frequent, as frequently as observed in demented patients, but they differed in being more often of the types of word intrusion and unrelated misnamings (Wallesch and Hundsaltz 1994). Word intrusion is in part explained by perseveration. The patient repeats a previously pronounced word (therefore perseverating) in place of the expected word that he is unable to find or pronounce. Unrelated misnaming is the use of a word that wildly differs in meaning from the intended word and therefore has no relationship with the word appropriate for the context.

4.4.3 **Writing**

Several observations have pointed at the relative importance of writing disturbances in the course of widespread brain failure and in particular of delirium. The fragility of writing is due to the complexity of its functional demand which integrates motor, praxic, visuospatial, linguistic, and kinaesthetic abilities. The control of this complex behaviour requires therefore the integrity of higher cortical function, high attention levels, and intact arousal. Not many studies specifically describe the frequency and type of writing disturbance that can be found in patients with delirium. Although we lack sound epidemiological data, clinical experience supports that writing is practically always and precociously abnormal (Aakerlund and Rosenberg 1994; Chedru and

Geschwind 1972b; Macleod and Whitehead 1997). The following list and examples can be used to classify writing abnormalities found in delirious patients.

◆ Motor impairment ranging from thin tremor affecting lines (Figure 4.1), to unreadable grossly deformed graphic elements.

◆ Visuospatial control abnormalities. Letters are poorly aligned, aligned upwards, downwards, or diagonally or written too close to the margins of the sheet of paper, making it impossible to conclude the word (Figure 4.2). Also characteristic is the contamination of a letter or a word by another.

◆ Reluctance to write. Chedru and Geschwind (1972b) in their classic paper found that 19 out of 34 patients hesitated and tried to refuse writing, excusing themselves in someway ('you know I am not much of a writer'). We observed this tendency of reluctance to participate in a complex task as a general phenomenon in examining confused patients. It is probably a sign of preserved insight and emotional involvement of the patient, due to his or her perception of inadequacy and fear of acknowledging to themselves the failure of their mental integrity.

◆ Syntactic changes. When asked to spontaneously write a sentence, agrammatic or simplified phrases are preferred with the extreme being the use of single or a few words in place of a complete sentence.

◆ Spelling mistakes involve mainly omissions, substitutions, and reduplications or perseverations often affecting the end of the word. In a recent hospice series reduplication of letters was the single most frequent sign of dysgraphia (Macleod and Whitehead 1997) (Figure 4.3).

In one study of the occurrence of postoperative delirium writing abnormalities were a very sensitive sign of the development of acute confusional state and a very specific index since they were not found in any patient who did not develop delirium (Aakerlund and Rosenberg 1994). A very recent study on 56 delirious patients observed that the detection of writing abnormalities was not very sensitive to the presence of delirium. By using a global rating of writing 32.7% of delirious patients made errors, but almost no patients with a psychiatric diagnosis but without delirium had pathological writing, leading to very a high specificity for writing evaluation (98.3%) (Baranowski and Patten 2000).

It is worth noting that the Mini-mental State Examination includes the production of a written complete sentence, after command but not dictated, and the duplication

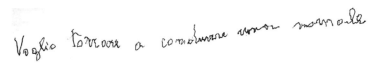

Fig. 4.1 Sample of spontaneous writing.
The patient wrote 'Voglio [I want] tornare [to go back] a condurre [to have] una normale [a normal]'. Tremor and lack of spatial control is evident and one word is missing [life] as the complete phrase should read 'I want to go back to have a normal life'.

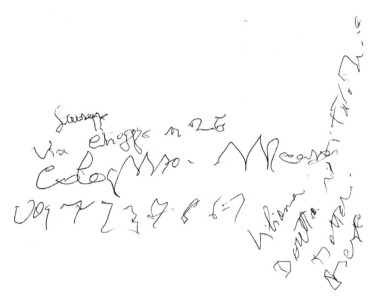

Fig. 4.2 Sample of spontaneous writing showing gross derangement of reasoning, and spatial control. The patient started to write most probably his address (Via Chioggia n 25 Cologno Monzese), followed by phone number, then went on with a list of names difficult to read, but he lost spatial control of his writing within the limits of the sheet of paper, going upwards across the lines he had already written when reaching the end of the sheet of paper.

of a drawing. These simple tests can be very useful for assessing the presence of writing abnormalities and constructional apraxia.

Testing writing has therefore significant value in association with other clinical findings and can have importance in the differential diagnosis with other psychiatric diseases. According to one interpretation the fragility of writing could be secondary to a primary defect of attention in the pathogenesis of delirium, justifying errors, perseveration, and lack of spatial control in the performance (Chedru and Geschwind 1972a, b).

4.5 **Perceptual disturbances**

Disorders of perception are frequent in acutely confused patients but not invariably present. Earlier clinical description of the syndrome reported a high prevalence of hallucinations ranging from 50 to 75% of patients (Farber 1959; Wolf and Curran 1935).

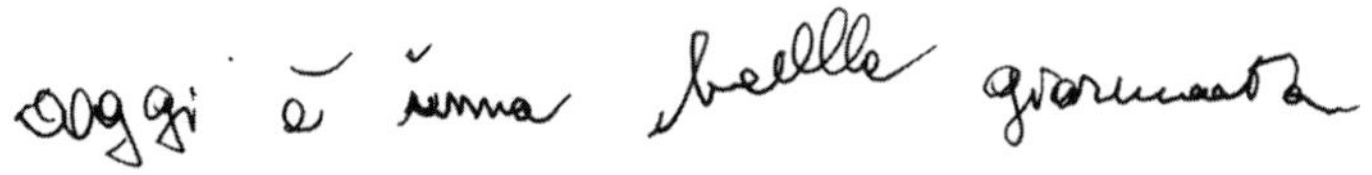

Fig. 4.3 Dictate writing. The patient was asked to write the sentence: 'Oggi [Today] e [is] una bella giornata [a nice day]'. Several perseverations can be seen.

These case series included many patients with delirium tremens (DT) (Wolf and Curran 1935) or alcohol abuse, head trauma, acute fevers, and drug toxicities (Farber 1959) and is more representative of the hyperactive agitated type of delirium than of the hypoactive variant. This type of delirium is found more commonly in younger patients who do not present complex symptoms such as multiorgan failure and metabolic derangement found in the elderly patients with long-term chronic disease. An historical change in patient referral, and use of clinical diagnostic criteria and more accurate study methods explain the difference with the old stereotype of the agitated, hallucinated patient. Also a study based on psychiatric referrals cannot be used to give definite prevalence data due to the likelihood of referral bias (Webster and Holroyd 2000). However, in this study, of 227 patients with a DSM-IV diagnosis of delirium, 32.6% had hallucinations, 27% of the visual type, 12.4 auditory, and 2.7% tactile hallucinations. No olfactory nor gustatory hallucinations were found. In prevalence studies perceptual disturbances were found in only 23% of acutely confused elderly in one hospital series (Levkoff et al. 1992), and hallucinations in 24% in another one (Francis et al. 1990). In a palliative care population perceptual disturbances were seen in 50% of 100 consecutive delirium cases (Meagher et al. 2007).

Recently Brown et al. (2009) showed that patients with delirium have specific visual perceptual deficits that cannot be accounted for by general cognitive impairment, suggesting possible neural mechanisms underling delirium and supporting the hypothesis that cognitive perceptual deficits may have a causal role in eliciting psychiatric symptoms of perceptual disturbance. These data can be partly in line with the results reported by Leentjens et al. (2008), who attempted to compare the phenomenology of delirium in children ($n = 46$), adults ($n = 49$), and geriatric patients ($n = 70$). The authors found childhood delirium is characterized by more severe perceptual disturbances and more frequent visual hallucinations, as well as a more acute onset, more severe delusions, more severe lability of mood, greater agitation, less severe cognitive deficits, less severe sleep–wake cycle disturbance, and less variability of symptoms over time. Perceptual changes associated with delirium include the following possibilities:

♦ *Perceptual distortions* usually involve visual modality and can cause changes in the number, shape, and magnitude of the perceived objects of the external world or parts of them or of own body parts

♦ *Illusions* are misinterpretations of inner or external perceptions; they can be simple, such as folds on the bedcover mistaken for objects or animals, or more complex and fading into interpretation and delusional thoughts, as in the case of a nurse misidentified as a maid, or doctors as ghosts.

♦ *Hallucinations* will be discussed in the next section.

4.5.1 Hallucinations

Hallucination is a perception in the absence of an object. The definition of hallucinations covers a wide range of clinical phenomena, from simple sensations such as the vision of lights and geometrical shapes (photopsia, teicopsia, vision of fortifications) or the perception of single-tone sounds (tinnitus; also referred to as unformed hallucinations) to seeing people, animals, or complex scenes, or hearing music or voices (also referred to as formed hallucinations). Hallucinations are at times, but not always, associated with complex emotional experiences. In its broader definition phantom limb phenomena and synaesthesia can also be considered hallucinations.

Hallucinations can be part of a primary psychotic disorder or be found as the effect of substance toxicity or of an identifiable structural brain pathology. Beside the quality and type of the hallucination, we can also distinguish hallucinations occurring with a clear sensorium and hallucinations with consciousness compromise, as those occurring in delirium.

Every type of lesion on a specific sensory and perceptual system from the peripheral receptor, for instance, in the retina, to the cortical areas responsible for conscious perception and cognition can evoke abnormal perceptions. The same is true for other sensory modalities; one patient, for instance, had musical hallucinations in the context of a brain metastases as an effect of partial seizures (Fenelon et al. 1993). When delirium is associated with hallucinations a more general affection of different brain functions is likely to occur, as already discussed. Some cases are, however, intriguing due to the overlap of different clinical conditions.

Cyclosporine toxicity, for instance, is an interesting condition mainly seen in organ transplant recipients treated with cyclosporine for immunosuppression (Craven 1991; Gijtenbeek et al. 1999). Visual hallucinations are typical when neurotoxic levels of the drug are reached (Katirji 1987) and have been associated with a transitory lesion of the occipital white matter (posterior leucoencephalopathy), loss of vision (Strouse et al. 1998), delirium, and coma.

A similar clinical course has been observed in cases of centrally acting drug toxicities (Rosenbraugh et al. 2001). Visual hallucinations indeed (unformed or formed) can be the only sign of opioid toxicity or be prodromal to the onset of opioid-induced delirium (Caraceni et al. 1994; Jellema 1987).

The phenomenology of hallucinations in course of delirium has been described only in the early case series. In general, visual hallucinations predominate in the delirious states (Wolf and Curran 1935), they tend to occur at night, and in some cases they can appear during the day as soon as the patient closes his eyes. The content of the hallucination tends to be simple, at times just colours, lines, or shapes (metamorphopsia or teikopsia). In comparison with the more structured experiences of the psychoses, hallucinations in the course of deliria tend to be short-lived and poorly defined. Patients sometime report seeing lots of people and confused scenes as if watching a fast-played movie, at times intruding upon their vision only when they close their eyes. Hallucinations, on the other hand, can be part of a delusional experience and can be coloured by negative emotions, such as fear and anxiety. Hallucination of small animals with an aversive emotional content are considered typical of DT.

Auditory and tactile hallucinations are possible. Auditory hallucinations are reported by about 40% of patients in older series (Farber 1959; Wolf and Curran 1935), but are probably more frequent in DT and alcohol toxicity.

The clinical rationale of this discussion is confirmed by a paper on 100 patients admitted to hospice, showing that 43 had hallucinations and only 23% had delirium (Fountain 2001). The more simple hallucinations, such as visions of lights, shapes, and people standing at the bedside, occurred more often alone and were not frightening. The vision of people occurred in about 40% of the hallucinations recalled, and half of them were of the hypnagogic (arising when going asleep) or hypnopompic (arising when awakening) type. Complex scenes occurred in 22% of the cases. The vision of complex scenes and animals could be frightening and were more often recalled after a delirious episode. The occurrence of hallucinations in this study was associated with the use of opioids; the relevance of other factors could not be ascertained due to the small population under study.

Among the explanation given of hallucinations in the course of delirium we identified a few useful theories:

♦ The reduction of the level of arousal is possibly important, together with sleep–wakefulness cycle abnormalities, in producing a cortical defect in judging or evaluating the reality of inner flow of consciousness, imagery, memories, and dreamlike activity (the oneiric consciousness or dreamy state of the French authors).

♦ Dreamlike cerebral activity can occur because of pathological condition and be facilitated by closing eyes or through a change in external stimuli (putting lights off). In the past delirium has been described as a waking dream. Indeed dreams, nightmares, and hallucinations were connected with the content of patients' experience, which reproduced the content of previous vivid dreams (Wolf and Curran 1935).

In line with the interpretation that reality may be distorted due to reduced arousal are those cases of disperception and delusion that follow the rule of the 'known for the unknown': foreign places or people are interpreted as more familiar ones, the hospital as a house, the nurse as a waiter. and so forth.

4.6 **Thought**

4.6.1 **Thought process**

Thought process, that is the organization, flow, and production of thought, is affected by delirium in several ways. The patient seems blocked on some internal perplexity, unable to focus on, access, and marshal his own thoughts. This condition, together with the lack of accurateness in retrieving memories and information, has been often alluded to with the term clouding or narrowing of consciousness. Thinking can be rambling, irrelevant and redundant, and incoherent. At times though, the process can be abnormally slow or fast. Abstract concept formation is more difficult than focusing on concrete experiences. The patient with mild delirium is partially aware of the difficulties in thinking and can report it to the examiner.

4.6.2 **Thought content**

Thought content can be completely deranged and delusional. The patient is totally unable to criticize his/her delusional experience and acts accordingly. Delusions were reported more frequently up to 54% of cases in the past (Farber 1959), and in around 30% in more recent prevalence studies (Schor et al. 1992, Meagher et al. 2007). The available descriptions of delusions come from a case series of patients with agitated delirium referred for psychiatric management (Wolf and Curran 1935). They are invariably transient and poorly systematized. Interestingly delusions suffered in the course of delirium can have a relationship with the patient's premorbid personality, involving important life events or conflicts, including previous psychopathology. In these cases often persecutory and paranoid ideas of imprisonment, homicide, poisoning, and jealousy are present, probably facilitated by the unfamiliar hospital environment. One of our patients was convinced that during the night she had been abducted with the whole bed, and taken home where she found her husband with another woman. The patient was right only as far as the bed had had to be moved to clean the room, and some conflict, about her family life, was also real. Another patient was very suspicious about the possibility that people wanted to poison him with some pills, after physicians examined him and talked about the efficacy of oxycodone for his pain. In other cases the delusion has a quiet occupational everyday quality (as in our patient who was busy milking his cow in the barn). Patients undergoing several separate delirium episodes due to different causes experienced similar delusional reactions. Amnesia can follow the delirious delusional episode but not always as patients' reports of their delusions are available (Lipowski 1990b; Wolf and Curran 1935).

4.6.3 Suicidal ideation

Suicidal ideation or attempt has been reported in 7% of cases during delirium in early studies (Farber 1959). Premorbid psychiatric conditions are extremely important. In their own case series, Wolf and Curran (1935) described one patient with a likely underlying psychopathology who was delirious due to barbiturate toxicity and throughout his delirium made several suicidal attempts. The acute episode was solved and the patient was discharged and went back to work. A few years later he committed suicide.

In the palliative care population with advanced cancer the risk of suicide is likely higher than in the general population (Akechi et al. 2004; Robson et al. 2010). Among the few studies available Farberow et al.'s (1963) study suggest that delirium is a protecting factor against suicidal acts in the population with cancer. Breitbart (1987, 1990) suggests instead that delirium can facilitate impulsive behaviours and loosen control and can be important in explaining cases of suicide in hospitalized patients with advanced cancer. The theory is interesting but nobody has yet assessed the relevance and consequences of suicidal ideation in delirious patient affected by a terminal disease. One study reported conversely that suicidal ideation in cancer patients was associated with depression in 57% of cases and with delirium in 29% (Akechi et al. 1999). Considering the possible association between delirium and depression (see the section Affectivity) and the vast literature regarding the issue of suicide in cancer and its relationship with depression (Robson et al. 2010), the risk of suicide in delirious and depressed patients should be evaluated in a more comprehensive way.[1]

Also in the case of thought pathology, the symptoms and the clinical course of delirium are compounded by abnormality of arousal, attention, and fluctuations in

---

[1] The important and debated area relative to request for euthanasia-hastened death, physician-assisted suicide, suicide ideation, and depression in palliative medicine is beyond the scope of this book. The number of studies have increased enormously over the past years and interested readers are referred to specific reviews (e.g. Hudson et al. 2006b; Hurst and Mauron 2006; Wasteson et al. 2009).

the short time. In a unitary view this can explain different levels of awareness and perhaps justify impulsive actions, such as harming oneself or other people.

4.7 **Psychomotor behaviour**

The observation of overt behaviour can give important information. Restlessness and agitation often combines with an abnormally fast and pressured thought process, delusions, and hallucinations. Hypoactive patient are confused in a more defective way with less positive symptoms and signs. By combining the assessment of the level of arousal with the quality of observed behaviours it is possible to classify patients as suffering hypo- or hyperactive or mixed variants of delirium. (Liptzin and Levkoff 1992; Ross et al. 1991). These definitions are, however, at present not univocal. Behavioural evaluation always includes the assessment of arousal level, which is linked, but not equivalent, to the concept of hyper/hypoactivity. Hypoactive patients are often lethargic. More importantly, patients often evolve from hyperactive states into lethargic hypoactive deliria, and in some cases this stage precedes stupor and coma.

Extreme hypoactivity can be confused with lethargy while it could be better explained as depression, catatonia, or frontal lobe dysfunction, due to the fact that arousal compromise may be difficult to evaluate (see Figure 6.6 and related case report). The inconsistent association of causes with clinical manifestations can be explained by the evolving nature of the process in many cases.

Typical behaviours associated with delirium include signs originally described by Hippocrates and Soranus:

- *Jactitatio*: purposeless movement of the hands in the air; other similar behaviour may involve searching under the bed, or in the closet;
- *Carphology*: picking at bedclothes; and
- *Crocydismos*: picking at the walls.

Interestingly moving away from old semeiotic knowledge more recent operationalized systems to describe motoric behaviour in delirium proved quite imprecise and unable to consistently classify patients (Meagher et al. 2008). Recent attempts to examine the use and feasibility of accelerometry-based monitoring (e.g. periods of sitting/lying, standing, stepping, number of postural transitions) in order to determine motoric subtypes in delirious patients in palliative care have given some promising results. Although more research is needed to understand the complex phenomena underlying motor behaviour in advanced physically ill patients, motor subtypes of delirium defined by observed ward behaviour seem in fact different in electronically measured activity levels (Godfrey et al. 2009, 2010).

In general, behaviour and emotional expression are modified from the patient's usual habit. The impression of change is often the first sign reported by relatives and people knowing the patient well before florid signs can be observed. Psychomotor slowing, apathetic attitude, repetitive gestures, lack of interest in the environment are common and can be misinterpreted as signs of depression (Farrell and Ganzini 1995). These symptoms are far more common than the overly agitated picture in the early phase. Agitation with purposeless behaviours that can, at the extreme of the spectrum, be aggressive and dangerous for the patient and caregivers can follow or characterize a minority of cases since the onset. Preliminary observations by means of motor activity recordings made it possible to classify demented patients with delirium into different groups according to their motor activity, e.g. nocturnal delirium type, wandering type, hypoboulic type, and lying-down type (Honma et al. 1998).

4.8 **Affectivity**

As already mentioned, perplexity is probably the most frequent mood colour appearing to the examiner. Patients look very often apathetic as if lacking drive or motivation. This would be considered as a failure of frontal lobe functions. Fear, anxiety, and anger can dominate the clinical picture of the hypoactive conditions at times associated with DT or toxicity of some drugs. Mood lability with sudden unexplained hilarity or sadness can be found. Emotions are often consonant with the impact of the underlying illness and can be influenced by the painful awareness of mental impairment. In some cases depressive symptoms mislead the diagnosis from delirium to depression (Nicholas and Lindsey 1995). Earlier clinical descriptions reported depression in 53% of cases and constricted or flat affect in 30% (Farber 1959). In a study on an elderly population, depressive symptoms were frequent with 60% of patients showing low mood, 68% worthlessness, and 52% thoughts of death (Farrell and Ganzini 1995). More recently McAvy et al. (2007), in a study of 416 elderly inpatients found that patients who developed delirium within the first five days of hospitalization (8.6%) had higher scores on the Geriatric Depression scale at admission with respect to patients who did not develop delirium. By using a Cox proportional hazards model, the authors showed that depressive symptoms assessing dysphoric mood and hopelessness were predictive of incident delirium, controlling for measures of physical and mental health, while symptoms of withdrawal, apathy, and vigor were not significantly associated with delirium. In a study of 459 elderly patients admitted to the hospital, Givens et al. (2009) also reported that 23 (5.0%) had the overlap syndrome of coexisting depression and incident delirium, 39 (8.5%) delirium alone, 121 (26.3%) depression alone, and 276 (60.1%) neither condition. Patients with the overlap syndrome had higher odds of new nursing home placement or death at 1 year and 1-month functional decline than patients with neither condition (Givens et al. 2009).

Patients with delirium under specialized palliative care were found to invariably fulfil the criteria for major depression and patients with depressive symptoms had delirium or subsyndromal delirium in about 50% of cases (Leonard et al. 2009).

4.9 **Early clinical findings**

Delirium episodes often occur suddenly but can be heralded by subtle symptoms and signs often recalled after the episodes are full-blown, by carefully interviewing family members or caregivers. Table 4.2 summarizes a list of potential warning signs. The value of such a list is probably higher if combined with the careful monitoring of the risk factors (baseline vulnerability) and potential causal factors characterizing the high-risk populations demonstrated by recent studies (see Chapter 3). No study has specifically addressed the relevance of these observations that are so consistently found in everyday clinical practice.

One article on patients admitted to a coronary care unit showed that delirium was preceded by anxiety, slight agitation, EEG slowing, and changes in eye movements (Matsushima et al. 1997), but it is unclear whether these signs can be related to the classic clinical observations mentioned above and listed in Table 4.2.

4.10 **Subjective perception**

Systematic assessment of subjective awareness or consciousness during a delirious episode has been lacking, although some recent data have focused attention to this area. Anecdotal reports, many of which discussed patients recovering from a febrile illness or a postoperative delirium, have indicated that recall of delirium is often characterized by unpleasant experiences, horrible dreams, waking experiences merging with dreams, and a lack of control on the waking state intruded by hallucinatory or dream-like experiences (Lipowski 1990b). Following the suggestion for a better documentation of patients' perceptions and of the subjective awareness and recall in the fluctuating phases of the disease (Crammer 2002), Breitbart et al. (2002) found that 53.5% patients recalled their delirium experience. Short-term memory impairment, delirium severity, and the presence of perceptual disturbances were significant predictors of delirium recall (Breitbart et al. 2002).

Table 4.2 Prodromal presentations of delirium

Symptoms and signs
Insomnia
Vivid dreams or nightmares with difficulty in distinguishing dream from reality when awake
Restlessness
Irritability
Distractability
Hypersensitivity to lights and sounds
Anxiety
Subjective sense of difficulty in marshalling own thought
Difficulty in concentrating
Behaviours
Unaccustomed behaviours
Change in behaviour
Hyper- or hypoactivity
Inappropriate behaviours

In our experience the characteristic fluctuations of severity and of the level of consciousness have significant impact on a patient's affective experience. Phases of greater
lucidity may make it possible to understand the potential occurrence of further mental
changes, generating anxiety, anguish, and fear. Emotional reactions can include
apathy, depression, and perplexity when the clinical situation is perceived as worsened
and cognitive compromise as part of inevitable grim course; this can influence the
elaboration of suicidal thoughts. The quality of individual experience about one's
delirium is not easy to predict and depends probably, as already mentioned, on the
patient's personality structure and previous experiences (Wolf and Curran 1935).

Frequently personal feelings are associated with themes related to the severity of the
actual disease (death, torture, kidnapping). It should be significant for the medical
culture that most, or at least many, of the illusional or delusional interpretation of the
medical environment, reported to us by acutely confused patients, had very bad, and
hostile qualities. One patient perceived physicians around the bed as ghosts, and
therapies were seen as attempts to poison her. Another patient believed that she was in
a 'lager' with a friend of hers, who was also a patient in the same ward. She recalled that
they were both bald (as they indeed were due to chemotherapy), and that people (doctors and nurses) were coming to laugh at them and torture them. This patient, in
particular, had never had war or imprisonment experiences in her life.

Other experiences are possible in different situations; for instance, in the post-liver
transplant deliria the relationship with the donor and donor's family is often present:
one patient hallucinated that the donor came to him to request the restitution of the
organ. The subjective experience was very negative. Another patient had the vision of
a kaleidoscopically coloured forest inhabited by a fantastic flora and fauna; on recall
he found it a very positive and interesting experience that he connected with his curi-
osity in the 1960s as to the effect of hallucinogenic drugs popular among his peers and
that he never tried. These two opposite reactions may reflect different ways of living
the transplant experience.

It is therefore likely that present circumstances together with personality structure and
more profound relationship between life events and personal feelings play a role in producing the final quality and emotional impact of delirium. These considerations should
be valid also for delirium at the end of life but empirical data about the medical, psychological, existential, or spiritual issues characterizing delirium in this particular condition
is limited (Block 2001; Kelly et al. 2006; Kubler-Ross 1969; Massie et al. 1983).

It is also interesting to evaluate how patients are aware of being confused, and again
published experiences are not useful in answering this question, In a study on delirium
in patients with cancer, we asked the patients whether they felt confused and to rate
their perceived level of confusion on a four-point scale from 'not at all' to 'very much'.
While a group of patients reported to feel not confused at all while fulfilling the diagnostic criteria for delirium, subjective report of confusion correlated, at a low level of
statistical significance, with the DRS and MDAS scores for delirium, but the patients
with more severe symptoms were not able to answer the questionnaire (Bosisio et al.
2002). These observations have been substantially confirmed also in the palliative care
setting (Bruera et al. 2009) and indicate that delirium is 'per se', in most cases, a source
of suffering, justifying the need for palliative treatment.

4.11 **Involuntary movements and other neurological signs**

It should be said, at least once, in a book on delirium, that the diagnosis of delirium always requires a complete neurological examination. Typically then the diagnosis of delirium does not require the presence of any specific neurological sign. However, some neurological signs, in particular involuntary movements, are common in patients with delirium. Tremor, myoclonus, and asterixis are considered typical of some clinical conditions. We will see that the specificity of these and other neurological signs is low but their presence has significant clinical value as it can contribute to the differential diagnosis.

4.11.1 **Tremor**

Tremor is a classic finding in DT. Tremor is by definition an involuntary movement involving one joint characterized by a periodic swinging of a body segment according to the joint range of motion due to alternate contraction of antagonist muscles. Tremor is characterized by its frequency, amplitude, occurrence, and provocative conditions. The tremor of DT is a thin, high-frequency tremor thought to be due to overactivity of the adrenergic system, inducing a pathological exacerbation of the physiological tremor.

A thin tremor can be found also in course of uraemia and other metabolic abnormalities (metabolic tremor) but it is not specific to any clinical condition. In states of emotional or organic excitement increased tremulousness can be seen as part of an adrenergic activation as the enhancement of physiologic tremor (Elble 2000).

4.11.2 **Myoclonus**

Myoclonus is an involuntary sudden, brief, shock-like movement caused by muscle contraction (positive myoclonus) or inhibition (negative myoclonus) sufficient to displace a limb or a body segment (Fahn et al. 1986). It is different from a fasciculation, which is the contraction of only some fascicles in a muscle unable to move the limb, and from tremor, because the contraction is not rhythmic and will affect antagonist muscles at the same time. This confers to myoclonus its 'jerky' feature. Myoclonus is characteristic of some neurological diseases. It can be segmental (only one muscle or muscle group is involved), multifocal (different muscles are involved randomly), or generalized (all body muscles are involved). Myoclonus can also be classified according to its pathophysiology as cortical, subcortical, spinal, and peripheral. By this classification it is recognized that myoclonus can originate at many different levels in the peripheral and central nervous system. Myoclonic jerks are typical of several toxic-metabolic encephalopathies and often present together with delirium. Renal failure, hyponatraemia, and drug toxicity can cause myoclonus. Usually in these types of encephalopathies myoclonus is multifocal or generalized and has a cortical subcortical aetiology; at times it can precede or be complicated by seizures. Generalized myoclonus has the appearance of the muscles fits experienced randomly by anybody in the phases preceding sleep. A typical example is holding a book when lying down in bed and suddenly finding oneself jumping from sleep with the book still in the hands. A similar reaction can be obtained by waking somebody up briskly (Startle reaction). The same contraction in a fully awake state is usually pathological.

Opioid-induced myoclonus is increasingly reported in the palliative care literature perhaps due to the more liberal use of higher doses of opioid drugs (Daeninck and Bruera 1999). Its pathophysiology has to do with excitatory effects of opioids at the CNS level able to produce also hyperalgesia and seizures but needs to be studied at greater depth (see also Chapter 6).

4.11.3 Asterixis

Asterixis, also known as flapping tremor or hepatic tremor, is a negative myoclonus. With the patient keeping his arms and hands extended at the level of its eyes, the first movement to be seen is a coarse tremor in the horizontal plan, giving a kind of rotation to the hands; after a little while (the position should be held for at least a minute) the hands drop due to the resolution of the anti-gravitary muscle tone and abruptly rise back as the muscles automatically correct the position in response to the tone resolution. This failure of maintaining the muscle tone is due to central inhibition and is considered a negative myoclonus. Asterixis is seen in hepatic failure but also in other metabolic derangements and drug toxicities (ifosfamide, opioids, acyclovir); it can be shown in the legs by having them in hip, leg flexed position, foot against foot with the knees in a external suspended posture. For the very ill and exhausted patient, it is more comfortable to try to observe asterixis by just having him or her extend their index finger; the flapping movement of the finger is equivalent to the more demanding traditional manoeuvre.

4.11.4 Aspecific motor signs

These signs are thought to be related to cortical damage, often referred to as frontal liberation signs, as they are often associated with frontal syndromes. They are also referred to as primitive reflexes that would be released under pathological conditions, affecting the cerebral cortex and consciousness, by the control of higher structures in Jacksonian terms. They are frequent in different types of dementias, while physiological in newborn babies. Their finding in a patient known for not manifesting such reactions previously is valuable for diagnosing the recent onset of encephalopathy. A list of these signs follows.

- *Palmomental reflex*: by gently but firmly scratching with a blunt instrument against the palm of the hand, a contraction of the mental mimick muscle is evoked homolaterally to the stimulation side.

- *Sucking reflex*: by presenting a tactile stimulus to the lips and mouth, lip protrusion, as if in the process of sucking, is evoked.

- *Grasping*: tactile stimulation of the palm causes the patient to grasp the examiner's hand. The response cannot be inhibited voluntarily by the patient.

- *Snouting*: tactile stimulation or the perioral area evokes a mimick reflex comparable with animal snouting.

- *Paratonia* or *gegenhalten*: it is a paradoxical reflex increase of the muscle tone by semi-voluntary contraction in opposition to passive stretching of the muscles, usually tested on the arm flexory muscles. It is not easy to distinguish from true voluntary opposition.

♦ *Glabella*: when gently tapping the glabella area in the forehead a physiological blink-ing of the eyelids results, which usually disappears after a number of trials. The inability to naturally block this reflex in time is pathological.

4.12 Clinical course

Delirium was traditionally considered an acute event, with a fluctuating course that should lead to a relative quick recovery, or a transitory condition on the worsening course towards coma and death. This is still true for deliria developing in young rela-tively healthy individuals due to acute conditions or stressing events, which have a favourable course and it lasts usually for a few days. Duration is longer in the elderly with stroke, metabolic disorders, and structural brain disease (19.5 ± 15.4 days in one study; Koponen and Riekkinen 1993). Other studies suggest that duration is shorter in postoperative delirium (mean 7.6 days) than in medically ill cases (13.2 days; Manos and Wu 1997) and that longer duration is associated with dementia (Manos and Wu 1997), poorer functional recovery (Kiely et al. 2006), and threefold risk of mortality within one year (Kiely et al. 2009). Persistence of delirium is also associated with increasing numbers of medical conditions, increasing severity of delirium, hypoactive symptoms, and hypoxic illnesses (Dasgupta and Hillier 2010). Recent data (Basinski et al. 2010) show also that patients with a delirium episode within the four weeks fol-lowing haematopoietic stem cell transplantation had significantly more distress and fatigue at 6 months and at 1 year than patients without delirium. At 1 year, patients with delirium also had worse symptoms of depression and post-traumatic stress, worse physical health on a quality of life instrument (SF-12) at 6 months, and worse mental health on the SF-12 at 1 year, as well as worse memory and executive function-ing at both at 6 months and 1 year.

In a study by Levkoff et al. (1992), mentioned in the Section 3.2.1, on delirium out-comes in an elderly population showed, full recovery was shown to be rare before discharge. Only 4% of cases and more than 50% of the patients diagnosed according to DSM-III criteria during their hospital stay still fulfilled criteria for delirium after 6 months. In such cases the differential diagnosis with dementia can be difficult (Lipowski 1990b). It is possible that cognitive symptoms that persist after the delirium episode resolves are due to an underlying structural brain disorder (Hill et al. 1992). Indeed in a series of cases, an episode of delirium in the elderly was followed by a diagnosis of dementia either immediately or within the subsequent 2 years in 55% of 51 patients (Rahakonen et al. 2000). As already mentioned in patients admitted to a specialized palliative care unit, 49% of the delirious episodes were reversible (Lawlor et al. 2000b), while lower rates of reversibility in palliative care were reported by Leonard et al. (2008).

Chapter 5

Differential diagnosis

The most important differential diagnoses of delirium are dementia; psychoses (Table 5.1); focal neurological disorders affecting higher brain functions such as attention, memory, and language; psychogenic reactions, and epilepsy.

5.1 Dementia

The clinical picture of dementia can be very similar to delirium due to the widespread failure of higher cerebral functions, and to the overlap of some pathogenic mechanisms involving the failure of cortical activity and in particular of cholinergic transmission (Perry et al. 1999).

Conversely patients with dementia, as already discussed, are at increased risk of developing delirium. In a thematic symposium on delirium in the elderly, some authors (Blass and Gibson 1999; MacDonald 1999) challenged the need to distinguish between the clinical concepts of delirium and dementia, at least in the special population of the elderly demented patients.

The classic distinction between dementia and delirium is based on the acute onset and the derangement of the consciousness level (in the ICD-10, 'clouding of consciousness') characterizing delirium, as opposed to the chronic process sparing the level of consciousness, at least initially and for a period that potentially can be very long, which is typical of dementia.

The underemphasis of the transitory failure of the arousal system and therefore of consciousness in delirium can lead to a de-emphasis this clinical distinction (Lindesay 1999) and can lead to the conclusion that the global dysfunction of cognitive process can affect the elderly brain via different processes leading to a similar final condition. This view can be supported by clinical observations in the elderly with severe dementia, but also in other states of failure of the brain functions such as the preterminal phases of chronic debilitating illnesses, and in patients with severe but fluctuating compromise of state of consciousness. Yet we think that the distinction between dementia and delirium is very useful and nosologically sound for at least two reasons:

- Delirium can affect many different clinical conditions, acute illnesses as well as chronic, besides dementia as considered in this book, and some acute conditions can be well recognized also when superimposed on chronic co-morbidities.

- Delirium can be reversible: the effect of psychotropic drug toxicity so common among the elderly can acutely impair their function and be promptly reversed even in demented or terminally ill patients, confirming the therapeutic usefulness of the concept of delirium in these cases (Lawlor et al. 2000b),

Table 5.1 Main differential diagnoses of delirium

Clinical features	Delirium	Dementia	Acute psychosis
Onset	Acute	Slow	Acute
Circadian course	Fluctuating	Stable	Stable
Level of consciousness	Affected	Spared unless in severe cases	Spared
Attention	Impaired	Initially spared	Can be impaired
Cognition	Impaired	Impaired	Can be impaired
Hallucinations	Usually visual	Often absent	Often auditory
Delusions	Poorly systematized and fleeting	Often absent	Sustained and systematized
Psychomotor activity	Increased, reduced mixed with alternating course	Often normal	Can vary with bizarre behaviour depending on the psychosis
Involuntary movements	Asterixis, myoclonus, or tremor can be present in some subtypes	Absent in most forms	Absent
Electroencephalography (EEG)	Abnormal[a]	Abnormal[a]	Normal

[a] See text for more details

The case of the patient with dementia, however, is a special one and poses specific clinical difficulties. As described earlier many elderly demented patients have prolonged courses after delirious episodes with incomplete reversibility of symptoms and functional compromise. The diagnosis of delirium may apply, but in some cases the change in mental status is the manifestation of cognitive failure heralding the onset of dementia, or the worsening of an already established dementia. These challenging cases notwithstanding, we see very good reasons in agreement with the available and up-to-date diagnostic systems to maintain a clear-cut distinction between delirium and dementia.

5.2 **Psychoses**

An acute behavioural change with altered cognition and attention can be the result of a psychosis. Often the patient has a history of psychiatric disease but he or she could present for the first time with a dramatic bizarre course (*poussee' delirant*). Toxicity from amphetamines or amphetamine-type street drugs often can mimic this type of reaction.

A particular challenge is posed by the patient with a psychiatric diagnosis who develops delirium. This event is not totally rare: in one study of psychiatric admissions over three years, delirium was found in 10.4% cases most often due to drug toxicity (Huang et al. 1998). A good knowledge of the patient's pre-delirious behaviour and the observation of the sudden change of this behaviour, especially if associated with a change in the level of consciousness, can guide the diagnosis, which, however, can still be difficult. A very informative example was reported by Buchman et al. (1999) of a schizophrenic patient who developed acute psychotic symptoms after pneumonia and was found to be deficient of B12 and folic acid. After the appropriate vitamin therapy, the acute symptoms disappeared. Another case report highlighted the need to suspect toxic effects, in this situation from the reoccurrence of psychiatric disease (Brown and Rosen 1992).

Another important differential psychiatric diagnosis is the possibility of a fully psychogenic condition mimicking delirium or altered states of consciousness. The range of acute psychogenic reactions goes from epileptic pseudostatus (Makker and Yanny 2000) to psychogenic unresponsiveness (Plum and Posner 1980a). Psychogenic excitement with bizarre behaviour and movements can be mistaken for delirium with hyperactive characteristics. Alternatively, catatonia or unresponsiveness can be confused with stupor or coma. The most important aspect of these conditions is that they are quite rare and that organic causes need first to be accurately ruled out, as delirium is far more common. Psychiatric advise is required as the treatment of catatonia with benzodiazepines can resolve otherwise difficult cases (Hung and Huang 2006; Taylor and Fink 2003). In all of these cases the history of psychiatric disease is very important, and episodes, in association with new severe medical conditions, can be precipitated a long time after previous and often resolved psychiatric problems. In one very interesting case report the postoperative delirium diagnosis was compatible with the initial presentation, which evolved in a state of 'unresponsiveness' finally diagnosed with catatonia and successfully treated with lorazepam (Kalivas and Bourgeois 2009). In the past very interesting cases were described by using the amytal interview (Plum and Posner 1980a).

Depression must be considered also among the important differential psychiatric diagnoses of delirium. As already documented, many delirious patients, perhaps up to 50%, report depressive symptoms and more importantly, in the elderly medically ill, up to 42% of the patients referred for depression were finally diagnosed with delirium (Farrell and Ganzini 1995; Leonard et al 2009).

Case report

A patient of 75 years of age with a known history of manic psychosis was admitted for pain management because of advanced intrapelvic recurrence of rectal cancer with infiltration of the pelvic bone and sciatic nerve compression on the right. He had been on lithium (300 mg/day) for 12 years. On oxycodone 5mg every 6 hours pain was not controlled; because of his psychiatric disease, antidepressants were not tried; and carbamazepine had not been tolerated previously. Therefore mexiletine was added for the neuropathic component of the pain. At 1200 mg of mexiletine per day he started to be ataxic, pain was not much better, and mexiletine was discontinued. Oxycodone was substituted with morphine slow-release tablets at the dose of 40 mg b.i.d. During the night the patient started to have hallucinations and to present delusions and grandiose behaviours (he wanted to invite all the staff to a dinner with the son of the ex-king of Italy and his ministers). This type of behaviour was not totally new for him and characteristic of his manic phases and the night-shift nurse considered it to be part of his chronic psychiatric illness. In the morning he was disoriented to time but not to space and person although he had some difficulties in naming objects and no focal neurological signs. A computerized tomography (CT) scan of the head was immediately taken and showed a cortical atrophy. Morphine was stopped and changed to oxycodone with complete recovery of cognitive function. Subsequently, due to insufficient pain control, a young fellow in the pain service prescribed methadone at the dose of 10 mg t.i.d., a very high dose if compared with his previous opioid exposure (= 20 mg per day of oxycodone and 40 mg per day of morphine). After 12 hours he was acutely confused, he started to be agitated again and the grandiose delusion previously observed (the patient's wish to invite the staff to a party with the ex-king of Italy and his ministers) reappeared. Shortly afterwards stuporous, respiratory frequency decreased to 9 per minute. Naloxone was administered (0.05 mg IV) with recovery of consciousness and of respiratory rate, but the confusional state persisted for a few hours. Laboratory exams showed no metabolic nor haematologic abnormalities and lithium levels were within therapeutic ranges (0.84 mEq/L, therapeutic range 0.4–10.5 mEq/L). Therapy was modified again to oxycodone 5 mg every 6 hours plus p.r.n. (*pro re* nata; 'as circumstances may require'), and palliative radiation therapy was started on the tumour mass with analgesic benefit.

Several considerations can be raised by the circumstances of this case report:

1. The differential diagnosis of the initial presentation of delirium, which was interpreted initially as a manifestation of psychosis; indeed the night-shift nurse did not even call the physician on duty;

2. The potential metabolic interference of lithium causing toxic effects with morphine and with methadone but not with oxycodone (Brown and Rosen 1992); and

3. The presence of brain atrophy, which is also common in psychiatric patients, and may be another risk factor for toxic reactions to opioid drugs.

5.3 **Focal neurological syndromes**

Both vascular- and tumour-related focal damage of the central nervous system (CNS) can be associated with delirium (see Chapter 6) or can be confused with it, especially when focal neurological deficits affect language, memory, attention, and thought, making the assessment of the patient level and content of consciousness very difficult. In fact, patients with fluent aphasia and a preserved level of consciousness are not delirious, while patients with severe amnestic syndromes and attention failure may be confabulating and apparently very confused. Also a selective impairment of attention not associated with a change in the level of consciousness should not be diagnosed as delirium. A frontal lobe lesion can cause attention failure, perseveration, and inappropriate behaviour (Deutsch and Eisemberg 1987; Deutsche Lezak 1995). All these symptoms are often found in delirium. However, a clear-cut diagnosis can be difficult,

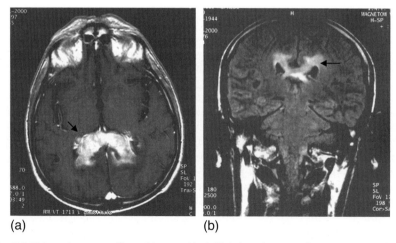

Fig. 5.1 This patient was affected by non-Hodgkin's lymphoma and metastases to the splenium of the corpus callosum. (a) Axial view of MRI with contrast (gadolinium) showing the lymphomatous lesion at the level of the splenium (arrow). (b) Coronal view showing the diffused periventricular white matter infiltration (arrow). This type of lesion is interfering with the main circuits of short-term memory.

but we would recommend being as clear as possible about the relative role of focal neurological impairment on one side and consciousness impairment on the other, recognizing that clinical overlap exists. Some acute cerebral events can present with delirium (see below) and it is important to identify and correct general metabolic or nutritional factors that might contribute to or complicate the neurological condition. Typical of this situation is the Wernicke Korsakoff syndrome, which is due to a deficit of thiamine that manifests as failure of recent memory and eye movement abnormalities, and is often associated with confabulation.

Selective, severe impairment of short-term memory can impair function and be superficially confused with delirium as in the following very short case example.

Case report

A patient with non-Hodgkin's lymphoma with a lesion of the corpus callosum (Figure 5.1) presented with amnesia and was not able to recall the whereabouts of his room in the hospital, the date, or why he was there. He was often found wandering in the hospital, apparently confused. Consciousness was preserved and he was able to perform adequately most cognitive tests, if his memory was not challenged, but he was immediately labelled as 'confused' by the medical and nursing staff of the oncology ward.

5.4 Epilepsy

Most cases of epileptic seizures cannot be confused with delirium when clinical presentation includes clear-cut convulsive generalized or partial seizures. Medical history will be helpful in patients who have suffered from a seizure disorder independently of the present illness.

On the other hand, any type of seizure is usually followed by a post-ictal confusional state that can last for hours and can be associated with headache. Seizures secondary to metastases or other general medical conditions are more often partial than generalized. If consciousness is compromised we talk of partial complex seizures, as opposed to partial simple seizures, which imply a normal level of consciousness.

Partial complex seizures and petit mal seizures can be more difficult to distinguish from delirium because they present with an altered state of consciousness and may be associated with limited and poorly defined motoric abnormalities such as visuofacial automatism. The specific clinical features are that consciousness is compromised while vigilance is apparently retained and the duration is short, lasting only a few seconds.

Non-convulsive status epilepticus (NCSE) is a situation of continuous or discontinuous but very frequent seizure activity, as documented by electroencephalographic (EEG) recordings, that does not allow consciousness recovery and lasts for hours or days. It is not totally rare in patients who are in markedly poor physical conditions and in those who have had brain injury due to metabolic disorders (Towne et al. 2000b). There are two main types of NCSE relevant to delirium: the petit mal type NCSE and the partial complex NCSE. Both manifest with an altered state of consciousness, bizarre behaviours, and/or psychotic symptoms. The substantial difference is that petit mal status implies a generalized EEG abnormality typical of petit mal seizures, while partial complex status is due to prolonged epileptic activity in discrete brain areas, often the temporal lobe, which produce behavioural and psychomotor symptoms without convulsions. At the other extreme of consciousness compromise there are cases of coma explained by NCSE (Towne et al. 2000a). Seizure activity can be continuous or discontinuous. In this last case partial seizures are recorded in cycles but no complete consciousness recovery is seen between single seizures. The clinical findings will completely overlap with the continuous type.

The possibility of partial complex seizures or NCSE should not be disregarded when considering altered states of consciousness in palliative care and in patients with complex structural, toxic, and metabolic abnormalities affecting the CNS. The diagnosis can be made only by EEG recordings. One well-described case of NCSE is ifosfamide toxicity (Figure 5.2). Ifosfamide toxicity manifests with confusion and myoclonus and is caused by subsequent partial seizures activity that can be abolished by the use of diazepam. Methylene blue proved to be an effective antidote for ifosfamide central toxicity (Kupfer et al. 1996).

Case report

The case whose EEG is reported in Figure 5.2 presented was a 65-year-old woman affected by a pelvic carcinosarcoma who underwent a course of chemotherapy with adriamycin 25 mg/m^2 (total dose = 41 mg) and ifosfamide 3 g/m^2 (total dose = 5 g). Within 12 hours after administration, she developed perseveration, inappropriate behaviours, and reduction of vigilance; she did not have abnormal movements, convulsions, or focal signs. The EEG recordings taken during the confusional state showed continuous periodic spike-type activity (mainly triphasic) compatible with the diagnosis of epileptic status.

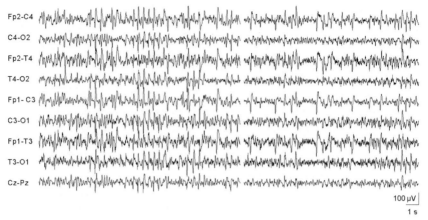

Fp2-C4

C4-O2

Fp2-T4

T4-O2

Fp1-C3

C3-O1

Fp1-T3

T3-O1

Cz-Pz

100 μV

1 s

Fig. 5.2 EEG recording during acute ifosfamide toxicity (see text). Periodic diffused peak groupings can be see on most derivations. This recording is compatible with epileptic status (Courtesy of Dr Franceschetti.)

5.5 **Incomplete syndromes**

Epidemiological studies have highlighted the frequency of partial syndromes. In a study on elderly (≥ 65 years old) hospitalized patients, some cognitive symptoms of disorientation, disturbance of consciousness, psychomotor abnormalities, speech disorders, sleep problems, and perceptual disturbances were found as often as the full syndrome without fulfilling the criteria for delirium (Levkoff et al. 1992). In a validation study of delirium scales in 105 cancer patients referred for neurological or psychiatric opinion for suspected delirium, 66 patients received the diagnosis of delirium, whereas, of the remaining 39, 13 had acute mental symptoms without fulfilling all the criteria for delirium (Grassi et al. 2001b).

The finding of symptoms of acute confusion without fulfilling the criteria for delirium is not therefore uncommon. Hallucinations are often reported as one effect of opioid toxicity that may be part of a developing delirium. One patient of ours with moderate renal failure developed visual hallucinations after increasing the morphine dose, and recovered after renal function improved (Caraceni et al. 1994). The findings of Fountain (2001) have already been reported in Chapter 4 and show a prevalence of 30% for hallucinations in the hospice patient population.

The DSM-III allowed the use of the terminology, 'organic hallucinosis', for a patient with these characteristics. The condition would have been classified under the organic brain disorders. In the DSM-IV the classification of such symptoms is more complicated, requiring that they be identified within either the mental disorders related to a general medical condition or a substance-related disorder and therefore lack of generality.

Partial syndromes represent, at times, cases at risk of developing the full syndrome, 'quasi delirious', or the more selective ability of some causal factor to induce a symptom (Trzepacz 1994a).

5.5.1 **An illustrative case report**

The patient is a 72-year-old lady affected by breast cancer and non-Hodgkin's lymphoma with spinal cord compression at D1–D2 level admitted for radiation therapy, chemotherapy, and symptom control. Pain in the legs and dorsal spine was treated with tramadol initially 50 mg in oral drops t.i.d., which was substituted at admission by transdermal fentanyl 25 µg/h patch. Therapy included dexamethasone 16 mg/day. After about 24 hours on this regimen she developed first hallucinations described as bees entering her room through the window and Talibans on top of her TV set. Durogesic and dexamethasone were stopped and tramadol given as IV infusion at the dose of 300 mg/day with morphine 5 mg rescue dose for p.r.n medication. Hallucinations disappeared for 2 days. Chemotherapy for her lymphoma was given, including prednisolone 100 mg/day for 3 days. At this time a new episode occurred and she saw her friends in the room who were changed into salt statues, and people coming in the room who fell asleep in strange positions. When examined and questioned about what was going on, she reported that, due to some radio waves still persisting within the room, the people coming in were very pale with black lips. The only way to solve this problem was that she put on a special suit that you could buy in the hospital and that she had bought the evening before for about 15 Euros. At the same time, she pointed at the TV set on top of which one nurse was asleep. Her vigilance was intact, visuospatial orientation perfect, memory and cognition not affected, and she could write and copy designs properly. No neurological signs were found and a head CT scan and laboratory examinations were normal.

Her drug regimen was kept unchanged regarding the intake of opioids, while steroids were tapered. In the following days hallucinations and delusions were absent, she was disoriented to time and had night-time insomnia and agitation. For her symptoms she received also haloperidol 2 mg at night with benefit. When asked again about the complex hallucinations experienced she was quite irritated and replied shortly that, although what had happened was real, it was not happening anymore. She developed febrile neutropenia and pneumonia and died about a week after the first hallucinatory episode.

In conclusion, the role of opioids in this case in uncertain. The episodes are characterized mainly by hallucinations and the patient report about them is still delusional when examining her after the full-blown episode was finished. Other areas of cognition were not affected and consciousness was not compromised. It would be possible to emphasize the role of corticosteroids, perhaps in combination with fentanyl, in the first episode and to classify the case as steroid psychosis, using an old definition. Using DSM-IV language one should talk of a 'substance-induced psychosis'. The subjective reaction of the patient to the episodes underlines the need for a better understanding of this area of subjective feelings and to be prepared to help patients in coping with this type of experiences.

5.6 **Role of the EEG in differential diagnosis**

EEG recordings can be used to differentiate delirium from seizures and from psychoses. The main EEG features found in delirium are the increase of the percentage of slow frequencies, possibly finding delta (< 4 Hz) and theta (4–8 Hz) rhythms together with the disruption of the physiological alpha rhythm (= 8–13 Hz). These characteristic features can be used to differentiate the delirious from the non-delirious and from demented elderly patients (Jacobson et al. 1993a, b; Koponen et al. 1989; Sidhu et al. 2009). The slowing of the EEG in the range of the alpha frequency that is still considered normal would be a significant sign of encephalopathy, but its usefulness is limited because the normal appearance of the alpha before the onset of delirium is usually unknown unless an EEG under 'control conditions'. This situation is clarified in the following case example. See also Chapter 8.

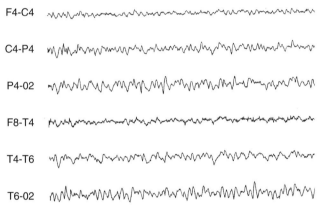

F4-C4

C4-P4

P4-02

F8-T4

T4-T6

T6-02

Fig. 5.3 This patient had chemotherapy toxicity with delirium and probably non-convulsive status epilepticus. The EEG shown corresponds to phase of recovery of the mental status, several days after the acute episode shows a persistent slowing (8 Hz) of the physiological alpha rhythm (13 Hz), mainly over the occipital areas where this type of frequency is physiologically mostly represented. The traces represent electrical activity recorded from only the right hemisphere. A significant slowing of the EEG frequency (8 Hz) can be seen principally in the recordings from the occipital areas (P4-02 and T6-O2).

Case report

A 22-year-old patient affected by medulloblastoma of the posterior fossa that was surgically resected had a course of chemotherapy that included high-dose IV thiotepa. She developed consciousness impairment associated with complex forelimb movements and eye rowing. Lorazepam 5 mg IV was given in several doses and fenitoin 18 mg/kg infusion was started; consciousness improved and pathological movement stopped but psychomotor slowing persisted for a few hours. After 6 hours she started to be confused again, and, later on, became stuporous. For better monitoring of her vital function, the patient was transferred to the ICU where,

despite antiepileptic medications, she had more episodes of involuntary movements and disturbances of consciousness. Brain MRI showed no change, in comparison with her previous imaging. In two days the level of consciousness improved
and the patient was awake and oriented but, however, somnolent and slow in
performing mental tasks. The EEG, taken on two different occasions, when the
patient consciousness was only slightly impaired, showed that the alpha rhythm on
the occipital derivations was relatively slow 8–9 Hz (Figure 5.3). On one occasion
during spontaneous sleep the EEG showed the onset of slow waves in the delta
rhythm range and of peaks. Thiothepa-induced encephalopathy was the final
diagnosis. Consciousness compromise was attributed to potential NCES (although
seizure activity was never recorded) on the basis of the sparse ictal activiy (peaks)
seen in the EEG, with intercurrent phases of recovery associated with delirium and
encephalopathy as documented by slow waves and slowing of the physiological
alpha rhythm.

Chapter 6

Frequent aetiologies

In this section a more detailed description is given of some clinically defined delirious syndromes. Not every cause or condition is examined but only those that are more frequent or can be particularly relevant in the palliative care settings. The clinical conditions that follow are grouped according to aetiology or to a particular patient population.

6.1 Alcohol withdrawal delirium (delirium tremens) and other withdrawal deliria

Withdrawal from substances is a frequent cause of delirium. As already indicated in Chapter 2 the most recent classification of delirium indicate that delirium can occur as a consequence of withdrawal from alcohol or substances with sedative, hypnotic, or anxiolytic properties. It is important to recognize that although full-blown withdrawal syndromes (such as delirium tremens) are relatively rare, symptoms of withdrawal are more common and can be associated with delirium (Norton 2001).

6.1.1 Delirium Tremens

Alcoholism is recognized throughout the world as an important public health problem. Individuals who excessively and continuously consume alcohol have been drinking for years and maintain a high alcohol intake, shifting from alcohol abuse to alcohol dependence (Ashworth and Gerada 1997; Langenbucher et al. 2000; McKeon et al. 2008). They commonly experience withdrawal symptoms one or two days after substantial reduction or complete withdrawn from alcohol (Chang and Steinberg 2001; Hall and Zador 1997).

Symptoms include general malaise, signs of autonomic hyperactivity (i.e. tremors, especially hands, legs, and trunk tremors; tachycardia and hypertension; sweating; nausea; insomnia), and psychological symptoms (i.e. anxiety and agitation, irritability and mood lability, transient perceptual disturbances, such as illusions, visual and tactile hallucinations) in a condition in which reality testing is, however, intact. These symptoms may last about 1 week and are rapidly relieved by alcohol intake. However, in some forms, alcohol withdrawal can be complicated by the onset of seizures, 6-48 hours and a peak at 24 hours after the last consumption of alcohol. Seizures actually represent a major complication of delirium tremens (DT), which has been the focus of careful attention for their consequences (Hillbom et al. 2003). They are related to several mechanisms, including modification of the calcium and chloride flux through the ion-gated glutamate N-methyl-D-aspartate (NMDA) and gamma-aminobutyric acid (GABA) receptors, and concurrent metabolic, toxic, infectious, traumatic, neoplastic, and cerebrovascular diseases (Hughes 2009; Rogawski 2005).

In these cases, the onset of a full-blown delirium state, diagnosed as alcohol withdrawal delirium, or delirium tremens, is not uncommon (30%). Thus the onset of DT is usually gradual (2–3 days after cessation of alcohol intake, with a peak at 4–5 days), with early and prodromic symptoms represented by uncomplicated alcohol withdrawal syndrome, although sudden forms of DT are also possible (Erwin et al. 1998).

Risk factors for developing DT in patients with alcohol withdrawal syndrome have been suggested to be concurrent infections, tachycardia (heart rate above 100–120 beats per minute at admission), signs of alcohol withdrawal accompanied by an alcohol concentration of more than 1 g/L of body fluid, a history of epileptic seizures, a history of delirious episodes, and, possibly, thrombocytopenia (Berggren et al. 2009; Lee JH et al. 2005; Monte et al. 2009; Palmstierna 2001). It has also been suggested that patients with alcohol dependence who present prefrontal atrophy and frontal cortical and temporal (sub)cortical atrophy at CT scan may be at higher risk of developing DT (Maes et al. 2000). Some recent studies have tried to demonstrate a possible genetic predisposition for DT, with data suggesting positive associations of DT with neuropeptide and cannabinoid gene, and in candidate genes involved in the dopamine transmission and in the glutamate pathway (Adamis et al. 2009; van Muster et al. 2007). More studies are, however, necessary in this complex area of research.

The clinical features of DT are represented by alcohol withdrawal symptoms, complicated by the typical symptoms of delirium: reduced level of consciousness, disorientation in time and place, impairment in recent memory, and insomnia. In DT significant perceptual disturbances and thought disorders are present. The patient appears agitated and frightened by visual, but also tactile and auditory, vivid hallucinations (mostly insects or small animals) and misinterpretations of environmental stimuli. Marked autonomic arousal is also a typical feature of DT, with tremors, tachycardia, hypertension, sweating, and mild fever, complicated sometimes, as already mentioned, by seizures. DT usually lasts 3 days, followed by a deep sleep from which the patient frequently awakes with no memory of the delirium. However, it has also been reported that DT may fluctuate for several weeks. Metabolic disorders, infections, poor general physical conditions, and concomitant physical illness are all risk factors for more severe complications associated with DT (Wojnar et al. 1999).

Mortality ranges from very low percentages to a maximum of 5%, according to clinical severity of delirium, predisposing factors, and response to treatment (McCowan and Marik 2000). It has been indicated that use of restraint and hyperthermia in the first 24 hours of DT diagnosis were associated with increased mortality (Khan et al. 2008).

Thus, obtaining an alcohol consumption history, identifying possible risk factors, recognizing alcohol withdrawal symptoms, and initiating early treatment are significant steps in the prevention of DT among hospitalized patients, especially those in advanced stages of physical illness (Mayo-Smith 1997; Schumacher et al. 2000).

Driessen et al. (2005), by using hierarchical cluster analysis and discriminant analysis in the study of alcohol withdrawal syndrome in 217 alcohol-dependent patients, found five clusters representing increasing severity of alcohol withdrawal, each of the clusters being characterized by a combination of the two maximum subscores (vegetative and psychopathological subscore) and three additional psychopathological symptoms (anxiety, disorientation, and hallucination). The authors showed that relevant symptoms were not observed in 18.4% of the patients (cluster 1), 18.9% developed mild or moderate vegetative symptoms only (cluster 2), and 40.6% developed the additional symptom of anxiety (cluster 3). In cluster 4 (11.1%) the most frequent psychopathological symptoms were disorientation and anxiety but no hallucinations, which could be observed only in cluster 5 (11.1%). The maximum subscores at the first day of treatment as independent variables correctly predicted 89.9% of the five clusters.

6.1.2 **Other forms of withdrawal delirium**

As indicated in both the DSM-IV-TR and the ICD-10, other forms of delirium can develop because of withdrawal from several substances (Olmedo and Hoffman 2000).

The persistent use (or abuse) of anxiolytics and hypnotics has been reported to favour the onset of delirium at abrupt discontinuation (Heritch et al. 1987). However, Bruera et al. (1996) showed that, among cancer patients in an advanced phase of illness, a rapid decrease in the doses of hypnotic drugs was not followed by withdrawal syndrome nor rebound phenomena, as expected. This experience will not, however, suffice, in our opinion, to avoid caution in withdrawing benzodiazepine therapy in patients who have been using it for significant periods of time. We saw several cases presenting with signs of withdrawal, including delirium, after abrupt discontinuation of benzodiazepine that had been habitually taken for months or years.

Nicotine can also be considered a possible cause of withdrawal delirium. Mayer et al. (2001) reported five cases of nicotine withdrawal delirium among patients with a history of heavy tobacco usage who were treated in a neurologic intensive care unit for brain injury. Transdermal nicotine replacement showed to be effective in recovering patients from delirium within a few hours (Gallagher 1998).

Cases of withdrawal from gamma-hydroxybutyric acid (GHB) and gamma-butyrolactone (GBL), as new drugs of abuse for their similarities to sedative-hypnotic or alcohol intoxication, have been reported. These substances not only determine disturbances of consciousness due to overdose, but delirium-like symptoms at rapid discontinuation, among high-frequency users. Withdrawal syndrome that presented with anxiety, agitation, tremor, and delirium was shown in a study carried out by Miotto et al. (2001) in GHB abusers. Sivilotti et al. (2001) reported cases of delirium, with tachycardia, hypertension, paranoid delusions, hallucinations, and rapid fluctuations in sensorium, secondary to abrupt GBL discontinuation. While high doses of lorazepam proved to be ineffective, pentobarbital resulted in excellent control of behavioural, autonomic, and psychiatric symptoms.

Recent reports have repeatedly registered withdrawal syndrome after abrupt discontinuation of the commonly used centrally acting muscle relaxant carisoprodol (Reeves et al. 2007; Reeves and Burke 2010), including the onset of delirium (Ni et al. 2007). Delirium has been reported in association with withdrawal from many different drugs and case reports of this type are increasing. Clinical observations have reported withdrawal from valerian root (Garges et al. 1998), alprazolam (Zalsman et al. 1998), zopiclone (Wong et al. 2005), amantadine (Factor et al. 1998), clozapine (Stanilla et al. 1997), selective serotonin re-uptake inhibitors (SSRIs), such as paroxetine (Hayakawa et al. 2004) and fluoxetine (Blum et al. 2008), gabapentin (Norton 2001; Pittenger and Desan 2007), and baclofen (Leo and Bader 2005), to give a non-comprehensive list.

6.2 Delirium due to metabolic causes

Together with drug-induced toxic deliria, metabolic abnormalities are likely to account for the most common group of aetiologies encountered in medically ill patients. This condition is one of the most common diagnoses in consultation or liaison psychiatry and neurology at general and tertiary care hospitals (Tuma and DeAngelis 2000). The term 'metabolic encephalopathy' is often used as a synonym for metabolic delirium and can be considered to be, in the neurologist's vocabulary, its neuropathogenic equivalent (Lipowski 1990b; Plum and Posner 1980b). In palliative care metabolic encephalopathy is often found in the very terminal phases of disease, as shown in a postdoctoral thesis dissertation on the result of a home-care program for advanced cancer patients, where metabolic encephalopathy was considered the main final cause of coma and death in 56% of cases (Groff 1993).

Metabolic encephalopathy is the result of several general metabolic abnormalities producing diffused brain damage through mechanisms that finally cause dysfunction of the brain cellular metabolism. Brain metabolism is particularly sensitive to oxygen and glucose demand. In general all the causes of metabolic encephalopathy result in a reduction of oxygen and glucose consumption by the brain, leading to initially reversible cellular damage and finally to cell death. An accurate mechanistic classification of metabolic encephalopathies is reproduced, in its general terms, from Plum and Posner (1980b) in Table 6.1. Table 6.2 summarizes instead a few principles that hold valid through the review of most metabolic encephalopathies.

6.2.1 Hepatic encephalopathy

Hepatic encephalopathy occurs either in patients with advanced liver disease and evidence of hepatic failure or when for different reasons, including liver disease, the bloodstream from the enteroportal cycle due to portosystemic shunt bypasses liver circulation. The clinical picture of hepatic encephalopathy can range from mild cognitive failure, drowsiness, and memory laps to full-blown delirium. Delirium due to hepatic failure is more often of the hypoactive type (Ross et al. 1991) with lethargy evolving into a comatose state if not treated. However, this is only partially true, as hallucinations and hyperactive delirium are reported in up to 10–20% of the cases (Plum and Posner 1980b). Asterixis can be seen in many metabolic encephalopathies and has been described first in liver failure—hence the denomination 'hepatic tremor' (Adams and Foley 1953). Preclinical changes in the EEG and evoked potentials have been shown preceding more pronounced clinical findings, and the combined use of EEG and cognitive testing has been shown to improve the accuracy of the clinical assessment (Trzepacz et al. 1989a, b). The pathogenesis of hepatic encephalopathy is not completely understood. Most explanations refer to the neurotoxic activity of substances coming from the portal circulation system that would normally be inactivated by the liver. Only in extreme cases (Muller et al. 1994) and in newborn babies can bilirubin cross the blood–brain barrier and be toxic for the brain.

Table 6.1 Classification of metabolic encephalopathies

A. Deprivation of oxygen, substrate, or metabolic cofactors

    Hypoxia (reduction of brain oxygen supply of pulmonary or haematologic origin)

    Ischaemia (of cardiac, circulatory, or rheologic origin)

    Hypoglycaemia

    Cofactor deficiency (thiamine, niacine, pyridoxine, cyanocobalamin, folic acid)

B. Diseases of other organs

    Liver

    Kidney

    Lung

    Pancreas

    Endocrine hypo-/hyperfunction (pituitary, thyroid, parathyroid, adrenal)

C. Exogenous toxic substances (poisons and drugs)

D. Ionic or acid–base imbalances

    Water and sodium imbalances hypo-/hypernatremia

    Acidosis

    Alkalosis

    Hyper-/hypomagnesaemia

    Hyper-/hypocalcaemia

    Hypo-phospahtaemia

E. Temperature dysregulation (hypothermia, heat stroke, fever)

F. Infections and inflammation of CNS

G. Primary neuronal or glial disorders

H. Miscellaneous disorders

    Seizures postictal state

    Post-traumatic encephalopathy

    Sedative drug withdrawal

    Postoperative delirium

Data from Plum and Posner (1980b).

Recent studies have valued the role of endogenous benzodiazepine-like substances in causing sedation, cognitive dysfunction, delirium, and eventually coma in patients with hepatic failure. The use of the benzodiazepine antagonist flumazenil was therefore proposed to improve cognitive functions and treat comatose patients in the advanced phases of hepatic failure. The most recent evidence shows that, although an increase in the GABA-ergic tone is likely in the pathogenesis of hepatic encephalopathy (Meyer et al. 1998), administration of flumazenil gave conflicting results in humans and had no effect on animals (Meyer et al. 1998), therefore bringing into question the

Table 6.2 General principles of metabolic encephalopathies

- The more rapid the development of the toxic state, the less perturbed the chemical findings need to be to produce symptoms

- No morphological brain abnormalities are found and when found are due to secondary effects

- Non-specific motor signs are common paratonia or gegenhalten, snouting, sucking, palmomental reflex, grasping

- Characteristic motor signs are asterixis and multifocal myoclonus; seizures can be found independently of the underlying etiology

- In coma resulting from metabolic encephalopathy pupillary reactivity is preserved

- Focal signs, eye deviation, and asymmetrical extensor plantar responses cannot rarely be found and do not rule out metabolic encephalopathy versus brain structural disease

- Hyperventilation is not always present but is rather specific, compensating for metabolic acidosis, or primary, driven by toxic state (respiratory alkalosis)

pathogenic role of benzodiazepine-like ligands (Macdonald et al. 1997). Randomized trials on patients with hepatic encephalopathy of different severities show that only a minor percentage of patients–about 30%–have clinical or EEG improvement (Annese et al. 1998; Barbaro et al. 1998; Groeneweg et al. 1996; Laccetti et al. 2000), and no improvement was seen on cognitive and neurophysiological assessment of patients with subclinical cognitive impairment (Amodio et al. 1997). Also recently no correlation was found between benzodiazepine-like substances levels and degree of encephalopathy (Venturini et al. 2001). Traditional chronic management relies on lactulose, neomycin, and protein restriction with an uncertain role for the administration of branched-chain amino acids.

In progressive hepatic failure encephalopathy will present as an inevitable progressive final evolution. When the portosystemic shunt of the venous intestinal blood is the main pathogenic mechanism, an acute excess of nitrogen due to increased alimentary intake, bleeding of esophageal varices, and protein catabolism can acutely precipitate encephalopathy. The speed of the change may be more important than the actual ammonia level, which only partially parallels the severity of the encephalopathy (Venturini et al. 2001). There is a considerable degree of overlap between the levels of ammonia recorded in patients with liver disease and hepatic encephalopathy and those without signs of encephalopathy (Plum and Posner 1980b). Although absolute ammonia levels do not correlate well with the degree of encephalopathy (Venturini et al. 2001), ammonia remains, however, the best biochemical correlate of hepatic encephalopathy. The evidence reported, however, must lead to the conclusion that it is not ammonia per se that causes brain toxicity. Interestingly, magnetic resonance imaging (MRI) spectroscopy may help to find more accurate metabolic counterparts of clinical finding but results are at the moment only in progress (Jenkins and Kraft 1999).

Liver failure is not uncommon in advanced cancer due to metastatic disease and ammonia should be tested when cognitive symptoms are found, also when other liver function tests are not excessively abnormal or different from usual. The contribution of liver failure to the mortality of palliative care patients is unknown; in one series of patients with advanced cancer followed up to death by a home-care-based palliative care service hepatic failure was considered the main cause of death in 18% of cases (Groff 1993).

6.2.2 Uraemic encephalopathy

Renal failure is known to cause delirium but the cause of brain dysfunction in the course of uraemia is unknown (Tyler 1968). Urea is not responsible of brain toxicity and the relationship between blood levels of uraemia and encephalopathy is not linear. In general plasma urea levels should be above 200 mg/dl to produce signs of encephalopathy but delirium has been seen in cases where levels were as low as 48 mg/dl, as in the case reported by Plum and Posner (1980b). Also in this situation the rapidity of the metabolic change is very important, more than the absolute abnormality level. EEG changes correlate with uraemia (Hagstam 1971; Hughes 1980). Parathormone and brain calcium abnormalities are one potential pathogenic mechanism that probably accounts for some clinical phenomena. Several guanidine compounds, e.g. creatinine, may also play a role in uraemic encephalopathy. These substances accumulate in uraemia and have excitatory effects at the central nervous system (CNS) level by activation of NMDA receptors (De Deyn et al. 2001).

Multifocal myoclonus is typically associated with uraemic encephalopathy and seizures are also frequent. Renal failure can be associated with electrolyte imbalance, metabolic acidosis, hypertensive encephalopathy, and in the medically ill patient not affected by a primary renal illness, other complications of the underlying main pathological process. Therefore it can be difficult to identify the aetiology of the delirium. Non-convulsive epileptic status should also be suspected in patients acutely confused or stuporous in the terminal phases of renal failure (Chow et al. 2001). In patients with advanced terminal illness, dehydration, oliguria, or anuria are common terminal events. Some patients will have specific causes of renal failure, such as bilateral hydronephosis, infections, or drug toxicity. Low renal perfusion pressure is likely to intervene in most cases due to hypotension and low systolic stroke volume. The role of renal failure in characterizing the final phases of many progressive diseases is unknown, although Bruera and co-workers (1995) suggested that moderate hydration can be useful to preserve the renal clearance of drugs and metabolites in order to prevent agitated deliria.

6.2.3 Pulmonary encephalopathy and acid–base imbalances

Pulmonary encephalopathy is also defined as hypercapnic encephalopathy and it is characteristic of advanced pulmonary disease, such as chronic obstructive pulmonary disease (COPD). In this respect, it is worthwhile considering that COPD and tobacco smoke are very frequent co-morbidities in the palliative care patient, and extremely frequent in patients affected by lung cancer.

In pulmonary encephalopathy, the relative roles of hypercarbia, hypoxia, and respiratory acidosis may be difficult to ascertain. In general CO_2 is a narcotic due to its effect on the brain pH. Posner et al. (1965) suggested that neurological symptoms are probably related to the degree of brain cellular acidosis. Acute hypercarbia is less tolerated than a slow increase in pCO_2 as develops in cases of COPD. In patients with acute hypercarbia, 70 mmHg of pCO_2 is sufficient to produce cerebral symptoms while the same level of hypercarbia can be well tolerated in COPD patients (Dulfano and Ishikawa 1965). The best correlate of encephalopathy in the derangement of acid–base balance is cerebrospinal fluid (CSF) pH, which is controlled by homeostatic mechanisms that are very efficient especially in metabolic acidosis, metabolic alkalosis, and respiratory alkalosis, and less so in respiratory acidosis (Posner and Plum 1967; Posner et al. 1965).

Intercurrent minor events can be crucial for the fragile balance of compensatory systems in the compromised patient. One typical example of this situation is the use of sedative drugs. Respiratory failure can develop in the progression of incurable illnesses in different patterns, depending on patient history and present disease. Acute dyspnea can be suddenly caused by pleural effusion or superior vena cava syndrome or more slowly by progressive pulmonary parenchyma metastatic substitution or carcinomatous lymphangites. Pulmonary infections are very common in both cancer and AIDS patients. Lawlor and co-workers (2000b) found that hypoxia associated with lung cancer or infection was a factor associated with irreversible deliria in advanced cancer patients. Dyspnoea is a severe and particularly distressful symptom associated with hypoxia, and has a compensatory role by stimulating ventilation in the attempt to keep pO_2 and pCO_2 within physiological limits. In the advanced patient with irreversible dyspnoea who is in high distress, palliative therapy with opioids and/or neuroleptics is often considered. One must be aware that the delicate balance between respiratory frequency, pCO_2, and acidosis can be affected by the use of opioids or neuroleptics and by any modification of the internal milieu that decreases the respiratory centres' response to pCO_2 (Mercadante 1997). The relief of dyspnoea may parallel a slow increase of pCO_2 and acidosis, although this is not clinically evident, and hypoxia will not occur in most cases (Bruera et al. 1990). Hypercapnic encephalopathy can ensue and a vicious irreversible cycle can lead to a coma due to respiratory failure. The control of this situation would be possible by careful monitoring of arterial pO_2, pCO_2, and serum bicarbonate. The clinical conditions (prognosis, suffering, patient's will, goals of care) will dictate the choice between optimizing patient comfort and maximising respiratory function and biochemical control (Ventafridda et al. 1990b).

Respiratory failure together with the metabolic abnormalities already discussed is a common scenario in the last days or hours of life for many terminal patients but also in these cases the prevalence of respiratory failure as a cause of death is not known (Lawlor et al. 2000b). The only data available to us report a 15% frequency of respiratory failure as the main cause of death in terminal cancer patients under hospice home-care (Groff 1993).

Pure metabolic changes due to systemic metabolic causes are probably more rare in palliative care than respiratory failure, but should not be discarded, in cases with concurrent diabetes, hyponutrition, or malabsorption, and renal failure. Diabetic ketoacidosis is the most common cause of encephalopathy of primarily metabolic origin (Posner and Plum 1967). Other more rare conditions, such as in cases of abnormal absorption of carbohydrates in short bowel syndrome combined with a dysmicrobic colonic flora, can be found (Gavazzi et al. 2001).

6.2.4 **Cofactor deficiency**

Nutritional reduced intake of vitamins is typical of patients with abuse of alcohol and it is not uncommon in the elderly or in patients with advanced cancer and anorexia. Thiamine (vitamin B1) deficiency is probably the most frequent vitamin deficiency that can manifest with an acute change in the state of consciousness, gross impairment of recent memory, and coma, for the endogenous reserve of this vitamin is easily depleted by relatively short-lived periods of insufficient intake. The full-blown syndrome associates dementia, abnormalities of eye movement, peripheral neuropathy, and hypotension, but partial presentations with normal eye movements, modest peripheral neuropathy, and initial cognitive impairment or delirium are possible.

Thiamine has a key role in carbohydrate metabolism and its daily intake should be of at least 1 mg but it increases when carbohydrates become the main source of energy. Thiamine bodily reserves are not abundant and strictly dependent on alimentary intake. A number of factors can predispose to a relatively fast exhaustion of thiamine deposits: surgery followed or preceded by hyponutrition (Vidal et al. 2000), emesis associated with treatment with glucose IV solutions, and chemotherapy interfering with hepatic synthesis of thiamine. A significant association has been found between thiamine deficiency and neoplasms in a series of 31 paediatric patients (Vasconcelos et al. 1999). Early signs of thiamine deficiency occur after a week of thiamine deprivation.

For these reasons the role of thiamin deficiency has been investigated to explain the increased risk of developing delirium in patients with poor general health, the elderly, or the malnourished, but results have been not homogeneous (Barbato and Rodriguez 1994; O'Keeffe et al. 1994; Papersack et al. 1999). The addition of thiamine to the therapeutic regimen of a confused patient with poor general condition can be empirically recommended (1000 mg/day to start).

Another vitamin often neglected but has been associated with mental changes in hyponutrition and in alcoholic encephalopathy is nicotinic acid (pellagra-protecting (PP) vitamin; Serdaru et al. 1988). It could be supplemented in 250 mg tablets once a day in cases of severely reduced food intake and obscure encephalopathy (Checkley et al. 1939).

Vitamin B12 deficiency causes anaemia, polyneuropathy, spinal cord degeneration, and encephalopathy (Buchman et al. 1999). Cases of encephalopathy without anaemia have been described (Lindenbaum et al. 1988). Patients with gastric disease and malabsorption are at risk of B12 deficiency.

6.2.5 **Electrolyte and water imbalances**

In the medically ill, water balance can be easily affected because of insufficient attention to input and output of fluids; particular attention must be paid to renal function especially when IV fluids or diuretic therapy are instituted. Hyponatraemia is the most common condition. It is also frequently an effect of the syndrome of inappropriate antidiuretic hormone secretion (SIADH), which is a complication of many drugs (morphine, cyclophosphamide, vincristine) and brain lesions. When hyponatraemia develops rapidly brain oedema and change in neuronal membrane excitability cause encephalopathy, ranging from delirium with asterixis and multifocal myoclonus, to coma and seizures. Figure 6.1 shows the relationship between sodium plasma levels and brain dysfunction from an early study by Arieff et al. (1976).

In patients with advanced cancer, it is very common to find that sodium levels are slightly or moderately below normal limits (between 130 and 120 mEq/L). The role of this finding in the pathophysiology of other complications–the so-called 'deterioration of general conditions'–that we commonly see in the clinical picture of PC patients is not known. All electrolytes should be checked including magnesium. In rare cases even hypophosphatemia is a possibility (Hall et al. 1994).

Electrolyte abnormalities are, however, always to be considered in acute changes of mental status. Rare causes can be sought in particular conditions, but sodium, potassium, calcium, and magnesium should never be left out of a diagnostic screening (Hall et al. 1994). Hypercalcaemia is frequently associated with bone metastases or as result of paraneoplastic secretion of endocrine active substances. When serum calcium levels are above 12 mg/dl, cognition can be impaired. Hypoalbuminaemia is frequently associated with advanced patients where the fraction of calcium ions bound to albumin is decreased; therefore, it is important to calculate the actual calcaemia by correcting it for hypoalbuminaemia.

6.3 Toxic causes of delirium

The most clinically relevant toxicity affecting the CNS and causing delirium is drug toxicity, usually associated with medical therapy or abuse. The ability to identify one drug as a cause for delirium depends on anecdotal clinical observation, pharmacological knowledge, and clinical studies. One recent systematic review of the literature confirmed that scientific evidence supports the association of psychoactive medications and use of opioids with an independent increased risk of developing delirium (Gaudreau et al. 2005c).

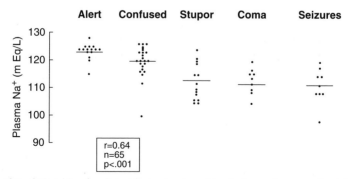

Fig. 6.1 The relationship of sodium plasma levels and level of consciousness. A relationship between severity of clinical findings and hyponatraemia is quite evident, but so is a wide degree of overlapping of laboratory values across very different clinical condition. Reproduced from Arieff et al. (1976) with permission.

6.3.1 **Anticholinergic drugs**

Since ancient times it has been known that anticholinergic drugs have the ability to cause delirium. Belladonna alkaloids were described as delirogenic by Theofrastus as long ago as the fourth century BC. Experimental human studies on anticholinergic delirium have already been summarized in Chapter 2 (see Itil and Fink 1968) and show that drugs such as scopolamine, ditran, and atropine can cause delirium, depending on dosage. Lower doses usually produce somnolence (scopolamine 0.3–0.8 mg), higher doses (atropine $\geq$ 5 mg, scopolamine = 1 mg) agitated florid delirium; paradoxical effect of low doses have also been demonstrated. The following observations are relevant to the understanding the toxic CNS effect of these drugs:

1. Attention and cognition are diminished by the administration of anticholinergics;

2. Pharmacokinetics changes in the elderly and in children enhance bioavailability of these drugs;

3. In the aging or demented brain the anticholinergic system is already compromised as part of the pathogenesis of global cognitive deficit;

4. The elderly and children are more susceptible to delirium when comparable lower doses of these drugs are administered;

5. Serum anticholinergic activity has been studied as one of the factors that might explain different clinical conditions such as drug toxicity and postoperative delirium; and

6. A list of the drugs in which CNS toxicity is believed to be related to their anticholinergic activity is given in Table 6.3.

True anticholinergic delirium should be reversible with physostigmine. The use of physostigmine is restricted to cases of proven anticholinergic toxicity (although cases of miscellaneous deliria are reported to respond to cholinergic stimulation), because there is the risk of inducing cholinergic toxic effects by using physostigmine. Anticholinergic toxicities should be associated with some of the physical signs reported in Table 6.4. The recent introduction of cholinergic drugs for the therapy of dementia offers an interesting opportunity to test these drugs in some acute confusional states.

6.3.2 **Opioids**

Opioid therapy for pain, dyspnoea, and terminal sedation is a mainstay of palliative medicine. Delirium can be the result of some effects of opioids on the CNS (Stiefel and Morant 1991). To understand opioid-induced delirium, it is necessary to review the sedative activity of opioids and other toxic effects on the CNS (Lawlor 2002).

Opioid-induced sedation

Among the central side effects of opioids, the modification of cognition and vigilance is the most important limitation in dose titration (Portenoy et al. 1990). The subjective sensation of mental clouding and sedation ('foggy, obtunded' in patient's words) is the single most disliked component of opioid therapy by patients and, in our experience, it is the most important reason to resist dose escalation, usually before sedation or cognitive impairment is clinically evident to an external examiner. Subjective sedation is commonly related to sleepiness. Subjectively patients feel as they

Table 6.3 Drugs with anticholinergic activity

Prototypical anticholinergics
Belladonna alkaloids
Atropine
Scopolamine
Tricyclic antidepressants
Marzine
Diphenidramine
Promethazine
Biperidene
Trihexiphenidile
Chlorpromazine
Hyoscine buthylbromide
Robinul
Hypnotics
Barbiturates
Chloral hydrate
Paraldehyde
Bromides
Benzodiazepines
Antibiotics
Antimalarian
Antituberculous
Antiviral
Antifungal
Anticonvulsants
Antiparkinsonian
Amantadine

might easily fall asleep especially while reading or lying in bed in a quiet environment. Sleepiness can be considered objectively as the subject's propensity to fall asleep or alternatively as the subject's subjective sensation of sleepiness (Johns 1993). The two concepts do not necessarily overlap (Johnson et al. 1990). Opioid drugs induce sleepiness but have never been studied systematically in this regard by using a specific definition of sleepiness. While looking at the central side effects of opioids it is therefore important to distinguish between subjective sedation, objective sedation, cognitive impairment, and delirium.

Table 6.4 Syndrome of anticholinergic toxicity

Dilated pupils with reduced light reactivity
Hot, dry skin, and mucous membranes
Flushed face, peripheral vasodilation
Blurred vision, impaired accommodation
Tachycardia
Urinary retention
Hypertension
Tachypnoea
Fever

Patients' subjective sensation of opioid-induced sedation does not correlate with the impairment of cognitive performance as, at formal testing, patients report sedation while cognitive tests can still be performed efficiently (Caraceni et al. 1993). Sedation is dose-related and is a pharmacological phenomenon that shows dynamic and kinetic related changes. The only human data available on this subject comes from the EEG changes induced by potent opioids used for anaesthesia. In this setting opioids increase the power in the range of low (1–10 Hz) EEG frequencies, and specifically the percentage of delta rhythm (< 4 Hz) (Scott et al. 1991). With this method the EEG slowing to the delta frequency was related to the drug plasma level and EEG sensitivity was also reversely related to age, showing a pharmacodynamic change due to ageing (Scott and Stanski 1987), demonstrating that the elderly brain is more sensitive to opioid effects. Slowing of EEG frequency is a common finding also in delirium as expected in a condition that shares with sedation a lowered level of consciousness. The relationship between these EEG changes and the clinical condition of chronic or acute opioid administration for pain is practically unknown. In the only study available patients who were taking opioids alone for pain did not show cognitive failure nor EEG changes while patient taking benzodiazepines alone or in combination with opioids had both cognitive disturbances and EEG changes (Hendler et al. 1980).

In animal models, opioids changed the EEG organization of normal sleep of which the most constant finding was a reduction of REM sleep. A similar finding has been shown in humans but in an experimental model which involved ex-addicts (Kay et al. 1969). These observations have never been reproduced in patients with opioid-induced delirium.

Opiods and cognitive performance

Cognitive performance is diminished when opioids are acutely given to normal volunteers (Zacny 1995; Zacny and Gutierrez 2009), while in patients with pain the situation is more complex. Cognitive impairment has been documented after increasing dosage (Bruera et al. 1989, 1992c). It is reasonable to think that cognitive impairment is likely to occur when vigilance is compromised to an extent that the performance of complex tasks and thought are affected (Bruera et al. 1987). In chronic use a balance between the therapeutic analgesic effect and the sedative effect seems to occur, favouring a more functional cognitive situation that can be compatible with car driving (Galski et al. 2000). When pain is controlled by adequate opioid dosing the failure of cognitive performance is more related to the pain and the underlying general conditions than to opioid therapy effects (Sjogren and Banning 1989; Sjogren et al. 2000). Tolerance to the sedative effects is also likely to develop in chronic dosing as has been demonstrated in studies on opioid addicts (Zacny 1995). A systematic review confirms that cognitive performance is reduced also in patients with cancer pain by opioids but also, otherwise, that the clinical significance of this evidence is not established (Kurita et al. 2009).

Opioids sedative action and delirium

Objective sedation is by definition a reduced level of consciousness that can increase to the point of inducing sleep (morphine is named after the Greek god of sleep). A patient who has a significant degree of sedation and fails in keeping his attention on external stimuli and in performing cognitive tasks fulfils the clinical definition of delirium (Bruera et al. 1987). In our opinion it is therefore possible to talk of dose-related, opioid-induced delirium of a somnolent form that can be readily induced in every patient depending on the dose employed. This type of effect is likely to be mediated via the interaction with opioid receptors, and be part of the opioid sedative properties discussed earlier. This effect can obviously be worsened by concomitant CNS depressive therapies or co-morbidities often encountered in the advanced phases of terminal illnesses (Leipzig et al. 1987). The immediate predecessor of this condition could be sleepiness when the arousal and attention are still sufficient to allow adequate cognitive performance.

The sedative effect of opioids, and of morphine in particular, has been associated with their inhibitory action on the cholinergic activating system. Peripheral anti-cholinergic effects of opioids are well known. As we discussed in Chapter 3, central cholinergic neuromodulation is essential for the regulation of arousal, the sleep–wakefulness cycle, and also respiratory function. Opioids have an inhibitory effect on cholinergic transmission at many CNS levels deemed relevant in controlling these functions. It is therefore possible that some central effects of opioids relevant to the syndrome of delirium–hallucination, disruption of the sleep–wakefulness cycle, diminished arousal and attention, and cognitive failure–are mediated at least in part through the cholinergic system. Recently some clinicians, favouring this hypothesis, tried to enhance cholinergic transmission with acetylcholinesterase (AchE) inhibitors to improve sedation and delirium-like symptoms related to opioids (Slatkin et al. 2001).

Opioids hallucinations, myoclonus, and delirium

A different set of opioid-induced CNS symptoms have been also reported: hallucinations, myoclonus, hyperalgesia, delirium, and seizures. These symptoms are found at times in isolation or can be part of the syndrome of delirium (Caraceni et al. 1994; Gregory et al. 1992).

In one of our patients, delirium and visual hallucinations were present when 60 mg of oral morphine was prescribed daily, changing to visual hallucinations without delirium when the dose of morphine was reduced to 40 mg per day. In another patient, visual hallucinations occurred in a totally clear state of mind with 90 mg of oral morphine a day. In this last patient the same type of hallucinations were reported after switching the therapy to oral methadone and titrating the dose to 18 mg per day (Caraceni et al. 1994); see also the cases reported by Jellema (1987), and Bruera et al. (1992d). These cases demonstrate that delirium can manifest, in a paradoxical way, with or without associated hallucinations and myoclonus, with low to moderate doses of opioids. Some cases are facilitated by other concurrent toxic or metabolic factors (Bortolussi et al. 1994; Caraceni et al. 1994), but others as shown by the examples seem to reflect a true specific opioid toxicity.

Of the three cases of myoclonus reported by McDonald et al. (1993) with high systemic opioid therapy (hydromorphone IV infusions of 200, 200, and 65 mg/h), two were also delirious. At high levels of opioid administration this type of excitatory toxicity seems to occur very often, provided that a high enough dose can be reached without the onset of sedative or CNS depressive limiting effects. In some patients myoclonus evolved into generalized convulsions without other signs of encephalopathy or delirium in between (Hagen and Swanson 1997). Patients reporting myoclonus and eventually seizures have often reported generalized hyperalgesia and allodynia as well (Sjogren et al. 1993b). Myoclonus and hyperalgesia or their association seem to be the results of an excitatory CNS effect of opioid on some non-opioid neural circuits. With systemic administration, multifocal generalized myoclonus and total body hyperalgesia have been described (Sjogren et al. 1993a, b, 1994). Seizures can occur at very high doses (Bruera and Pereira 1997; Hagen and Swanson 1997), and delirium with hallucinations has also been reported (Bruera and Pereira 1997; MacDonald et al. 1993; Sjogren et al. 1993b). In one case myoclonus, allodynia, and delirium were observed in association with the use of transdermal fentanyl (200 μg/h) and disappeared when the treatment was changed to a weak opioid (Okon and George 2008).

With the use of spinal opioids, both intrathecal and epidural, hyperalgesia and myoclonus can be seen with a segmental distribution without signs of encephalopathy (Cartwright et al. 1993; De Conno et al. 1991a; Glavina and Robertshaw 1988; Kloke et al. 1994). Different opioids have been associated with symptoms of CNS hyperexcitability, morphine (Stiefel and Morant 1991), hydromorphone, sufentanyl (Bowdle and Rooke 1994), fentanyl (Steinberg et al. 1992), and methadone (Mercadante 1995).

The most credited pathophysiologic mechanism for these effects implies a non-opioidergic disinhibition of glycinergin and/or GABAergic control systems, which would affect an activation of the NMDA receptors. Hyperalgesia and seizures can be induced in animal models and are not reversed by naloxone (Frenk et al. 1984; Yaksh et al. 1986). Spinal cord neurons respond with paroxysmal depolarization with the application of opiates antagonizing postsynaptic glycine and GABA inhibition in a way that resembles strychnine (Werz and MacDonald 1982). It is therefore possible that this peculiar non-opioid action is responsible, when high doses are employed or for idiosyncratic reasons, of segmental or generalized myoclonus and hyperalgesia, hallucinations, delirium, and seizures, depending on the neural system involved.

A more complete and complex view of the interaction of opioid and non-opioid systems has been reviewed by Frenk (1983; Van Praag et al. 1993), showing that some convulsive effects are also opioid-receptor mediated. This possibility is confirmed by at least one human case of encephalopathy with generalized myoclonus and hallucinations secondary to fentanyl overdosing who responded dramatically to naloxone (Bruera and Pereira 1997).

The role of morphine metabolites morphine-3- and -6-glucuronides in producing these effects is unsettled. Their accumulation in renal failure may be relevant for the development of toxicity (Sjogren et al. 1998), but it has been very difficult to define when and how morphine glucoronides have a role, if any, in the pharmacological effects of morphine in humans (Anderson et al. 2002; Lotsch et al. 1997; Morita et al. 2002; Teseo et al. 1995). Glare et al. (1990) have suggested that normorphine may also have a role to play. Other opioids such as fentanyl produce, as shown, similar effects and do not have known active metabolites. Meperidine, on the other hand, has more neuroexcitatory side effects due to the accumulation of normeperidine (Szeto et al. 1977). Recently a case has been reported with anileridine associated with delirium (Moss 1995). However, oxycodone seems to be less often associated with toxic reaction (Maddocks et al. 1996). Meperidine and tramadol also have serotonergic effects that could justify some symptoms of toxicity mediated by serotonergic mechanisms.

The mechanisms underlying what is commonly seen in clinical practice are therefore likely to be multiple and still poorly understood. The contribution, for instance, of this type of excitatory toxicity to cases of terminal restlessness is unknown. The role of opioid- and non-opioid-mediated effects, concomitant drugs, or active opioid metabolites is still unknown. The presence of myoclonus, seizures, and other symptoms in such cases should be better documented (Potter et al. 1989).

Recent data confirm that opioid-increasing doses bear a definite risk for developing delirium both in cancer and in the postoperative period (Gaudreau et al. 2005c; Leung et al. 2009). Therefore careful strategies to reduce this risk should be developed. Specific management recommendations for opioid-induced delirium are difficult to establish at the present state of knowledge; however, several guidelines can be tentatively offered to reduce the risk of this type of reaction (Cherny et al. 2001), some of which are reviewed elsewhere in this text and in particular in Chapter 9.

6.3.3 Serotonin syndrome

The availability and popularity of selective serotonin reuptake inhibitors (SSRIs) for the treatment of depression has contributed to the slow epidemic diffusion of a previously rarely recognized toxic reaction due to overstimulation of serotonin receptors in the CNS (Gillman 1995, 1998, 1999; Sternbach 1991). This syndrome, originally described in 1960, has been reported more and more frequently in the past 10 years. It is characterized clinically by signs of encephalopathy (confusion, restlessness, myoclonus, hyperreflexia, rigidity, coma) and of autonomic instability (fever, diaphoresis, diarrhoea, flushing, tachycardia, tachypnoea, blood pressure changes, midriasis, shivering, and tremor). It can be fatal or have a more benign course. It is usually seen after the addition of a serotonergic drug to a drug regimen already containing serotonin-enhancing drugs. Table 6.5 (Bodner et al. 1995; Bonin et al. 1999; Chambost et al. 2000; Daniels 1998; Gill et al. 1999; Hamilton and Malone 2000; Karki and Masood 2003;

Table 6.5 Anti-depressant drugs and drug combinations associated with serotonin syndrome

Drug	Combinations
Fuoxetine	Carbamazepine
	Pentazocine
	MAOIs
	Moclobemibe
	Nefazodone
	Tramadol
	Mirtazapine
Fluvoxamine	Alone
	Nefazodone
Paroxetine	Risperidone
	Moclobemide
Sertraline	Isocarboxazide
	Nortriptyline
	Tranylcypromine
	Erytromycine
	Buspirone
	Loxapine
Tryptopan	Fluoxetine
	Nonselective MAOIs
	Clomipramine
Venlafaxine	Alone
Trazodone	Buspirone
	Nefazodone
Moclobemide	Citalopram
	Imipramine
Meperidine	Iproniazid
	MAOIs
	Moclobemide
Phenelzine	3,4 Methylenedioxy-methamphetamine
Dextrometorphan	nonselective MAOIs
Dothiepine	Alone

Derived from Bodner et al (1995)

Kesavan and Sobala 1999; Lee and Lee 1999; Margolese and Chouinard 2000; Perry 2000; Rosebush et al. 1999; Smith and Wenegrat 2000; Weiner 1999) reports the drugs and the combinations that have been associated with the syndrome. For the palliative care setting it is interesting to note that in general SSRIs are now more often found in the therapeutic regimens in patients with advanced illness for their beneficial effects on mood and night-time sleep and that in the complex polypharmacy so common in these patients unexpected reaction can become less rare. Table 6.5 enlists cases involving meperidine, tramadol, and dextrometorphan. At least these two last drugs are likely to be commonly used in palliative care. Cases of delirium following the use of SSRI have been reported already and may represent manifestations of partial serotonin syndrome or of a different toxic effect from the same drugs (Rothschild 1995).

Case report

A 72-year-old man, affected by a laryngeal carcinoma with local relapse and lung metastases, tracheostomy, and enteral nutrition via PEG tube, had pain in his throat radiating bilaterally to both ears, insomnia, depression, cough, and dyspnoea due to the formation of mucous and necrotic material into the tracheostomy cannula. His drug regimen included tramadol 50 mg every 8 h, citalopram 5 mg at night, ketorolac 30 mg *pro re nata* (p.r.n.; 'as circumstance may require'), gabapentin 200 mg every 8 h. When the tramadol dose was increased up to 100 mg every 8 h he developed generalized myoclonus, rigidity, diaphoresis, and delirium. When he was admitted to the hospital palliative care ward the therapeutic regimen was switched to morphine subcutaneous (SC) infusion alone (30 mg/day) with progressive recovery of the neurological status. The clinical symptoms fulfil the characteristics of serotonin syndrome. The pathogenesis may involve a metabolic interaction of tramadol with citalopram or a pharmacodynamic potentiation of serotonergic effects by the combination of the two drugs.

6.3.4 Steroid-induced delirium

This is also commonly described as steroid psychosis. Since steroids are so commonly used in palliative care it is worth reminding that the possibility that corticosteroid therapy is the direct cause of delirium should be considered with a dose equivalent to at least 40 mg of prednisone per day (see also case report in Section 5.5). Usually at least a week or two of therapy are needed to develop psychiatric complications (Stiefel et al. 1989). The symptoms can range from depression to mania and psychosis. The true incidence of mental changes related to steroid administration in palliative care is unknown. High doses are often reported to cause euphoria. One study comparing cancer patients receiving high-dose dexamethasone (100 mg IV and then a tapering schedule) for spinal cord compression with a group of patients not receiving steroids found an higher incidence of depression and a tendency for greater incidence of delirium in patients treated with steroids (Breitbart et al. 1993).

Also steroid withdrawal can cause delirium together with other symptoms of hypocortisolism (Campbell and Schubert 1991). It is a useful measure to taper slowly and discontinue steroids in any patient who does not need them for specific indications (Twycross 1992).

6.3.5 **Miscellaneous drugs**

A very extensive number of drugs are continuously reported in the literature because of their potential or actual association with delirium. Practically every drug with known CNS activity can potentially cause delirium with mechanisms only sometimes understood. In some cases anticholinergic properties are likely and are the first to be blamed. For most drugs, however, mechanisms are unknown or hypothetical. Table 6.6 lists the old and new drugs that continue to be reported as causes of delirium.

6.3.6 **Drug interactions**

The role of metabolic interactions as a cause of toxicity in palliative care is more and more likely as the number of drug increases and the patient general condition deteriorates (Bernard and Bruera 2000; Cheng et al. 2002). The induction or inhibition of hepatic enzyme metabolism is an important source of variability in drug effect and can lead to unexpected toxic reactions. The P450 system is made of a family of more than 20 isoenzymes, among which the CYP 2D6 and the CYP 3A4 metabolize 80% of know drugs. The article by Bernard and Bruera (2000) reports on a number of drugs of common use in palliative care that have high or moderate probability to interact with the same metabolic pathways and to lead to unexpected high or low levels of a drug with the consequence of under- or overdosing (methadone, codeine, oxycodone, haloperidol, TCAs, SSRIs, MAO inhibitors, benzodizepines, macrolides, azoles, rifampin, antifungines).

In particular CYP 3A4 metabolizes fentanyl, alfentanyl methadone, alprazolam, midazolam, and dexamethasone and can be inhibited by most antifungal drugs, fluoxetine and norfloxacin, while it is induced by dexamethasone, phenytoin, carbamazepine, phenobarbital, rifampicin, erythromycin, omeprazole, and cyclophospamide. CYP 2D6 metabolizes codeine, oxycodone, tramadol, haloperidol, risperidone, fluoxetine, paroxetine, venlafaxine, and desimipramine. It is inhibited by cimetidine, desimipramine, fluoxetine, paroxetine, haloperidol, and sertraline and induced by carbamazepine, phenobarbital, and phenytoin.

These examples can be integrated with the available literature and may explain also cases of so-called serotonin syndromes as serotonergic drugs have significant interaction as already evident from the brief list provided (Bernard and Bruera 2000).

However, the clinical role of drug interaction in producing specific effects may be very difficult to ascertain, laboratory *in vitro* data may not be applicable to the clinical situation, while *in vivo* other circumstances may be operating to change the effect that was expected on the basis of laboratory data (Bernard and Bruera 2000).

The case of flecainide-induced delirium when administered together with paroxetine is didactic as it shows that due to CYP 2D6 inhibition paroxetine can cause toxic flecainide levels and in turn delirium (Tsao and Gugger 2009).

Case report

An interesting case of a patient affected by an advanced head and neck carcinoma presented with oral candidiasis, pain, and dysphagia. The patient received fentanyl transdermally (50 mg/h patch) and itroconazole 200 mg b.i.d., and 24 hours after starting this therapy developed an agitated delirium with myoclonus.

Table 6.6 Case reports of drug toxicities manifesting with delirium

Amiodarone (Barry and Franklin 1999)

Benzodiazepine and clozapine combination (Jackson et al. 1995)

Clarithromycin (Mermelstein 1998)

Clozapine (Szymanski et al. 1991; Wilkins-Ho and Hollander 1997)

Ciprofloxacin (McDermott et al. 1991)

Cyclosporin (Steg and Garcia 1991)

Donepezil (Kawashima and Yamada 2002)

Ethanol and niacin coingestion (Schwab and Bachhuber 1991)

Diet pills Phentermine (Bagri and Reddy 1998)

Mefloquine (Hall 1994)

Diphenydramine (Agostini et al. 2001; Tejera et al. 1994)

Diphenhydramine linezolide combination (Serio 2004)

Famotidine 6 cases (Catalano et al. 1996)

Flecainamide and paroxetine combination (Tsao et al. 2009)

Fluoxetine (Leinonen et al. 1993)

H-2 receptor blockers (Nickell 1991)

Herbal medicine loperamide, theales, valerian (Khawaja et al. 1999)

Levodopa (Delmas et al. 2008)

Lithium neuroleptic combination (Normann et al. 1998)

Lithium (Shibasaki Warabi et al. 2006; Wilkinson et al. 2009)

Mianserin (Bonne et al. 1995)

Nizatidine (Galynker and Tendler 1997)

Ofloxacillin (Fennig and Mauas 1992)

Omeprazole (Heckmann et al. 2000)

Paclitaxel (Ziske et al. 2002)

Paroxetine benztropine combination (Amstrong and Schweitzer 1997)

Promethazine (Page et al. 2009)

Ranitidine (Eisendrath and Ostroff 1990)

Ranitidine and cimetidine (Kim et al. 1996)

Risperidone (Tavcar and Dernovsek 1998)

Tacrine (Trzepacz et al. 1996)

Tacrine ibuprofen interaction (Hooten and Pearlson 1996)

Sertraline haloperidol benztropine combination (Byelry et al. 1996)

Steroids (Stoudemine et al. 1996)

Ziconotide (Levin et al. 2002)

Zolpidem (Freudenreich and Menza 2000)

All laboratory exams and head CT were normal. The fentanyl patch was stopped and changed with oral methadone 7 mg t.i.d. without any change in the following 48 hours. Methadone was also stopped and changed to morphine IV with resolution of the neurological symptoms. After a few days also itroconazole was discontinued and transdermal fentanyl reinstituted at the same dose (50 mg/hr) without further complications (this case is reported courtesy of Dr Oscar Corli, personal communication). The most likely explanation involves the interaction of both fentanyl and methadone with itroconazole. Morphine, which is metabolized by glucoronization and does not interact with the P450 enzyme system (see list and literature), did not cause toxic effect and nor did fentanyl when administered alone.

6.4 Delirium and structural brain lesions

Structural brain lesions that can often cause delirium are vascular lesions and tumors. We can classify these lesions into two broad categories: lesions that cause widespread brain damage and focal lesions. All of these conditions, whether vascular, or due to tumor or to other causes, can produce reduced cerebral blood flow, raised intracranial pressure, and decreased brain metabolism.

6.4.1 Vascular causes of delirium

In cases of cerebrovascular disease, delirium can be potentially caused by focal or widespread cerebral damage (Table 6.7). Ischaemic stroke, without signs of intracranial hypertension, is the only condition where a precise focal aetiology of delirium can be explored and crucial brain areas for the development of this syndrome should manifest themselves.

Delirium frequency in ischaemic strokes is uncertain. Two recent prospective studies found a prevalence of 24.3% (Henon et al. 1999) and 48% (Gustafson et al. 1991b), respectively, whereas cerebral haemorrhage is more frequently associated with delirium in up to 53% of cases (Dunne et al. 1986). Case reports have associated some focal ischaemic lesions with the onset of delirium. These lesions affected the right middle cerebral artery territory, left posterior cerebral artery territory, hippocampal area, lingula and fusiform gyrus, or thalamus (Lipowski 1990b; Trzepacz 1994a). Acute agitated deliria have been reported after an infarction of the right medial cerebral artery (Mesulam et al. 1976). In general some observations suggest a higher frequency of delirium with right-sided lesions. On the basis of the attention deficit associated with these lesions, some authors have put forward the theory that delirium is primarily due to a derangement of attention. With respect to these observations, most of the old case series do not offer a specific definition of delirium (Dunne et al. 1986).

In an article that used DSM IV criteria for diagnosing delirium in stroke patients, the authors were able to define several important clinicopathological aspects associated with the onset of the syndrome (Henon et al. 1999). Pre-existing and concurrent morbid factors associated with delirium at univariate analysis were older age, alcohol consumption, previous cognitive decline, leukoaraiosis, more severe cerebral atrophy scores on CT scan, and metabolic or infectious disorders. The stroke location did not predict the onset of delirium, but a negative association with posterior fossa lesion was found. After logistic regression analyses the only factors that retained independent association with the presence of delirium were pre-existing cognitive impairment and metabolic or infectious disorders. When only the patients with previous cognitive impairment were considered, the presence of a right superficial lesion was independently associated with the onset of delirium. While in-hospital mortality was not affected by the presence of delirium, overall functional recovery and neurological outcome was worse for the patients who had delirium (Ferro et al. 2002; Henon et al. 1999; Sandberg et al. 2001).

If a strict clinical definition of delirium is used, a single brain lesion is very rarely sufficient to produce the full syndrome per se, and, more importantly, although some clinical observations suggest that at times a lesion of one brain area will produce delirium, there is no evidence that this type of lesion is invariably associated with it. Deficit in attention, language, and cognition commonly associated with focal brain lesions are not sufficient to cause delirium. Delirium can again be seen as a multifactorial syndrome that can also be precipitated by a focal brain lesion in predisposed patients or when concurrent precipitating factors are present. Right-sided lesions affecting attention and orientation are more likely to cause delirium when unfavourable underlying conditions are already operating.

The differential diagnosis of focal cerebral disorders causing selective failure of higher brain function versus delirium has already been discussed in Chapter 5.

Lesions in the hypothalamus have been associated with hypersomnia, a condition that may largely overlap with the clinical definition of delirium (see also Figure 6.4).

Other cerebrovascular diseases, such as hypertensive encephalopathy, subdural hematoma, brain haemorrhage, multiple brain embolisms (Figure 6.2), DIC, and vasculitis (Table 6.7), can cause delirium via their interference with brain metabolism and function. In these cases is very difficult to say whether the pathogenetic mechanism has to do with the 'diffused' cerebral hypometabolism or with the 'specific' failure of those hypothalamic and brainstem structures crucial for maintaining a normal state of consciousness.

Table 6.7 Cerebrovascular diseases that can be associated with delirium

Cerebral thrombosis or embolism

Cerebral haemorrhage

Subdural haematoma

Hypertensive encephalopathy

Cerebral vasculitis

Diffused intravascular coagulation (DIC)

Other coagulopathies (e.g. Moscowitz syndrome)

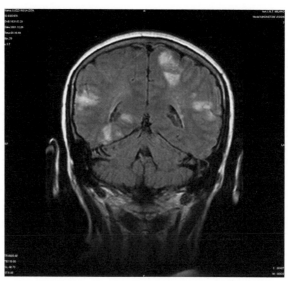

Fig. 6.2 Multiple ischaemic cortical areas are visible in this coronal MR image of the brain as white areas within the different grey appearances of the normal brain tissue. This patient had metastatic colon carcinoma and multiple chemotherapy courses. Personality change and vigilance abnormalities were the first sign of brain ischaemia. The clinical picture progressed to coma and death. Multiple embolisms are likely to be the cause of such diffused ischaemic disorder probably due to predisposing factors associated with the primary disease or therapy, such as non-bacterial thrombotic endocarditis.

6.4.2 **Tumours**

Altered mental status and psychiatric symptoms can be found in association with brain tumours, whether primary or metastatic, due to two main causes: direct effect of the tumour on the brain or due to the effects of therapies. The clinical findings will be compatible with a diagnosis of delirium or dementia depending on the time course of the operating mechanism, potential reversibility, and the type of cognitive decline (see also Section 7.3). The differential diagnosis will not always be easy or clear-cut.

Brain tumours

Brain tumours often present with changes in cognition and personality, depressed mood, apathetic behaviour, memory failure, and disorientation to space and time. Clinical findings can develop subacutely but at times the onset is acute as in delirium. Attention as well as the level of consciousness can be affected. Findings will depend on the site and type of cerebral lesion. The principal mechanisms that cause mental changes and compromised consciousness due to the presence of intracranial tumour can be focal, due to compression (direct or due to oedema) on structures important for cognition and regulation of consciousness level (the hypothalamus and the brainstem; Figures 6.3, 6.4), or diffuse due to intracranial hypertension, hydrocephalus, or

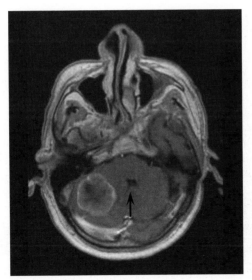

Fig. 6.3 Cerebellar metastases from small-cell lung cancer.
The lesion is compressing the fourth ventricle and the underlying brainstem (arrow). The patient presented with somnolence, inattention, and delirium. In this case compression on the ventricle could interfere with CSF circulation, or direct compression on the brainstem could be the cause of consciousness compromise.

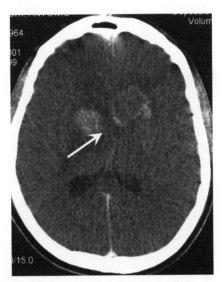

Fig. 6.4 Cerebral metastases from non-small cell lung cancer.
CT scan with contrast. Two sizeable lesions can be seen in the deep cerebral areas surrounded by oedema and compressing the thalamus and likely the underlying hypothalamus. A significant shift of the midline structures towards the right can be seen (arrow). A pronounced reduction of vigilance was the main symptom. The patient was oriented when awake but tended to go asleep very easily if not stimulated.

interference with brain metabolism and nutrition. The patient in Figure 6.4 had a specific hypersomniac disorder characterized by easily falling asleep if not stimulated, even while talking to the examining physician, but with preserved cognitive functions when fully awake. In view of this it is very helpful to remember again the distinction between assessing the level of consciousness and assessing the content of consciousness.

When tumour causes oedema and intracranial hypertension, fluctuations of intracranial pressure (plateau waves) can be responsible for unexpected, reversible, acute changes of mental status. (Posner 1995). The association of headache and papilloedema greatly facilitate the diagnosis, but these findings can be absent.

Tumours can widely diffuse to the brain and cause global cognitive failure by miliariform or bulky metastatic lesions, or white matter diffuse infiltration such as in the case of glioblastoma multiformis.

Case report

A 45-year-old woman presented with progressive difficulties of attention and of memory. Physical examination showed no focal neurological signs but short-term memory and calculation failure with slight constructional apraxia as shown by reproducing simple design. Brain MRI with contrast (Figure 6.5) showed a lesion of the corpus callosum. In this case the mild compromise of vigilance, slight disorientation with more pronounced and specific, short-term memory deficit would make the diagnosis of delirium controversial. Cases like this not uncommonly progress with widespread white matter infiltration, leading to profound dementia and other neurological impairment (aphasia, paralysis) before dying.

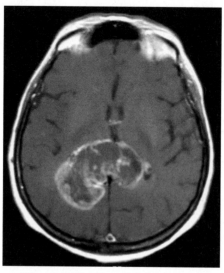

Fig. 6.5 Gliobastoma multiformis (MRI with gadolinium) presenting with memory impairment and slight mental changes (see text).

Brain metastases

Brain parenchymal metastases and meningeal metastases from systemic cancer present with signs of altered cognition in about 50% of cases, even before giving rise to other symptoms or focal signs (Formaglio and Caraceni 1998; Posner 1995; Wasserstrom et al. 1982). In the advanced phases of cancer, brain metastases are statistically associated with an increased risk of developing delirium, together with other clinical factors such as dyspnoea, anorexia low performance, and clinical prediction of survival (Caraceni et al. 2000).

Case report

A case of a 56-year-old man with metastatic melanoma presented with disorientation to space and time, low vigilance, and perseveration, without other focal signs. No metabolic, biochemical, or haematological abnormalities could be found. CT scan of the head showed multiple brain metastases (at least 48 could be counted by the radiologist).

In another case, a 62-year-old woman with metastatic breast cancer was referred to the neurology unit because of depression and confusion. Her neurological examination was normal and her cognitive status examination showed only psychomotor slowing and apathy. This finding was reinforced by her husband's report of a major and sudden change in her mood and usually active behaviour. A CT scan with contrast showed multiple brain lesions with relevant brain oedema and frontal lobe involvement (Figure 6.6).

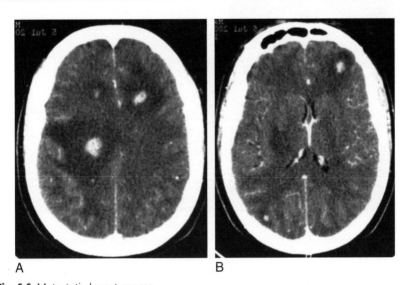

A   B

Fig. 6.6 Metastatic breast cancer.
The patient presented with depression, behavioural changes, and psychomotor slowing.
(A) The CT scan shows contrast-enhancing lesions with oedema and mass effect. (B)
One lesion is located in the frontal lobe and causes significant oedema.

Both cases show acute behavioural and cognitive symptoms. In the first case the diagnosis of delirium is relatively straightforward; in the second case it is more likely that the compromise of frontal lobe functions resulted in behavioural inhibition and loss of drive dominating the clinical picture.

Leptomeningeal metastases

Case studies show that microscopic meningeal infiltration can cause mental changes without focal signs and symptoms (Trachman et al. 1991; Weitzener et al. 1995). Seeding of malignant cells to the meninges can cause hydrocephalus (Figure 6.7), but, before imaging can show cerebral ventricle dilation, the CSF dynamics is often already altered and can by itself cause symptoms due to intracranial pressure changes (Grossman et al. 1982). Encephalopathy due to meningeal metastases can also be explained by tumour cell seeding to the meninges and interfering with CSF formation and reabsorption, competing with the brain parenchyma for essential nutrients, and/ or producing ischaemic damage by infiltrating the Virchow–Robin spaces.

The classic findings of papilloedema, severe headaches, or meningismus can be absent as in the case summarized in Figure 6.7 (Grossman et al. 1982). As already mentioned in the case of brain tumour, fluctuations of intracranial pressure (plateau waves) can be responsible for unexpected, reversible, acute changes of mental status (Posner 1995).

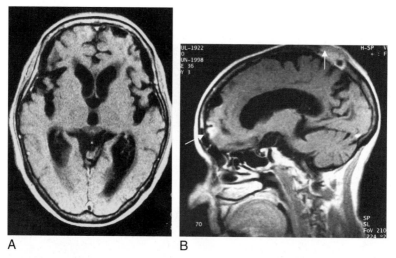

A   B

Fig. 6.7 (A) Meningeal metastases causing tetraventricular hydrocephalus. (B) The arrows show two contrast enhancement areas demonstrating a skull lesion (on the right) that invades the dura and is adjacent to the cortex and leptomeningeal covering and a typical leptomeningeal lesion of the frontal lobe (on the left). The patient had a lung carcinoma and presented with delirium with disorientation to space and time, perseveration and somnolence. Headache, meningismus, papilloedema and focal signs were absent. CSF examination showed malignant cells.

Brain tumour therapy

Radiation is commonly employed to treat brain tumours and intracranial metastases. Other therapies, such as chemotherapy concurrently or in sequence, are also used and can contribute to brain toxicity. The side effects of chemotherapy and remote effects of systemic cancer will be considered in Chapter 7. Whole brain radiation is more frequently followed by cognitive sequelae than focal radiation. Cognitive failure due to radiation can be acute or subacute or delayed. Three main clinical variants can be seen (Jennings 1995; Petterson and Rottemberg 1997; Posner 1995).

♦ Early radiation encephalopathy can manifest as delirium within hours or days of treatment delivery and can be difficult to distinguish from symptoms of tumour progression. It is a transient phenomenon due to increased oedema that may fulfill the diagnosis of delirium.

♦ Early delayed encephalopathy can be seen, more often in children, the so-called somnolence syndrome, and occurs a few months after therapy, usually in patients with no apparent active tumour. Patients usually recover from it.

♦ Delayed encephalopathy is equivalent to radiation-induced dementia (De Angelis 1989). It is progressive, associated with cortical atrophy or white matter degeneration, and can occur years after radiation in patients cured of the initial tumour (Petterson and Rottemberg 1997).

Radiation toxicity can be enhanced by concurrent chemotherapy. Studies have focused on the late cognitive sequelae so important for the intellectual development of children treated for leukaemias and other tumours (Spunberg et al. 1981; Suc et al. 1990).

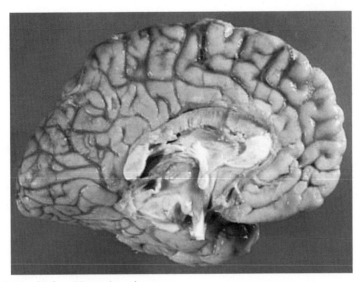

Fig. 6.8 Marchiafava Bignami syndrome.
The patient had a history of alcohol abuse and lung cancer, and was admitted to the hospital for neutropenia after chemotherapy but suddenly developed delirium with progressive deterioration to coma and died. At autopsy a clear-cut central necrosis of the corpus callosum was found.

The risk of acute encephalopathy, and therefore delirium, is also increased by concomitant chemotherapy treatments (Gerritsen van der Hoop et al. 1990).

6.4.3 Lesions of the corpus callosum

A relatively rare form of brain lesion is the degeneration of the axons interconnecting the two cerebral hemispheres within the white matter of the corpus callosum. These lesions can develop during the course of alcoholism either acutely or subacutely in the Marchiafava Bignami syndrome. More recently lesions of this kind were seen in children with infectious encephalitis and flu (Takanashi 2009). Delirium is a prominent clinical aspect of these syndromes, which are also complicated by rigidity and seizures; however, acutely altered mental status may be the only clinical finding. The diagnosis can be made with MRI but at times only autopsy can solve it, as shown in a recently published case (Figure 6.8; Caraceni et al. 2003).

Chapter 7

Delirium in special populations

7.1 Delirium in HIV-infected patients

Delirium has been reported to be a common psychiatric complication during the course of HIV infection, especially among patients in more advanced stage of illness and AIDS (Grassi et al. 1995; Khouzam et al. 1998; Snyder et al. 1992) and before the era of highly active antiretroviral therapy (HAART) and immune reconstitution (Cohen and Gorman 2008; Fernandez and Ruiz 2006). By analysing psychiatric co-morbidity among patients hospitalized with HIV infection versus non-infected patients referred for psychiatric consultation, a prevalence of delirium between 20 and 35% was found (Bialer et al. 1996; O'Dowd and McKegney 1990) and often under-diagnosed in many AIDS patients (Lalonde et al. 1996).

Delirium has been associated with medication changes, narcotics, benzodiazepines, anticholinergic/antihistamine, and steroid medications (Uldall and Berghuis 1997), antibiotic use (Salkind 2000), and cerebral opportunistic infections or metabolic encephalopathy (Alciati et al. 2001). The consequences of delirium in AIDS patients are multiple and severe. In a series of studies on the outcome of delirium in AIDS patients, Udall et al. (2000a, b) showed that patients with delirium were more likely to die during admission, had a longer hospital stay, and needed long-term care to a greater extent if discharged, than non-delirious patients.

For these reason, early identification of cognitive disorders, indicating possible pro-dromal symptoms of delirium, is of upmost importance in palliative care services dedicated to AIDS patients, in order to start appropriate treatment. This seems to be more significant in recent times, when new data are accumulating in regards to old patients, since HIV-infected individuals live longer than in the past thanks to long-term antiretroviral treatment. Neurocognitive disorders are, in fact, common in HIV-infected patients (Justice et al. 2004) and new evidence is accumulating on brain injuries and infiltration of the virus into the central nervous system (CNS) as responsible for cognitive dysfunction (Fuller et al. 2009). As indicated by several authors, the changing landscape of HIV-related cognitive impairment has implications in terms of both long-term effects of antiretroviral therapy and psychiatric treatment of possible delirium states and dementia (Brogan and Lux 2009). The problem is also becoming particularly important for HIV-infected patients showing psychiatric disorders and drugs abuse, where adherence to new treatments is low (Mellins et al. 2009) and mental health service utilization is not elevated (Weaver et al. 2008).

7.2 **Delirium in primary psychiatric disorders**

Since patients with severe psychiatric illness share many of the risk factors for delirium, especially medications with anticholinergic properties (e.g. tryciclic antidepressants, neuroleptics, anticholinergic drugs), delirium might be a possible complication of psychiatric illness (Gill and Mayou 2000). The diagnosis of delirium can be complex among psychiatric patients due to the overlap of symptoms between delirium itself and acute mental illness. For this reason it has been reported that delirium is under-recognized in mental health settings. A retrospective study of the charts of almost 200 patients admitted to a psychiatric unit was conducted by Ritchie et al. (1996). After exclusion of patients with alcohol or drug abuse, those with dementia, and those who developed delirium within 2 days of admission, the authors found a 14.6% prevalence of delirium by following DSM-III-R criteria. The highest prevalence was found among individuals with a diagnosis of bipolar disorders (35.5%), schizoaffective disorders (15.8%), and schizophrenia or other psychoses (12.1%). Delirium developed after a mean of 3 weeks from admission and virtually doubled the length of hospital stay (92.2 days among delirious versus 50.7 days among non-delirious patients). Anti-Parkinsonian medication and old age were the most significant factors associated with the development of delirium, being correctly recognized in only 48% of delirious patients. However, a different study carried out on 401 psychiatric admissions by using a more specific methodology (the Delirium Symptom Interview, the Confusion Assessment Method, and the Mini-mental State Examination (MMSE)) found a 2.14% incidence of delirium (Patten et al. 1997). The risk factors for delirium included anticholinergic medications, electroconvulsive therapy, lithium-antipsychotic combination, and high doses of low-potency neuroleptics and non-psychiatric medications capable of causing delirium. In a study carried out by Huang et al. (1998), a diagnosis of delirium was made in 1.4% of psychiatric in-patients and it was mostly related to the adverse effects of medication. However, in comparison with medical and surgical patients, the rate of mortality was lower among psychiatric patients in the short run (5.9%), but it increased during a 2-year follow-up period (39.4%).

Recently, a retrospective analysis of psychiatric patients who underwent surgery (Copeland et al. 2008) showed that the literature regarding this area is extremely scarce. In the few studies available, patients with schizophrenia, compared with those without mental illness, seem to have higher pain thresholds, higher rates of death and postoperative complications, and differential outcomes (e.g. confusion, ileus) by anaesthetic technique. Higher rates of postoperative delirium and confusion are also reported amongst patients with major depressive disorder. Furthermore, both patients with schizophrenia and those with depression experienced more postoperative confusion or delirium when psychiatric medications were discontinued preoperatively.

Delirium should also be considered a possible, sometimes unexpected, complication of treatment with or the discontinuation of psychoactive drugs in psychiatric patients affected by different disorders (Kruszewski et al. 2009; Lin and Ceo 2010). The differential diagnosis of delirium with acute psychoses is also discussed in Section 5.2. See also the case reported in Chapter 5 highlighting the differential diagnosis of delirium in a patient with underlying psychosis admitted to a palliative care facility.

7.3 **Postoperative delirium**

Postoperative delirium is quite a common complication of surgery, especially invasive cardiac, transplantation, orthopaedic, ophthalmic, and urologic surgery (Bitondo Dyer et al. 1995). As well as other clinical types of delirium, postoperative delirium needs a clear definition and operationalized criteria (van der Mast 1999), as well as well-designed prospective research (Winawer 2001). The term 'postoperative delirium' would seem to include either a temporal or an aetiologic relationship between surgery and the occurrence of the disorder. Clinically, the notion that 'emergence' delirium (developing within the first 24 hours) should be distinguished from 'interval' delirium (developing after 24 hours or more of lucid consciousness; Lipowski 1992) is considered inconsequential, although the term 'postoperative agitation' is still used and it is unclear whether it represents a specific condition (see below). Because of the number of different medical situations, types of surgery, population, pathophysiological mechanisms, and predisposing factors, postoperative delirium deserves to be further, and more specifically investigated.

A substantial underdiagnosis and under-reporting of postoperative delirium has been shown. In only 12% of cases suffering from postoperative delirium was it reported in their discharge documents (Glick et al. 1996). Postoperative delirium usually develops during the first four days after surgery, with a peak in the first or second day, and should be distinguished from transient and emergence excitement or somnolence as a result of anaesthesia (O'Keeffe and Chonchubhair 1995). Immediate agitated reactions following anaesthesia are common and not well studied as they may actually be delirious episodes. Interestingly this condition, usually described as postoperative agitation, is more frequent in children and with the use of volatile anaesthetics. Among anaesthetic gases desflurane and sevoflurane seem to produce more postoperative agitation than halothane (Lapin et al. 1999; Welborn et al. 1996). Preoperative or perioperative medication with benzodiazepines and opioids reduce the degree and frequency of postoperative agitation (Galinkin et al. 2000; Lapin et al. 1999). No study that we know links the concept of postoperative agitation with later-onset postoperative delirium.

Clinical features include the classic symptoms of delirium (e.g. impaired attention, hyperactivity or hypoactivity, progressive disturbance of thinking, with dream-like quality, illogical and incoherent speech, impaired capacity to judge, illusions, and vivid hallucinations), which tend to worsen at night. These symptoms are often associated with neurological symptoms such as asterixis, especially when metabolic alterations are present, multifocal myoclonus, and transient parietal signs, such as apraxia, aphasia, and agraphia. Postoperative delirium tends to be of shorter duration than non-postoperative delirium in medical patients and usually disappears in a week (Manos and Wu 1997). However, it has been reported that it can last from one to several weeks, especially in the elderly (Parkh and Chung 1995).

As already indicated (see Section 3.1) the incidence of the disorder varies across the clinical context (e.g. orthopaedics or cardiosurgery units) as well as the type of population (e.g. elderly or severely physically ill patients).

An accurate evaluation of potential aetiologies is necessary and sometimes a specific cause can be found in previous or concurrent drug toxicity or withdrawal reaction as shown in cases of prolonged benzodiazepine use interrupted suddenly due to surgery (Madi and Langonnet 1988), or in other specific factors, such as thiamine deficiency (Vidal et al. 2000). More often, however, it is difficult to pinpoint a single specific cause, and many cases are explained by a combination of preoperative risk factors and intra- and postoperative conditions (see Chapter 3).

A number of studies have substantiated that postoperative delirium is favoured by a series of factors (Duppils and Wikblad 2000; Galanakis el al. 2001; Litaker et al. 2001; Rolfson et al. 1999, 2007, 2008a). In a large study involving 1,341 patients 50 years of age and older admitted for major elective non-cardiac surgery, Marcantonio et al. (1998) found a 9% incidence of delirium and showed that delirium was associated with greater intraoperative blood loss, more postoperative blood transfusions, and, especially, a postoperative hematocrit less than 30%. Pain seems also a significant factor associated with delirium. In a study of patients undergoing non-cardiac surgery Lynch et al. (1998) showed that, after controlling for known preoperative risk factors for delirium (i.e. age, alcohol abuse, cognitive function, physical function, serum chemistries, and type of surgery), higher pain scores at rest were associated with an increased risk of delirium over the first 3 postoperative days. Factors associated with the development of postoperative delirium are listed in Table 7.1. Orthopaedic surgery in the elderly is at particularly high risk of this complication. The preoperative score by Marcantonio et al. (1994b) for predicting the risk of postoperative delirium accounts for multivariate analysis of commonly identified risk factors. This score gives an estimate of a patient's risk for developing delirium from 0 (low risk = 2%) to 1–2 (intermediate risk = 8-13%) to ≥3 (high risk = 50%); the following factors each contribute 1 point to the score:

◆ Age ≥ 70;

◆ Alcohol abuse;

◆ Cognitive impairment;

◆ SAS (specific activity scale) class IV;

◆ Non-cardiac thoracic surgery; and

◆ Aortic aneurism surgery (associated with 2 points on the score).

Cardiac surgery has been recognized at higher risk of delirium and a number of factors have been associated with this increased risk, such as old age, low-level albumin, poor physical condition, use of nifedipine, and a high ratio of the amino acid phenylalanine to the sum of isoleucine, leucine, valine, tyrosine, and tryptophan (van der Mast and Roest 1996). More recently a very accurate study demonstrated a model for predicting the development of delirium with this type of surgery and proposed a predictive score that took into account independent factors such as a MMSE score ≤ 23 (2 points) or = 24–27 (1 point); a Geriatric depression scale score > 4 (1 point), and a history of stroke or transient ischaemic attack (TIA; 1 point). In the derivation sample, the cumulative incidence of delirium for patients with a score = 0 or ≥ 3 was 19 and 86%, respectively, while in the validation sample, it was 18 and 87%, respectively (Rudolph et al. 2009).

Table 7.1 Risk factors for postoperative delirium

Predisposing factors
Aged ≥ 70
Cognitive impairment (dementia)
Functional impairment
High medical comorbidity
Markedly abnormal laboratory values
Alcohol abuse
Sensory impairment (vision, hearing loss)
Precipitating factors
High-risk surgery (cardiac, aortic aneurism repair, thoracic surgery)
Postoperative benzodiazepines
Postoperative meperidine
Poorly controlled postoperative pain and high-dose opioids
Low postoperative haematrocrit
Postoperative complications

Preoperative detailed cognitive assessment revealed that executive function impairment is more important than memory impairment in predicting the occurrence of delirium, pointing at the relevance of frontal lobe dysfunction in the cognitive failure observed in postoperative delirium (Rudolph et al. 2006).

It must be iterated that risk factors for delirium vary according to the population examined as well as to the clinical context. Aldemir et al. (2001), for example, by studying 818 patients who had been hospitalized for either elective or emergency services, showed a prevalence of postoperative delirium of 10.9%. The authors found that delirium was *not* correlated with conditions such as hypertension, hypo/hyperpotassaemia, hypernatraemia, hypoalbuminaemia, hypo/hyperglycaemia, cardiac disease, emergency admission, age, length of stay in the intensive care unit (ICU), length of stay in hospital, and gender. In contrast, respiratory diseases, infections, fever, anaemia, hypotension, hypocalcaemia, hyponatraemia, azotaemia, elevated liver enzymes, hyperamylasaemia, hyperbilirubinaemia, and metabolic acidosis *were* predicting factors for delirium. In a study carried out by Dubois et al. (2001) on over 200 consecutive patients admitted to ICUs it has been shown that, among the patients who developed delirium (19%), hypertension, smoking history, abnormal bilirubin level, epidural use, and morphine were statistically significantly associated with the disorder. Thus, the authors conclude that traditional factors associated with the development of delirium on general ward patients may be not significant or applicable to critically ill patients.

Gupta et al. (2001) indicated also that certain clinical conditions, namely obstructive sleep apnoea syndrome (OSAS), may represent a significant factor associated with the onset of adverse postoperative outcomes, including delirium, among patients who underwent orthopaedic surgery (hip or knee replacement).

The consequences of postoperative delirium are severe. Mortality is the most severe consequence with data showing an incidence of 4 to 40% among post-surgery patients who developed delirium (O'Keeffe 1994). Manos and Wu (1997) found a mortality over a 3½-year period of 46.8% among patients who developed delirium and postoperative delirium. Medical complications, such as increased risk for infections due to need of catheterization, increased falls with possible trauma, and bone fractures, are also important consequences of postoperative delirium. This can determine an increasing length of stay (LOS) in the hospital.

It is interesting to note that delirium is a predictor of poor functional recovery after hip fracture surgery, in the elderly, independent of prefracture risk factors such as age and poor cognitive and functional status. Furthermore, hip fracture outcome is worsened when patients present with delirium preoperatively (Dolan et al. 2000; Marcantonio et al. 2000, 2002). Also the risks of death and of developing dementia are increased in elderly patients experiencing an episode of postoperative delirium (Lundstrom et al. 2003).

As far as economic data, LOS is obviously associated with increased direct and indirect costs of care. Franco et al. (2001) have recently shown that both professional costs (i.e. those related to services provided by physicians and nursing) and technical costs (i.e. those related to non-medical services, such as number of medications, imaging, laboratory tests during admission) increased among 57 patients out of 500 (11.4%) who developed delirium during admission.

While it has been shown that about one-third of delirium secondary to orthopaedic surgery go unrecognized by the staff (Gustafson et al. 1991a), it is likely that regular assessment of the patients' cognitive function, early diagnosis of confusional symptoms, and early treatment of underlying causes are the key factor for postoperative delirium prevention and management. Indeed in a recent randomized controlled trial on hip fracture in the elderly proactive geriatric consultation reduced the frequency of delirium from 50 to 32%, and severe delirious cases from 29 to 12% (Marcantonio et al. 2001).

In a study of 296 patients undergoing elective cardiac surgery, van der Mast et al. (2000) have shown that plasma tryptophan (Trp) and the ratio of Trp with other large neutral amino acids were reduced, while the ratio of phenylalanine was increased in delirious patients. The former result could determine a decreased serotoninergic function, while the latter an increased noradrenergic and dopaminergic function, causing an imbalance in cerebral neurotransmission. With regard to the role of noradrenaline, Nakamura et al. (2001) measured the levels of plasma free 3-methoxy-4-hydroxyphenyl (ethylene)glycol (pMHPG), a major metabolite of noradrenaline (norepinephrine), in patients prior to surgery for cardiovascular diseases. The authors found that preoperative pMHPG levels were higher in patients who subsequently developed postoperative delirium than in the patients who were non-delirious, suggesting an hyperactivity of noradrenargic neurons as a possible risk factor of postoperative delirium.

The role of serotonin was evaluated by Bayindir et al. (2000), who analysed the effect of the 5-HT3-receptor antagonist ondansetron (8 mg IV) in 35 patients with postcardiotomy delirium. The authors found that the use of ondansetron was effective and safe, leading them to hypothesize that impaired serotonin metabolism may play a role in postcardiotomy delirium. Although the multiple aetiologies in postoperative delirium make it difficult to understand the role of the several mechanisms involved in it, Stanford and Stanford (1999) have described a case that suggests that alterations of cerebral 5-HT induced by drugs (e.g. selective serotonin re-uptake inhibitors (SSRIs) and ondansetron) can play a major role in causing postoperative delirium. This report shares similarities with what we have observed in a patient admitted to the hospital for surgery of colon cancer.

Case report

The patient, a 74-old-year woman, was admitted to the surgery department from the nursing home, where she had lived for five years. Reason for admission was a colon cancer that had caused intestinal occlusion. She underwent surgery and intravenous infusion of morphine was started to control her pain. After 2 days she developed symptoms characterized by severe agitation with disruptive behaviour, confusion, hallucinations, and pyrexia. A psychiatric consultation was immediately requested with the aim to transfer the patient to the acute psychiatric unit. Clinical evaluation confirmed a diagnosis of postoperative delirium due to multiple factors, including the patient's poor metabolic conditions, dehydration, and continuous use of opioids. By analysing the patient's chart, it was also noticed that she had used paroxetine 20 mg/day, which had been prescribed by the nursing house's physician 6 months earlier to treat the patients' depression. Paroxetine had been *ex abrubto* discontinued the day before surgery. The risk of SSRIs discontinuation syndrome, especially for paroxetine, has been repeatedly shown (Black et al. 2000), and the possible interaction of opioids with serotonin and dopamine has been suggested (Stanford and Stanford 1999). Aetiologic intervention (treatment of dehydration and metabolic imbalance), indicating to the medical and nursing staff on how to behaviourally treat the patient's confusional status, and prescription of risperidone 2 mg/day were followed by recovery from delirium within 4 days.

7.3.1 Prevention of postoperative delirium

Considering the general scheme of predisposing and precipitating factors for postoperative delirium (Table 7.1) it is possible to design pharmacological interventions potentially useful for reducing the incidence of delirium by modifying the intraoperative anaesthesia condition or, the postoperative use of analgesics and sedative drugs, or by introducing use of preoperative medications.

Intraoperative modifications

One study randomized 228 patients above the age of 65 undergoing non-cardiac surgery to nitrous oxide or oxygen inhalation. The frequency of postoperative delirium was 43.8% and it was not influenced by the administration of nitrous oxide (Leung et al. 2006).

The use of ketamine in inducing anaesthesia compared with placebo in a randomized trial of 58 patients was associated with a lower incidence of delirium in the ketamine-treated group (3%) than in the placebo group (31%) with an odds ration of 12.6

(confidence interval, CI 1.5–107.5; Hudetz et al. 2009). The authors discussed a potential antinflammatory effect showing lower levels of serum polymerase chain reaction (PCR) in patients treated with ketamine.

Postoperative interventions

The association of delirium with the postoperative use of opioids and benzodiazepines has been demonstrated in some studies (Leung et al. 2006a, 2009; Pandharipande et al. 2006); therefore the use of alternative sedative and analgesic protocols has been proposed in some clinical trials. One non-blinded random comparison of dexmedetomidine, propofol, and midazolam in 118 patients undergoing elective cardiac surgery observed a much lower incidence of delirium in the patient group that had dexmedetomidine as postoperative protocol. Dropout rate was significant in this study (Maldonado et al. 2009). See also Pandharipande et al. (2008). With a better study design Shehabi et al. (2009) compared dexmedetomidine (0.1–07 µg/kg) with morphine (10–70 µg/kg) for postoperative sedation in 306 patients of at least 60 years of age also after cardiac surgery. The incidence of delirium was not statistically different in the two groups (8.6% with dexmedetomidine and 15% with morphine) but the duration of delirium was shorter in the group treated with dexmedetomidine.

In managing postoperative pain a pilot study showed a promising effect of combining gabapentin with morphine. Patients receiving combination analgesia seem to have a reduced risk of delirium due to an opioid sparing effect of the co-administration of gabapentin (Leung et al. 2006a).

The use of regional (lumbar plexus and femoral nerve) blockade was also associated with less hydromorphone administration by patient-controlled anaesthesia (PCA) and a reduced incidence of delirium after hip surgery in 225 patients randomly allocate to peripheral block plus PCA IV hydromorphone infusion or PCA alone (Marino et al. 2009).

Preventative interventions

The anticholinergic theory of delirium and the availability of new cholinergic medication used in dementia suggested a few trials for testing their potential usefulness in preventing postoperative delirium in the elderly. In one trial donepezil was administered for 14 days before and after surgery in a random double-blind protocol in 80 patients of 50 or more years of age. Delirium developed overall in 18.8% of patients and no benefit could be demonstrated by the study intervention in either preventing or treating it (Liptzin et al. 2005).

A similar randomized, placebo-controlled trial addressed the role of rivastigmine for preventing delirium in a more selected group of patients, aged 65 year or older undergoing cardiac surgery. In this trial the drug was given only since the night before surgery until the sixth postoperative day. Delirium incidence was 30 and 32%, respectively, in the placebo and rivastigmine groups, and no difference could be demonstrated between the two groups in cognitive test results nor in the use of haloperidol or lorazepam (Gamberini et al. 2009).

One interesting study used haloperidol 0.5 mg t.i.d. preoperatively and for three subsequent days in comparison with placebo in a cohort of elderly (70 years old or more) undergoing hip surgery. The incidence of delirium was the same–15.1%

with haloperidol and 16.5% with placebo–but delirium severity and duration seemed improved in the group treated with haloperidol (Kalisvaart et al. 2005).

Conclusion

These studies confirm with different methodologies that benzodiazepines and opioids increase the risk of postoperative delirium. Although specific preventative effects could not be shown, a positive effect on delirium by the perioperative use of haloperidol, ketamine, and dexmedetomidine could be seen. In Chapter 9 these interventions will also be reviewed. It is worth noting that the preventative clinical trials are the only ethically feasible means for testing the effectiveness of treatments for delirium against placebo.

7.4 **Delirium in children**

Delirium in children and adolescents represents a challenge in many clinical context (de Carvalho and Fonseca 2008; Smith et al. 2009), although some data are currently available in the literature, coming especially from anaesthesia and the intensive care field (Schieveld and Leentjens 2005) and, to a less degree, from HIV infection literature (Hatherill and Flisher 2009).

In general, the incidence of delirium has been reported to be low (4.5%) in a study of 877 critically ill children and adolescents acutely, non-electively, and consecutively admitted to a hospital during a 4-year period (Schieveld et al. 2008). It seems that the incidence is, however, lower in little children (ages 0–3 years: 3%) than in adolescents (aged 16–18 years: 19%) (Schieveld et al. 2007). In a study by Grover et al. (2009), 46 children seen by consultation-liaison psychiatrists were found to be affected by infectious disease and cancer. The main common symptoms were sleep–wake cycle disturbance and impaired orientation, followed by impaired attention (89.5%), impaired short-term memory (84.2%), agitation (68.4%), and affect lability (60.5%), while delusions and hallucinations were quite rare. Most patients responded well to haloperidol.

A form of delirium that has been described in children is emergence delirium, also known as emergence agitation or postanesthetic excitement, a form of a confusional status characterized by severe restlessness, combativeness, thrashing, kicking, agitation with non-purposeful movements, disorientation, incoherence, and unresponsiveness (Voepel-Lewis 2003). In order to reduce the incidence of this adverse event, Vlajkovic and Sindjelic (2007) strongly emphasize the need to identify children at risk and take preventive measures, such as reducing preoperative anxiety, removing postoperative pain, and providing a quiet, stress-free environment for postanaesthesia recovery.

Clinical presentation of delirium in children and adolescents is characterized by classical form of hyperactive and hypoactive delirium, but a third form characterized mainly by anxiety in a study of 61 children with delirium admitted to paediatric ICU (Schieveld et al. 2007). By analysing the possible differences between delirium in adults and delirium in children, Turkel et al. (2006) found that sleep–wake disturbance, fluctuating symptoms, impaired attention, irritability, agitation, affective lability, and confusion were more often noted in children, while impaired memory, depressed mood, speech disturbance, delusions, and paranoia more often in adults. Other symptoms, such as impaired alertness, apathy, anxiety, disorientation, and hallucination occurrence, were similar among adults and children. The authors conclude that these data may actually represent true differences in the presentation of delirium across the life cycle, or may be attributable to inconsistent methodologies. However, as already reported (Chapter 4), by comparing delirium in children, adults, and geriatric patients, Leentjens et al. (2008) found more severe perceptual disturbances and more frequent visual hallucinations, a more acute onset, more severe delusions, more severe lability of mood, greater agitation, less severe cognitive deficits, less severe sleep–wake cycle disturbance, and less variability of symptoms over time in childhood delirium.

Regarding the aetiology, Karnik et al. (2007) hypothesized different mechanisms to explain the different responses to treatment. In the case of hyperactive/active delirium a high dopaminergic state leads to agitation and aggression, with features reminiscent of the positive symptoms of schizophrenia, which respond better to haloperidol. The hypoactive/mixed form of delirium seems to involve low or normal levels of dopamine and a notable cholinergic dysregulation accompanying the dopamine dysregulation, making this subtype of delirium more responsive to risperidone.

Schiveld et al. (2009) recently proposed an algorithm for assesing paediatric delirium that took into account the lack of instruments, the under-recognition of the phenomenon, and the specific clinical problems paediatric delirium poses to clinicians (e.g. the concept of 'disorganized thinking' in a very young child is difficult to assess, because mental processes in a child's very early years are frequently either not verbally assessable or 'unripe, illogical, magical'). By preferring an observational instrument that evaluates behavioural changes (as a sign of acute brain failure, i.e. delirium), the authors indicated some useful steps. This basically consists of observing some child parameters scored 0–4 on the Likert scale and given a Pediatric Anesthesia Emergence Delirium (PAED) scale score:

1. The child makes eye contact with the caregiver;
2. The child's actions are purposeful;
3. The child is aware of his/her surroundings;
4. The child is restless; and
5. the child is inconsolable.

This effort of clinical research is extremely helpful in all the contexts mentioned, but data are needed regarding paediatric delirium in palliative care, as well as in the whole area of paediatric palliative care (Knapp 2009; Korones 2007; McSherry et al. 2007).

7.5 Delirium in the elderly

The frequency of delirium in the elderly population and, above all, in the cognitively impaired elderly patient leads to the development of a specific interest on the side of the geriatricians in this syndrome (Carlson et al. 1999). Many different types of evidence concur to suggest that the process of aging of the brain, the occurrence of dementia, and delirium share some basic pathophysiological mechanisms.

Age and pre-existing cognitive impairment are independent risk factors for developing delirium as demonstrated by several well-conducted epidemiological studies (see Chapter 3 and tables therein). Age is a risk factor also when the population under study is over 65. The relevance of a failure of the cholinergic system as a consequence of age, dementia, or acute events is one of the core elements of these clinical conditions (Blass and Gibson 1999).

The differential diagnosis of delirium in the elderly with preceding and concurrent cognitive deficit and dementia is particularly challenging and already an object of debate. The diagnostic criteria in use may not be specific enough to distinguish between fluctuations in cognition related to a chronic underlying, slowly evolving condition and superimposed acute events acting on an already compromised system. Geriatricians are very aware of the fact that in many cases the boundaries between these two conditions are foggy or may have no clinical impact on subsequent patient management (Lindesay 1999; MacDonald 1999).

According to electroencephalography (EEG) results and phenomenological point of view, delirium in the course of dementia does not differ from the delirium not associated with dementia. A quantitative analysis of the EEG can help differentiate delirium from dementia in the elderly (Jacobson and Jerrier 2000; Jacobson et al. 1993a, b). Factor analysis of the Delirium Rating Scale showed that only subtle differences can be found between these two conditions and that the subtle differences due to dementia would require more study (Trzepacz et al. 1998). Delirium in the course of dementia seems to be of a longer duration than other types of deliria (Manos and Wu 1997).

The usefulness of a classification system obviously relies on its clinical impact. In the elderly the concept of 'acute confusional state' is still useful especially when exogenous causes or potentially correctable risk factors are identified (Treloar and Macdonald 1997a, b). This can be difficult but not impossible (Inouye et al. 1999a). Recognizing an unexpected worsening in the cognitive performances of a demented patient can impact on the clinical management and be a guide to the diagnosis of many co-morbidities and acute illnesses such as infection or myocardial infarction. This is even more important if it is recognized that the elderly, especially when cognitively impaired, are particularly prone to suffer from the toxic effects of drugs at doses usually thought safe for the general population (Tune et al. 1992).

The impact of the type of dementing illness on the likelihood of developing delirium and on its clinical aspects is unknown. Data on the demented population are preliminary and in part contradictory. In one study vascular dementias and late-onset Alzheimer's disease had a higher rate of delirium than early-onset Alzheimer's disease and frontotemporal dementias (Robertsson et al. 1998). According to the authors this observation could be due to the more widespread brain damage found in the more severe pathologies. Another study retrospectively correlated the presence of right hemisphere dysfunction with the risk of developing delirium (Mach et al. 1996), which would support the view of a particular role of the non-dominant hemisphere in the pathogenesis of delirium (Mesulam 1985). In a prospective study that distinguished the type of regional brain syndrome, but without considering right or left hemisphere functions, cases of delirium were more frequently associated with global brain dysfunction, more severe dementia, and older age, and were less frequent with predominant frontal lobe dysfunction, supporting the idea of delirium as a diffused affection of cortical functions (Robertsson et al. 1999). More recent data seem to suggest a possible genetic predisposition to delirium among the elderly, with a role played by the apolipoprotein E (APOE) sigma4-allele (van Munster et al. 2007b, 2009b).

Postoperative delirium has also a particular impact on the elderly populations that are at increased risk of hip fracture due to falls and osteoporosis (Noimark, 2009). As we have already described, delirium, whether present pre- or postoperatively, is a predictor of poor functional recovery after hip fracture surgery, independently of prefracture risk factors such as age and poor cognitive and functional status (Dolan et al. 2000; Marcantonio et al. 2000, 2002).

The recovery from delirium in the elderly is often slow and incomplete (Francis and Kapoor 1992), and the occurrence of delirium during hospitalization, independent of other factors, including dementia, is a predictor of mortality and long-term poor functional and cognitive status (McCusker et al. 2001b, 2002). Postoperative delirium in the elderly (≥ 65 years of age) was associated with the development of dementia and increased mortality in the 5 years following the postoperative episode (Lundstrom et al. 2003).

Infections are another common offender for the elderly hospitalized populations. Both respiratory and urinary infections in the elderly often present with delirium even with low-grade temperature or no fever at all. The sensitivity of the aging or demented brain and other predisposing factors with the addition of a metabolic or infectious cause of relatively modest severity can be crucial for the onset of delirium. The strong association of urinary infections and delirium in the elderly can be explained following this line of reasoning (Manepalli et al. 1990).

Furthermore, poor preoperative nutritional status (Tei et al. 2010), a very advanced age (more than 75-80 years), low preoperative scores on cognitive scales or cognitive impairment, and poor preoperative quality of life have also been associated with postoperative delirium in the elderly (Ansaloni et al. 2010; Hattori et al. 2009).

Case report

Mrs T. was a 64-year-old woman affected by a severe chronic obstructive pulmonary disease (COPD) that determined numerous hospital admissions. She lived alone, since the death of her husband 3 years earlier. Because of the worsening of her respiratory conditions she was readmitted to a Internal Medicine ward. The patient's home therapy was prednisone (12.5 mg m.i.d.), digoxin (0.125 mg m.i.d.), amiloride hydrochloride (5.7 mg), and hydrochlorotiazide (50 mg m.i.d.), ranitidine (300 mg m.i.d), and inhalatory fluticasone propionate (500 µg b.i.d). This therapy was maintained throughout hospitalization. Measurement of arterial blood gas showed a severe hypoxia (pO_2 38 mm g) with hypercapnia (pCO_2 66 mm g), which were normalized during the first few days of admission through proper cycles of O_2 therapy. Laboratory findings showed normal hepatorenal functions, no electrolytes imbalance, and no hypoglicaemia. The blood chemistry panel was normal, except a mildly increased erythrocyte sedimentation rate level (25 mm/h), as the only index of a possible inflammation process. In fact, chest X-ray showed a right basilar density, though there was a lack of fever, for which ciprofloxacin therapy (250 mg t.i.d.) was added (fifth day of admission). After 3 days, the patient became progressively depressed, inhibited, apathetic, and non-compliant with therapy and routine interventions. For these reasons, she was first assessed by a neurologist consultant who excluded CNS disorders and was then referred to the C–L Psychiatric service for 'depression impairing cooperation and compliance'. At mental status examination the patient appeared extremely inhibited and apathetic with decreased reaction to internal and external stimuli. Reduced ability to maintain and shift attention and impairment in short-term memory, mild perception disturbances (misperceptions, illusions, and fragmented auditory hallucinations), and thought disorders (paranoid thinking) were the main symptoms. Vital signs and physical examination were unchanged from her baseline state. Data collected from family members indicated no previous history of psychiatric disorders. A diagnosis of hypoactive delirium was made. By considering the absence of mental disorders at admission, the lack of concomitant factors (e.g. substance withdrawal, neurological disorders), which could have explained her symptoms, and the absence of any metabolic disturbances, and the striking temporal relationship between the onset of psychiatric symptoms and fluoroquinolone use, ciprofloxacin was considered as the most probable precipitant factor of the patient's delirium. Lorazepam 2 mg b.i.d. was started, in view of the literature indicating the possible inhibition of the binding of gamma-aminobutyric acid (GABA) to its receptor sites and the involvement of benzodiazepine (BDZ)–GABA–receptor complex (Unseld et al. 1990), and the efficacy of BDZ in the treatment of delirium secondary to fluoroquinolones (Farrington et al. 1995). Orientation gradually improved, hallucinations and thought disorders disappeared, and sleep–wake cycle was restored. Three days later her behaviour was nearly at baseline and mental status returned to normality. She remained in the hospital for 2 weeks, and, after discharge, a home-care assistance programme was set up. However, in a month, the patient's respiratory and cardiovascular conditions worsened and she was readmitted to the hospital where, because of multiple physical complications (cardiac insufficiency, respiratory infection), she died 10 days later.

In the practice of palliative care more and more elderly patients are likely to be seen in the future and cognitive impairment must be recognized in its manifold clinical aspects. A specific ability to manage risk factors, psychotropic drugs administration, and complex cases will often be required.

In a study of 43 hospitalized older patients with cancer with prevalent or incident delirium, Bond et al. (2006, 2008) found that a significant majority (70%) of patients had delirium at discharge. Patients who recovered were less functionally impaired before hospitalization and exhibited fewer aetiologic risk patterns at admission. Mild delirium was more likely to resolve than severe delirium. On this basis, it seems mandatory that hospitalized older patients with cancer should incorporate delirium prevention and intervention strategies (Boyle 2006; Milisen et al. 2004).

7.6 Delirium in cancer

Delirium is very frequent in cancer patients as already mentioned in Section 3.1. Metastatic aetiologies and brain radiation have already been discussed in Chapter 6, but cancer patients have many other risk and precipitating factors, partially in common with other severely ill patients, and partially specific to the diseases listed in Table 7.2.

Mental status change was the second most common reason for neurological consult in cancer (Clouston et al. 1992). In a series of 140 consecutive patients the most frequent

Table 7.2 Causes of delirium in cancer patients

Secondary CNS Tumor

  Brain metastases

  Meningeal metastases

Non-metastatic complications of cancer

  Metabolic encephalopathy due to hepatic, renal, or pulmonary failure

  Electrolyte abnormalities

  Glucose abnormalities

  Infections

  Haematologic abnormalities

  Nutritional deficiency (thiamine, folic acid, vitamin B12 deficiency)

  Vasculitis

Paraneoplastic neurological syndrome

Toxicity of antineoplastic therapies

  Chemotherapy

  Chemotherapy drugs

    Methotrexate

    Cisplatin

    Vincristine

    Paclitaxel

    Procarbazine

    Asparaginase

    Cytosine arabinoside

    5-fluorouracil

    Ifosfamide

    Tamoxifen (rare)

    Thiotepa

    Etoposide (high doses)

    Nitrosourea (high doses or via arterial route)

  Radiation to brain

Toxicity of other drugs

Other diseases not related to neoplasm with CNS involvement

Alcohol or drug abuse or withdrawal

diagnosis was toxic or metabolic encephalopathy in 64 and 53% of cases, respectively. A single aetiology could be found in 33% of cases while multiple aetiologies were likely in 67% and a structural brain lesion was the only cause of confusion in 15% of cases (Tuma and DeAngelis 2000). See also the case described below under terminal delirium.

Case report

The patient was a 75-year-old man. His past medical history showed that he had suffered from a subdural haematoma due to trauma and more recently right carotidectomy for thrombectomy. He worked as a technician with managerial experience and had a high education level including good knowledge of English. He was diagnosed with a bronchogenic carcinoma, with an hilar mass infiltrating the D9 vertebral body and causing epidural compression at this site. He was transferred from a neurological facility to an oncology ward with severe thoracic pain for radiation therapy and symptom control. Morphine infusion was started with a PCA pump at 1.5 mg/h infusion rate and 10 mg p.r.n. bolus available as needed. Pain was well controlled with moderate somnolence; infusion rate was reduced to 1 mg/h. After about 36 hours following the administration of morphine infusion the patient became agitated in the night; he started to hallucinate and to be violent. When examined the patient was awake; attention was compromised with perseveration and confabulation. Neurological exam showed many pathological reflexes: snout, palmomental, and grasping reflexes, and extensor plantar response on the left. He was asked to write a sentence (Figure 7.1). The two sentences made sense (Tomorrow I will go to school, today is a humid day). Although the first one could reflect some disorientation, the main mistakes are represented by letter repetitions (perseveration).

Haloperidol was started at the dose of 4 mg/day. Morphine infusion was kept constant at 34 mg/daily. Over the next 4 days delirium continued with nocturnal hallucinations and delusions. The patient reported seeing a man printed on the wall with threatening attitude, that the nurses wanted to kill him, and that during the night he was taken by the nurses to Piazza Castello (Piazza Castello, 'the Castle Square', is a very popular downtown location in Milan). These episodes usually took place overnight. The patient, when questioned about them the following morning, although apparently vigilant and coherent, reported these experiences as real. He was disoriented for space, saying that he was still at the Neurological hospital where he was initially admitted for spinal cord compression. He was also suspicious and believed that the nurses were not correctly administering the prescribed therapies.

Morphine infusion was stopped and substituted with a transdermal fentanyl patch (25 μg/h); mental status recovered within 24 hours. The patient completed a course of radiation therapy and was discharged after a week without further neurological complications.

Laboratory examination showed mild hyponatraemia (129 mEq/L), and hypercalcaemia (11.7 mg/dL). CT scan of the head was compatible with normotensive hydrocephalus and cortical atrophy (Figure 7.2).

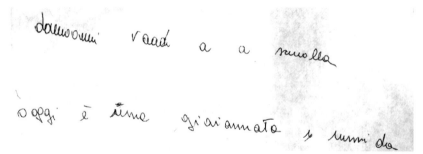

Fig. 7.1 Sample of spontaneous writing.
There are evident perseverations and mistakes. The correct spelling of the phrases should be: (first line) domani [tomorrow] vado [I will go] a scuola [to school]; (second line) oggi [today] e' [is] una [a] giornata umida [humid day]. Many a's are repeated (but also other letters) and 'giornata' is misspelled.

This case highlights several potentially important predisposing factors among which age, brain atrophy, and metabolic abnormalities may have facilitated a toxic effect from morphine administration. Fentanyl proved to have a more favourable therapeutic index in this case.

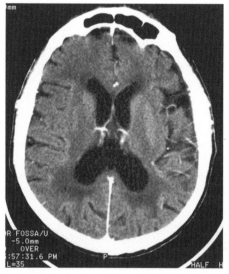

Fig. 7.2 CT scan of the head showing cortical atrophy and periventricular CSF reabsorption compatible with the diagnosis of normotensive hydrocephalus.

7.6.1 **Paraneoplastic neurological disease**

The case of paraneoplastic neurological diseases is specific of the cancer population. These diseases will usually cause dementia but their onset and clinical course can be characterized by acute mental symptoms and delirium. A paraneoplastic syndrome is a disease due to the presence of the tumour but not directly caused by it. The denomination of remote effects of neoplasia can also be found (Dalmau et al. 2008; Dropcho 2002; Rosenfeld and Dalmau 2001). The definition excludes also those indirect consequences of tumours that depend on metabolic, nutritional complications or are due to cachexia. Neurologic paraneoplastic disease can involve the peripheral and the CNS, often preceding by long term the diagnosis of cancer. They are usually severe and have a rapidly progressive and invalidating course. Paraneoplastic syndromes are rare diseases no more frequent than 1% of all neurological complications of cancer (Posner 1995).

In many of these syndromes specific autoantibodies that react against antigens common to the nervous and tumour tissue have been identified (Posner 1995). Neurological syndromes that can be paraneoplastic are the Lambert–Eaton myasthenic syndrome, encephalomyelitis, limbic encephalitis, dermato- and polymyositis, acute cerebellar degeneration, subacute sensory neuronopathy, and opsoclonus myoclonus in children.

Cognitive and psychiatric clinical presentation can occur in encephalomyelitis, limbic encephalitis, and opsoclonus myoclonus.

Limbic encephalitis can be found in association with microcytoma or testis carcinomas. The clinical findings can be of a subacute dementia, amnesia, personality changes,

Table 7.3 Main neurological paraneoplastic syndromes found in adults with the most common associated tumours and the characteristic autoantibodies

Neurological syndrome	Neoplasm	Antibody
Encephalomyelitis	SCLC*	Anti-Hu
Cerebellar	Breast, ovary	Anti-Yo
Degeneration	SCLC	Anti-Hu
	SCLC, others	Anti-CV2
	Hodkin's lymphoma	Anti-Tr
	Breast	Anti-Ri
Limbic encephalitis	SCLC	Anti-Hu
	SCLC	Anti-CV2
	Testis	Anti-Ta
Subacute sensory neuronopathy	SCLC	Anti-Hu
Lambert Eaton syndrome	SCLC	Anti-VGCC

Delirium can be found in encephalomyelitis and in limbic encephalitis. The associations listed here are typical but miscellaneous cases can be found with different combination of neoplasm and antibodies and with practically any known neoplasm. Unknown antibodies are often harboured in otherwise unexplainable cases
* Small cell lung cancer.

and psychotic features. The brain magnetic resonsance imaging (MRI) can be normal or show an abnormality of signal, and atrophy in the termporomesial cortical areas (Posner 1995; Voltz et al. 1999).

Encephalomyelitis is a syndrome of multilevel involvement of the CNS with complex clinical phenomenology. Altered mental status with delirium or dementia is frequent. The tumour most frequently associated is again microcytoma (Posner 1995).

Table 7.3 reports the most important paraneoplastic syndromes found in adult patients with their typical associated neoplasms and the autoantibodies most recently characterized. This field is in constant evolution and although a role for autoimmunity is highly likely, pathophysiological mechanisms are still under research. Paraneoplastic syndromes should not be forgotten in the differential diagnosis of delirium in patients with cancer while keeping in mind their rarity and their complex neurological presentations (Zeimer 2000).

7.6.2 Chemotherapy toxicity

The role of chemotherapy in causing delirium is often overlooked. A list of the drugs that have been associated with encephalopathy can be found in Table 7.2 (see also case reports in Chapter 5 and Figures 5.2 and 5.3). In general the use of high doses and intrathecal administrations increases toxicity. Newer drug combinations and dosages may lead to unexpected toxicities. The whole field suffers from under-reporting.

7.7 Terminal delirium

7.7.1 Delirium: 'a way of dying'?

The study of delirium in advanced diseases and in particular in the terminal phases of incurable illness is one of the developments of palliative care influenced by the changes witnessed in the way of dying in our modern or post-modern society. Delirium was a common sign of impending death when infectious, often epidemic, diseases were the first cause of death, frequently occurring at a very young age. The slowing of the dying process due to chronic progressive diseases, at a much older age than ever before, has implied the possibility of new prevalent morbidities. Delirium is still very common as an immediately pre-agonic condition but is also characteristic of a prolonged dying process with alternating abnormalities of the state of consciousness, at times with and at times without the potential for recovery. Nowadays the demand to die without suffering is growing and embraces concepts larger than the simple relief of pain (Clark 1999).

Our hypothesis is that the mental suffering of dying is dramatically embodied, in the view of lay people, by the behaviours characteristic of delirium in the terminal phase. Palliative care is expected to take an approach very different to the abandonment of dying patients depicted in Thomas Mann's (1994; English translation) *Buddenbrooks: The Decline of a Family* when describing the death of the old Lady Buddenbrook. She dies of pneumonia after a considerable period of dyspnoea and suffering. The doctors take no action to ease her subjective feelings and are strongly opposed to the request of giving a sedative drug that might worsen her respiratory conditions. She finally develops delirium, which is seen as a liberation by the family, and the writer, and dies without much help from official medicine.

Therapy today may mean dying without any perception, perhaps without the perception of mental impairment that precedes death. We are almost tempted to say 'dying without dying'. For many people dying without noticing it would be the goal of good palliative care in the post-modern society. In more pragmatic words the 'good death' that the contemporary palliative care patients expects from health providers would be peaceful, without pain, and in absolutely normal mental health until the end, with the alternative of being unconscious when these requirements cannot be fulfilled. However, these are only hypotheses since the perceived qualities of a good death are unknown (Gordon and Peruselli 2001; Morrison et al. 2000).

Another issue of debate is the degree of medicalization and the real needs of conducting research in the palliative care context. Criticisms have been raised about the possibility of applying traditional methods of research to the palliative care patient (Rinck et al. 1997). The subject of conducting research on delirium in terminal patients caused a heated debate on the limitations of the medical approach to research in palliative care, which deserves more space and more in-depth discussion (Davis and Walsh 2001; Lawlor et al. 2001).

A very important question is: How is it possible to help people with the aid of palliative care to have a 'good death'? What is a 'good death'? Research instruments for studying this approach are beginning to be discussed but have not yet been applied to empirical situations while the present difficulties of identifying outcome measurements for assessing the result of palliative care are well recognized (Kornblith 2001; Morrison et al. 2000). Qualitative methods of research may be more appropriate and their use in studying specific situations such as the impact of delirium at the end of life may be promising (Gordon and Peruselli 2001).

7.7.2 Clinical aspects

The hospice experience has contributed a number of important clinical observations to this subject. The term 'terminal restlessness' has been coined to describe a potentially specific condition of agitation and altered mental status often seen in hospices and that has been interpreted as the combination of a number of toxic and metabolic events (Burke 1997; Burke et al. 1991; Dunlop 1989). The proposed clinical characteristics of terminal restlessness are those of an 'agitated delirium in a dying patient frequently associated with impaired consciousness and multifocal myoclonus'. A more systematic description of this syndrome is lacking. In general there are no phenomenological data on the clinical features of delirium at the end of life, but terminal restlessness has remained a term relatively specific of the hospice culture. In the most recent reports, on a significant number of patients, agitated or hyperactive deliria were found in a significant number of cases but no specific assessment of the imminently dying deliria is attempted (Lawlor et al. 1998). In the study by Leonard et al. (2008) irreversible deliria were associated with a short survival and, likely, represented cases of 'terminal delirium'; in these cases a more severe impairment of cognitive functions (attention and vigilance) could be demonstrated. Earlier reports have suggested that the psychological content of deliria near to death is influenced by the unique existential meaning of the situation (Massie et al. 1983).

In our experience on the symptoms requiring sedation in the last 24-48 hours of life we identified delirium with agitation as the main reason in 19% of the patients requiring sedation (Caraceni et al. 2002). In a small number of cases agitation was a specific problem, clearly distinguished from hyperactive delirium. These patients had acute symptoms, due to rapid progression of the disease (often pain, dysphagia, and others), and extreme psychomotor agitation as a response to an unbearable physical and existential situation but they were not clinically delirious.

The prevalence of delirium in patients undergoing palliative care was about 30% in two recent studies in the hospice and home care populations with advanced incurable cancer (Caraceni et al. 2000; Minagawa et al. 1996) and 42% on admission in a specialized acute palliative care ward (Lawlor et al. 2000b). Terminal delirium, defined as delirium occurring at least 6 hours before death, occurred in 88% of 52 patients dying in hospital, and cognitive failure was reported in 83% of patients, occurring on average 16 days before death (Bruera et al. 1992b).

As already mentioned in Chapter 3 we now have data on risk factors for the development of delirium in palliative care (Caraceni et al. 2000; Lawlor et al. 2000b), on the potentially reversible aetiogical or precipitating factors (Lawlor et al. 2000b), and on its prognostic meaning (Caraceni et al. 2000; Lawlor et al. 2000b; Morita et al. 1999). Table 7.4 reports factors more frequently found in palliative care and therefore relatively specific of the high risk of delirium in this population and general risk factors also found in palliative care.

At the moment we lack studies that focus on delirium in the imminently dying that can identify the role of predisposing and precipitating factors with more detail in the palliative care situation.

Table 7.4 Factors facilitating delirium in palliative care

Factors more frequent in palliative care	General factors common with other medical conditions
Opioids[a]	Age
Psychotropic medication[a]	Previous cognitive failure
Cachexia/anorexia[b]	Dehydration
Low performance[b]	Environmental factors
Respiratory failure[a]	
Infections[a]	
Brain or meningeal metastases[b]	
AIDS brain pathology	

[a] Lawlor et al 2000b
[b] Caraceni et al 2000

7.7.3 **Assessment**

The systematic assessment of cognitive functions is very important in palliative care, for many reasons. Although the high prevalence and incidence of delirium in patients with terminal illnesses could be enough to recommend the routine use of some instruments for screening of cognitive function in patients admitted to palliative care programmes we see also many more specific reasons for adopting a systematic assessment of mental status:

◆ The aging population is an extremely significant proportion of the palliative care population. In these patients the frequency of dementia or other more subtle forms of cognitive failure is high; therefore a differential diagnosis between delirium, dementia, and adjustment disorders is often required (Farrell and Ganzini 1995).

◆ Symptom assessment is particularly difficult in patients with delirium. In one study patients admitted to a palliative care ward received higher p.r.n. opioid doses for pain when delirious than after recovering from the episode. Pain was rated as more severe by the staff during the delirious episode than by the patient himself after delirium had cleared (Bruera et al. 1992a; Coyle et al. 1994).

◆ This difficulty in interpreting symptom severity can cause conflicts within the staff and with the family. A compromised communication between patient and family can contribute to a compromised communication between staff and family in the terminal phases of life. This, in turn, can have a serious effect regarding therapeutic decision and can be a factor in family morbidity (see Chapter 10).

◆ One of the more baffling aspects of delirium is its symptom fluctuation and night worsening. For this reason, a codified assessment with written reports is essential. Nurse observation is a very valuable source of information that can be improved by specific education on delirium characteristics. Standardized assessment will improve communication that it is often limited to the poorly informative dialogue between staff members, such as nurses: nurse Jude: 'I saw Mr Smith yesterday night, he is confused'; nurse Angela 'No dear, I saw Mr Smith this morning and he is not confused!'

◆ Early detection and well-conducted assessment will enable the staff to inform family, encouraging communication and counselling on several critical issues (Borreani et al. 1997).

◆ Early detection of prodromal symptoms of delirium should help in preventing further worsening in reversible cases and has been proven useful as part of the strategy to reduce the risk of developing delirium in the elderly population (Inouye et al. 1999a).

◆ The whole process is aimed at understanding the dying process, easing suffering, and providing support for the family in a way that is proportionate to the actual clinical situation, being careful not to be caught unprepared and at the same time to not overemphasize excessive testing that could result in patient burden.

7.7.4 **Aetiological factors**

Multiple potential aetiological or precipitating factors are commonly found in palliative care with an average of 2.2 probable or possible causes attributed to 71 delirium episodes in a recent prospective study (Lawlor et al. 2000b). Similar observations can be found in older studies (Bruera et al. 1992b; Caraceni et al. 1994; Stiefel et al. 1992).

Reversibility is possible when delirium is not part of the failure of vital homeostatic mechanisms leading to death. This is suggested by recent findings showing that irreversibility is associated with hypoxia and respiratory failure, and metabolic factors (Lawlor et al. 2000b), while reversibility is related to the contributing effect of drug toxicity and dehydration (Caraceni et al. 1994; Lawlor et al. 2000b). Strategies that may reduce the incidence of reversible deliria have been suggested to improve the management of palliative care patients (Bruera et al. 1995), but their true impact on symptom control outcome cannot be clarified without performing controlled clinical trials which are hard to propose in palliative care.

While metabolic irreversible failures are often found as causes of both delirium and coma that precede many deaths in palliative, the exact contribution of these conditions as causes of death in terminal patients is not well established. In our experience on patients with advanced terminal cancer admitted to a home care programme, in 56% of patients death could be attributed to metabolic failure (Groff 1993). The complexity of the final events leading to death and the peculiarity of the home care setting are such that in a number of patients (17%), no specific cause could be attributed to the final clinical event. The case reported below shows how delirium can characterize the dying process in a modern palliative care unit, even though a specific cause cannot be found.

Case report

The patient was a 69-year-old university professor of chemistry still actively teaching before his recent clinical conditions deteriorated. The patient was affected by a locally advanced carcinoma of the pancreas and underwent prolonged chemotherapy with 5-FU and palliative local radiation. Abdominal and back pain was treated initially with oral morphine and then with subcutaneous morphine infusion. Worsening of pain suggested admission to an in-patient palliative care unit.

On admission the patient started to be delirious while on oral morphine and had a fluctuating course of delirium with phases of complete recovery (Memorial Delirium Assessment Scale [11] score = 12/30) and phases of severe delirium (MDAS score = 30/30), which lasted for 26 days before death.

His neurological examination never showed any focal sign, but bilateral palmomental reflexes and grasping reflexes were present.

Delirium was partially controlled with haloperidol; then the patient required prometazine and finally profound sedation in the terminal phase.

During the course of the last 4 weeks of life, respiratory, renal, and cardiac functions were within normal limits, with the exception of olyguria in the last 3-day phase. Temperature reached 38.5°C on one occasion but fever was remittent and usually of low grade. In the last days fever reached 39.5°C.

Laboratory findings showed no specific abnormalities that could justify delirium, but a very significant increase of specific tumour marker levels (Ca19.9, 142,290),

---

[1] See Section 8.2.2 and appendices.

low albumin, and high alkaline phosphatase. Brain MRI with gadolinium showed cortical atrophy, in particular at the level of the temporal lobes (Figure 7.3).

Finally a diagnosis could not be established as to the aetiology of delirium. Cortical brain atrophy could be due to a pre-existing beclouded or compensated dementia and could have facilitated the occurrence of delirium in association with the use of opioid analgesics and advanced cancer; the long-term 5-FU administration might have produced brain toxicity. Even paraneoplastic limbic encephalitis, although a rare event (specific tests were not felt necessary for the clinical situation), might explain irreversible cognitive decline.

The content and the subjective perception of terminal delirium, as already mentioned, are unknown. Extrapolating from other anecdotal reports, it is reasonable to conclude that the experience of delirium is usually unpleasant. The most authoritative opinion in this regards can be used to state that 'delirium itself is usually a highly disturbing experience that augments the sufferer's distress' (Lipowski 1990b). More specifically, it is likely that the content of delirium is influenced by the dramatic physical and emotional conditions associated with the disease progression: hospitalization, invasive therapies, painful procedures, fear of death, and existential and spiritual concerns. All these are hypotheses awaiting empirical confirmation. The possibility that pre-morbid psychologically distressful and significant past life events can be reactivated from unconscious processes within a delirium has been a given for a long time (Wolf and Curran 1935), but how these mechanisms impact on the very special case of terminal delirium is certainly a question worth considering.

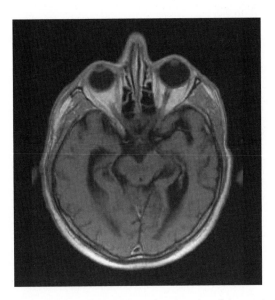

Fig. 7.3 Axial MRI view of the brain demonstrating atrophy of the cortical mantle mainly in the temporal areas. See text for patient's case report.

7.7.5 **Management**

There are little data on the specific management of delirium at the end of life. However, as already mentioned, a number of delirium episodes are reversible even in the advanced phases of disease. Therefore general principles of aetiology screening need to be followed if the goal of care is to improve the patient's mental status.

Some authors suggest that a systematic approach to reducing a number of potential risk factors could be implemented in the palliative care setting, with the aim of reducing the prevalent agitation and myoclonus characterizing the cognitive failure of terminal patients in hospice care experiences. The protocol that these authors suggest include intensive monitoring of cognitive functions, hydration, and opioid rotation to minimize toxicity due to uraemia and opioid toxicity (Bruera et al. 1995; Dunlop 1989). This approach recently created a controversy on its appropriateness in the model of hospice care (Davis and Walsh 2001; Lawlor et al. 2001).

We already mentioned that agitated terminal delirium is one of the situations that may require pharmacological sedation at the end of life (Cherny and Portenoy 1994; Stiefel et al. 1992). A discussion of the pharmacology of sedation can be found in Chapter 9.

The ethical implication of using sedation in the phases that precede death is beyond the scope of this chapter (Cherny and Portenoy 1994; Quill et al. 2000; Cherny et al. 2009). In a multicenter international trial, the frequency of delirium as an indication for sedation varied from 14 to 60% of cases (Fainsinger et al. 2000b), while in a Canadian series of patients who needed terminal sedation, this procedure was required in only 4% of cases and in most of them it was indicated because of delirium (Fainsinger et al. 2000a). In our experience delirium has been an indication for sedation in the terminal phase of cancer in 19% of the cases that required sedation (Caraceni et al. 2002). See also Section 9.3.

Chapter 8

Diagnostic assessment[1]

Delirium is viewed as a medical emergency and the guidelines recommended for its immediate assessment and management are available, usually from the experience of emergency medicine. Certainly the palliative care settings have different requirements but it is quite useful to recall some of these first line recommendations that maintain their practical and mnemonic usefulness. One popular acronym, I WATCH DEATH, is reproduced in Table 8.1.

In every setting of care delirium can be an emergency depending on its severity and on the occurrence of agitation and aggressiveness characterizing the individual cases.

8.1 Instrumental and laboratory findings

8.1.1 Diagnostic examinations

The onset of delirium should alert a series of diagnostic procedures that will be more or less aggressively pursued, depending on the clinical context. Table 8.2 summarizes one possible stepwise approach that can be followed to explore all the potentially correctable aetiologies. In our opinion, it is possible that, in many cases of the evolution of a quiet delirium as the terminal phase of metastatic cancer, none of these actions are undertaken. It should be obvious that the role of any further investigation must be weighted against the potential usefulness of the results to improve the patient's quality of life. As already discussed, in the severely ill population, it is often impossible to identify a single aetiology; a mean of 2 to 3 potential aetiological factors are common (Bruera et al. 1992b; Lawlor et al. 2000b; Tuma and DeAngelis 2000). See also the case reported in Section 7.5.

The last position of the EEG in Table 8.2 is probably not fair. The EEG can be a source of very useful information in some cases of delirium and reasonably economical when compared to many of the other procedures.

8.1.2 Electroencephalography

As already mentioned the EEG can be a sensitive and specific test for the diagnosis of delirium and indeed it was considered a candidate diagnostic criterion in the discussion that preceded the development of the DSM-IV (Tucker 1999). The relationship between consciousness level, EEG slowing, and the pathogenesis of delirium was

....

[1] Maria Giulia Nanni, MD, Section of Psychiatry, Department of Medical Disciplines of Communication and Behaviour, University of Ferrara, Italy, has contributed to the writing of this chapter.

Table 8.1 I WATCH DEATH A mnemonic for emergency assessment of the delirious patient

Infections
Withdrawal
Acute metabolic
Trauma
CNS pathology
Hypoxia
Deficiencies
Endocrinopathies
Acute vascular
Toxins or drugs
Heavy metals

originally described by Engels and Romano (1959). It clearly pointed out how the degree of slowing of the EEG corresponds to the degree of consciousness disturbance and parallels it, accounting for severity of the cause, reversibility, and implementation of therapeutic interventions.

Traditional electroencephalography combined with clinical findings can be used to diagnose delirium and differentiate it from functional psychoses (Brenner 1991; Trzepacz et al. 1988b) and from dementia (Jacobson et al. 1993a, b; Koponen et al. 1989), as well as to grade its severity and to follow up the patient's recovery (Niedermeyer et al. 1999). A recent grading system for the assessment of encephalopathies with altered level of consciousness has been published by Young et al. (1992).

EEG findings typical of metabolic encephalopathy, and of many cases of drug toxicity, parallel those seen with anaesthetic gases, showing a progressive slowing of EEG frequency with increase in amplitude (see Figure 5.3). Anaesthetic gases usually cause initial desincronization and the appearance of fast activity in the beta frequencies followed by progressive slowing of the EEG. Fast activity of low voltage is also typically seen in alcohol withdrawal delirium. This is the only type of delirium in which fast activity is reported to dominate the EEG pattern.

In case of toxic metabolic aetiologies EEG slowing can be compounded with triphasic waves or epileptiform discharges (Bortone et al. 1998). Suppression of the EEG and burst suppression pattern is seen when coma occurs (Young et al. 1992, 1997).

In selected cases the EEG recording may be the only way of demonstrating the occurrence of non-convulsive status epilepticus (Towne et al. 2000b; Wengs et al. 1993) (see Figure 5.2).

8.2 **Clinical assessment tools**

Although clinical evaluation according to the symptom phenomenology and the nosographic criteria (DSM-IV-TR and ICD-10) is the gold standard for the diagnosis

Table 8.2 Screening of main aetiologies and diagnostic process

Toxic factors	Bedside drug screening for present and recent medications
	Urine or blood drug screening
Sepsis	Temperature
	Blood/urine and other cultures for infection screen
	Leukocyte count
	Urinalysis
	Red cell count
Glucose-oxidative brain deficiency	Pulse oxymetry
	Blood gases and acid–base balance
	Blood glucose
Electrolyte imbalances	Serum electrolytes (Na, K, CL, Mg, Ca)
Renal failure	Urea, creatinine, creatinine clearance
Liver failure	Liver function tests
	Ammonia
CNS vascular, infectious, or structural lesion	Screening for disseminated intravascular coagulation (DIC) and coagulation profile
	CSF examination: blood, glucose, proteins, lymphocytes, leukocytes, malignant cells, culture
	Brain CT or MRI
Cofactor deficiency malnutrition	B12 levels–administer B1 1 g/day[a]
Endocrine dysfunction	Thyroid hormone and thyroid-stimulating hormone (TSH)
	Adrenal function
Seizures–Nonconvulsive status	EEG
Paraneoplastic neurological disease	Determination of specific auto-antibodies[b]

[a] The determination of B1 levels is problematic. Our practice is to supplement B1 to every elderly patient with poor nutritional status.
[b] See chapter 7.

of delirium (see Chapter 1), many instruments have been developed for this purpose in clinical practice and in research. The importance of correctly examining the symptoms of delirium for epidemiological reasons (e.g. prevalence and incidence in specific palliative settings), research (e.g. evaluation of the severity of delirium, description of subtypes, aetiologies, and identification of new treatments), and clinical aims (e.g. development of easiest ways to routine assessment) has been pointed out by a number of authors (Breitbart et al. 2009; Casarett and Inouye 2001; Hjermstad et al. 2004; Schuurmans et al. 2003; Smith et al. 1995).

Some concepts should be clarified when discussing the properties of assessment methods of delirium, since sound psychometric properties are necessary in order to have instruments that respect specific statistical constructs.

8.2.1 Validity of assessment tools

The first matter of importance regards *reliability*, which measures the accuracy and consistency of a specified instrument. More specifically, *test–retest reliability* indicates the stability of the test scores over time, as indicated by the correlation between the scores obtained in two different assessments; *inter-rater reliability* evaluates the degree of agreement in test scores (total score or individual items) as obtained by different raters; *internal consistency reliability*, usually measured by Cronbach's alpha coefficient, refers to the relationship between the instrument items.

A second issue regards the *validity* of the instrument. *Content validity* indicates the extent to which the content of the items adequately explores the specified psychological area or function. *Criterion-related validity* refers to the relationship between the scores and a reference criterion (e.g. clinical diagnostic criteria), which represents the true state of the patient. More particularly, within criterion-related validity it is possible to distinguish between *sensitivity* (i.e. correct identification of true positive cases: true positives/true positives + false negatives) and *specificity* (i.e. correct identification of true negative cases: true negatives/true negatives + false positives). Sensitivity and specificity tend to vary according to the cut-off scores used on the instrument to classify the patients:

Related concepts are the *positive predictive accuracy* (i.e. the probability that a patient who is 'positive' to the test receives a diagnosis of delirium) and the *negative predictive accuracy* (i.e. the probability that a patient who is 'negative' to the test does not receive a diagnosis of delirium).

Lastly, *construct validity* refers to the accuracy of the instrument to measure what it should measure, as indicated by high correlation with other instruments shown to measure the same construct (*convergent validity*) and low correlation with instruments shown to measure different constructs (*discriminant validity*).

Methods employed in clinical or research practice can be grouped into three broad categories: (1) general instruments for the evaluation of cognitive functions; (2) instruments specifically devised for the assessment of delirium; and (3) other instruments.

We will summarize herein the most important tools for palliative care professionals, sending the interested reader to more detailed revisions (Robertsson 1999; Smith et al. 1995; Trzepacz 1994b).

8.2.2 Instruments for the evaluation of cognitive functions

Among the several instruments belonging to this category, the Mini-mental State Examination (MMSE; Folstein et al. 1975) is one of the best known and used tests for cognitive disturbances that can follow organic mental disorders, such as dementia, delirium, or other cognitive disorders (Tombaugh and McIntyre, 1992). It has been translated into several languages and is widely applied in clinical settings.

The MMSE consists of 11 questions that evaluate several parameters, including orientation to time and space, memory (instantaneous recall and short-term memory), attention and calculation (serial subtractions or reverse spelling), language, and constructional abilities. The score ranges form 0 to 30, with three cut-off scores used to evaluate cognitive functions: 24–30 indicates no impairment, 18–23 mild impairment, and 0–17 severe impairment. The influences of age and education have been introduced to adjust the score obtained by using the MMSE (Crum et al. 1993).

Psychometric properties of the MMSE have been examined in several studies. As far as delirium is concerned, however, the MMSE has been criticized: first, because certain symptoms of delirium are not examined by the instrument (e.g. perceptual and thought disorders); second, because specificity/sensitivity and positive/negative predictive values varied across studies, with high percentages of clinically delirious patients not being recognized by the MMSE (Smith et al. 1995). In our experience with delirious cancer patients, MMSE had a sensitivity of 38% by using the classic cut-off of 24 over 30 for normal subjects (Grassi et al. 2001b). See Yue et al. (1994) for the example of a delirious patient with a normal MMSE. Furthermore, some tasks, such as writing a sentence and copying two intersecting pentagons, are difficult to perform in severely delirious patients or in certain clinical settings (e.g. intensive care units). The MMSE retains its importance for its simplicity and popularity as a bedside clinical tool. As is true for most instruments based on the assessment of orientation, short-term memory, calculation, and writing, the MMSE is particularly sensitive to attention deficit more than to other types of cognitive changes.

The clock drawing test has also been popular as a short way of assessing cognitive function; its use in delirium confirms that it can help in detecting cognitive dysfunction but that it cannot be used as a marker of delirium due to lack of specificity, as expected (Adamis et al. 2005).

8.2.3 Instruments devised for the diagnosis and assessment of delirium

A number of instruments have, however, been developed to more specifically assess delirium in clinical practice. They have different formats, such as algorithms, short interviews, and scales, that assist clinicians in screening for the presence of delirium or in evaluating the severity of the disorder.

Confusion assessment method (CAM) (Appendix 1)

The Confusion Assessment Method (CAM; Inouye et al. 1990) is an easy-to-administer instrument which has been repeatedly used as a tool for diagnosing delirium. The CAM consists of nine operationalized criteria from the DSM-III-R, with an a priori hypothesis (CAM algorithm) establishing the diagnosis of delirium according to four criteria: (1) acute onset and fluctuating course of symptoms; (2) inattention; and either (3) disorganized thinking or (4) altered level of consciousness. The CAM algorithm had the highest predictive accuracy for all possible combinations of the nine features of delirium. When validated against psychiatric diagnosis and used by trained health professionals, the CAM showed good psychometric properties, with high levels of sensitivity (94–100%), specificity (90–5%), and positive (91–4%) and negative predictive values (90–100%) (Farrell and Ganzini 1995; Inouye 1998; Inouye et al. 1990, 1999a; Zou et al. 1998). It can be administered in less than 5 minutes by clinicians, other than psychiatrists, and non-clinicians who, however, should have been trained in the method. The CAM was also shown to have convergent agreement with other mental status tests, including the MMMSE, and high interobserver reliability ($\kappa = 0.81$–1.0).

However, some reports have shown lower sensitivity, with values between 0.46 and 0.67, for the CAM when administered by a non-physician, in comparison with a physician, while specificity remained high (0.92–0.97; Pompei et al. 1995; Rockwood et al. 1994). A study carried out in an emergency room has shown that the coefficient of agreement between a trained non-physician and a geriatrician in the evaluation of delirium in 110 elderly patients by using the CAM was good (0.91), with remarkably high levels of sensitivity (0.86), specificity (1.0), and positive (0.97) and negative predictive values (1.0) (Monette et al. 2001).

The importance of the training of the operator administering the CAM in palliative care has been recently underlined by Ryan et al. (2009), who found that an 'enhanced' training programme was superior to the standard 1-hour training session based on the original CAM training manual. The sensitivity in diagnosing delirium significantly changed from 0.5 to 0.88.

In a recent review (Wei et al. 2008), the success of the CAM was demonstrated by the fact that it has been translated into 10 languages. CAM-rated delirium is most commonly used as a risk factor or outcome but also as an intervention or reference standard. As a recommendation, the CAM should be scored based on observations made during formal cognitive testing, and training is recommended in order to optimize performance.

A modified version of the CAM for use in intensive care unit patients (CAM-ICU) was applied, in a prospective cohort study, and compared against the reference standard, by a delirium expert who used delirium criteria from DSM-IV. The CAM-ICU ratings showed high inter-rater reliability ($\kappa = 0.79$–0.95) among the assessors (nurse and anaesthesiologist), with high sensitivity (95–100%) and specificity (89–93%) in comparison with DSM-IV diagnosis for patients who developed delirium (87%) (Ely et al. 2001). In a study of 96 mechanically ventilated patients, the same author (Ely 2001) showed that, among the patients who developed delirium (83%), critical care nurses were able to detect the disorder, by using the CAM-ICU, with high sensitivity (93-100%) and specificity (98–100%) in comparison with DSM-IV diagnosis by delirium experts. Inter-rater reliability was also high ($\kappa = 0.96$). The CAM-ICU is different from the original CAM in the assessment of some items, such as inattention (which is rated as positive if the patient reports less than eight correct answers on either the visual or the auditory components of the Attention Screening Examination) and disorganized thinking (which is rated positive if the patient gives at least three incorrect answers to four predetermined questions and is unable to follow three simple commands). The CAM-ICU showed the best validity of the evaluated scales for identifying delirium in a study of 156 surgical patients aged ≥ 60 years old admitted to ICU (Luetz et al. 2010).

Delirium Rating Scale (Appendix 2)

The Delirium Rating Scale (DRS; Trzepacz et al. 1988a) is one of the most frequently used instruments for the assessment of delirium. Its 10-symptom rating scale is designed to identify delirium in the medically ill and to measure its severity. Items are not based on any particular DSM system and measure the clinical characteristic of delirium, namely temporal onset of symptoms, perceptual disturbances (e.g. misperceptions, depersonalization, derealization), hallucinations, thought disorders (delusions), psychomotor behaviour, cognitive status, lability of mood, physical disorders, sleep–wake cycle disturbances, and variability of symptoms. The items are scored on different Lykert scales (most of them on a 0–3 scale). All available information from the patient interview, mental status examination, nursing observation, and family reports concur to the DRS rating, which is based on a 24-hour period of observation. The total DRS score is obtained by summing up the scores on the 10 items (range = 0–32). Although a cut-off score of 12 has been suggested to distinguish delirious from non-delirious patients (Trzepacz and Dew 1995), a cut-off score of 10 has shown a sensitivity of 94% and a specificity of 82% (Rosen et al. 1994), while another study, which used a less conservative cut-off of 7.5, showed a sensitivity of 90% and a specificity of 82% (Rockwood et al. 1996).

In our experience with the Italian version and validation of the DRS (Grassi et al. 2001b), 105 advanced cancer patients consecutively referred for cognitive disturbances were approached and a diagnosis of delirium was made in 62%. The DRS significantly differentiated delirious from non-delirious patients. Internal consistency was relatively high (Cronbach's alpha = 0.70). By using the proposed cut-off score of 10, the DRS showed a sensitivity of 95% and a specificity of 61%, whereas with the more conservative cut-off score of 12, sensitivity was 81% and specificity 76%. Factor analysis of the DRS showed the existence of three factors: the first regarding psychomotor behaviour, sleep–wake cycle, and cognitive status; the second consisting of psychotic items; and the third comprising other symptoms (temporal onset of symptoms, presence of causal physical disorder, lability of mood, and fluctuation of symptoms).

Delirium Rating Scale-Revised-98 (Appendix 3)

The DRS has been refined and revised by Trzepacz et al. (2001), by developing the Delirium Rating Scale-Revised-98 (DRS-R-98). It consists of a 16-item clinician-rated scale with 13 severity items and 3 diagnostic items. It covers some areas also assessed by the DRS items (i.e. sleep–wake cycle disturbance, delusions, lability of affect, temporal onset of symptoms, fluctuation of symptoms, and physical disorder); unlike the DRS, perceptual disturbances and hallucinations are combined into the same category and psychomotor behaviour is separated into two that assess motor agitation and motor retardation. Cognitive status is separated into five specific items (i.e. orientation, attention, short-term memory, long-term memory, and visuospatial activity), and two further items assess language and thought process abnormalities. Each item is rated on a 0–3 Lykert scale. The sum of the first 13 items provides a severity score (range 0–39), while the last three (temporal onset of symptoms, fluctuation of symptoms, and physical disorder) can be used to help clinicians in differentiating delirium from other disorders or for research aims. They can be added to the first 13 to provide a total score (range 0–46). The DRS-R-98 is used for initial assessment and repeated measures. In addition to the examination of the patient, all available sources of information (e.g. family, nurses, chart reports) are used to rate the items.

The authors administered the DRS-R–98, the DRS, the Cognitive Test for Delirium, and the Clinical Global Impression scale to 68 patients with diagnoses of delirium ($n = 24$), dementia ($n = 13$), depression ($n = 12$), schizophrenia ($n = 9$), and other disorders ($n = 10$). The DRS-R-98 significantly distinguished delirium from each other group. Significant correlations were also found between DRS-R-98 and the other instruments. High levels of the inter-rater reliability (0.98 for the DSR-R-98 total scale; 0.99 for the DRS-R-98 severity scale) and the internal consistency (Cronbach's alpha = 0.90 for the DSR-R-98 total scale; 0.87 for the DRS-R-98 severity scale) were also found. Cut-off scores of 17.75 on the DSR-R-98 total scale resulted in a 92% sensitivity and 95% specificity. Cut-off scores of 15.25 on the DSR-R-98 severity scale resulted in a sensitivity of 92% and a specificity of 93%. On the basis of these results, the authors point out that the DRS-R-98 is a valid measure of delirium severity over a broad range of symptoms and a useful diagnostic and assessment tool for longitudinal studies. In a study carried out to understand the phenomenology of delirium and the relationship between cognitive and non-cognitive delirium symptoms (Meagher et al. 2007), 100 patients with delirium were assessed using the DRS-R-98 and the Cognitive Test for Delirium (CTD). The authors found that the DRS-98 was a valid instrument for understanding delirium as a syndrome characterized in particular by inattention and sleep–wake cycle disturbance, where attention and comprehension together are the cognitive items that best account for the syndrome of delirium.

Memorial Delirium Assessment Scale (Appendix 4)

The Memorial Delirium Assessment Scale (MDAS; Breitbart et al. 1997) has been devised to assess delirium and to quantify the severity of the symptoms by experienced mental health professionals with minimal training. It is composed of 10 four-point observer-rated items, yielding a global score ranging from 0 to 30. The MDAS was developed to be consistent with the proposed DSM-IV diagnostic criteria for delirium, as well as earlier and alternative classification systems (e.g. DSM-III-R, ICD-9). Scale items explore arousal and level of consciousness, disorientation, short-term memory, digit span, attention, disorganized thinking, perceptual disturbances, delusions, psychomotor activity, and sleep–wake cycle disturbances. The MDAS integrates objective cognitive testing and evaluation of behavioural symptoms. It is rapid and easy to administer, requiring about 10 minutes for completion. It is also designed for repeated daily evaluation and to capture short-term fluctuations of symptoms and to document response to treatment. By using the suggested cut-off of 13 on the total score, the MDAS showed a sensitivity of 70.6% and a specificity of 93.7% in discriminating delirious from non-delirious patients in the cancer setting (Breitbart et al. 1997). The MDAS also accurately classified patients with different severity grades of delirium, in particular those with moderate and severe delirium.

In the above-mentioned Italian study of 105 advanced cancer patients, the MDAS significantly differentiated delirious from non-delirious patients. The MDAS showed high levels of internal consistency (Cronbach's alpha = 0.89). By using the cut-off of 13, the MDAS showed a specificity of 94% and a sensitivity of 68%. Factor analysis of the MDAS suggested the existence of two factors, one that explained 51.1% of the variance and consisted of cognitive items, and the other that explained a further 11.5% of the variance and consisted of psychotic systems (disorganized thinking, perceptual disturbance and delusions; Grassi et al. 2001b). Moreover, Bosisio et al. (2006) evaluated the ability of all DRS and MDAS items to discriminate delirium from non-delirium patients, testing the difference in the distribution of the individual MDAS and DRS item scores. The MDAS showed a greater number of discriminating items, while hallucinations and lability of mood were less discriminating on the DRS (Bosisio et al. 2006).

In a study of 104 patients admitted to an acute palliative care unit, Lawlor et al. (2000b) assessed cognitive functions by using the MMSE, a standardized semi-structured interview, and the MDAS. A DSM-IV diagnosis of delirium was made in 68% ($n = 71$) of the patients. Complete MDAS data were available for 56 patients. The authors found moderate to low correlations among the scale items. Two primary correlated factors emerged at the analysis of factor loadings: a global cognitive factor (Factor I) and a neurobehavioural factor (Factor II) with Cronbach's alpha coefficients indicating a relatively high level of correlation for items within each factor and a Cronbach's alpha for the MDAS (0.78), suggesting one general underlying factor. In a larger sample of complete MDAS ratings ($n = 330$), a cut-off score of 7 yielded the highest sensitivity (98%) and specificity (96%) for the diagnosis of delirium. The MDAS score moderately correlated with the MMSE score ($r = -0.55$) (Lawlor et al. 2000c). Matsuoka et al. (2001), in a study on 37 elderly Japanese patients, have confirmed the good internal consistency of the MDAS (Cronbach's alpha = 0.92) and its moderate correlation with the MMSE ($r = -0.55$).

The MDAS was applied to postoperative delirium by Marcantonio et al. (2002), in order to differentiate the hypoactive from the hyperactive subtypes. The MDAS showed a positive correlation between delirium severity and functional outcome.

Recently Fadul et al. (2007) showed that, through an adequate training and a guiding manual, the application of MDAS by palliative care health professionals and the recognition of delirium were enhanced, leading the authors to consider the MDAS as a screening tool in clinical practice. A study of cardiac surgery patients with delirium confirmed the MDAS cut-off score of 10, optimizing sensitivity and specificity with respect to DSM-IV and ICD-10 (Kazmierski et al. 2008).

Confusion State Evaluation

The Confusion State Evaluation (CSE; Robertsson et al. 1997) has been developed to assess delirium, with particular reference to the elderly. It consists of 22 items on a 5-point scale (0–4), with the possibility of rating each item on a half-point scale (e.g. 0–0.5-1-1.5–2). A group of 12 items measure the main clinical symptoms of delirium (disorientation to person, time, space, and situation; thought disturbance; memory disturbance; inability to concentrate; distractibility; perseveration; impaired contact; paranoid delusions; hallucinations) and their sum yields the 'confusion score'. A group of seven items deal with frequent symptoms of delirium (irritability, emotional lability, wakefulness disturbance, increased or reduced psychomotor activity, mental uneasiness, and sleep–wake disorders). The last group of three items regards the temporal characteristics of delirium (sudden impairment and/or fluctuations), the intensity of the current episode, and the frequency and intensity of the episodes of delirium. The authors report the usefulness of the CSE in measuring the severity of symptoms and their changes over time. It can be administered in a maximum of 30 minutes by nurses, physicians, and psychologists. In a study of elderly patients with a DSM-III-R diagnosis of delirium, the CSE showed an acceptable level of internal validity. The correlation between the CSE and the MMSE was –0.87. A confusion score of less than 25 is considered to indicate mild delirium, between 25 and 35 to suggest moderate delirium, and over 35 to show severe delirium. The authors acknowledge the need for further validation studies, including studies on different diagnostic and age groups.

Cognitive Test for Delirium

The Cognitive Test for Delirium (CTD) has been developed to identify delirium in critically ill patients admitted to ICU (Hart et al. 1996). The main aims of the authors in devising the CTD were to have an instrument that could be brief and easy to administer, that would focus solely on cognitive functions, and that could accommodate the severe medical conditions of ICU patients (e.g. intubation, motor restriction). For this reason, the patient's responses to the CTD are nonverbal (pointing, nodding head or raising hand). Following DSM-III-R-criteria, the CTD evaluates orientation, attention span, memory, comprehension/conceptual reasoning, and vigilance. Scores for each of these areas range from 0 to 6 and are added together, yielding a maximum total score of 30. Time of test administration is between 10 and 15 minutes. In a study of patients with delirium, dementia, depression, and schizophrenia the CTD showed a sensitivity of 100% and a specificity of 95%. The authors indicate that in almost half of ICU patients who completed the CTD, the MMSE could not be administered. More recently the same authors (Hart et al. 1996) have found that an abbreviated form of the CTD, consisting of two content scores (visual attention span and recognition memory for pictures), maintained a good reliability index and an ability to discriminate between delirium, dementia, depression, and schizophrenia.

Delirium Index

The Delirium Index (DI) (McCusker et al. 1998) has been developed to measure changes in the severity of symptoms of delirium over time. According to the authors, the DI has been designed for use in conjunction with the MMSE, the first five questions of which represent the basis of observation. The DI investigates seven symptoms of delirium, adapted from the CAM, namely attention, disorganized thinking, level of consciousness, memory, perceptual disturbance, and motor activity. The symptoms are assessed through direct observation and questions at the patient's bedside, without any need for additional information from the family, the staff, or the patient's chart. Each symptom is rated on a 0–3 scale (from absent to severe), with a total score ranging from 0 to 21. It takes 5–10 minutes to be completed and can be administered by research assistants and nurses. The authors used the DI in 27 delirious patients, showing a good agreement between the psychiatrist's and research assistant's ratings (0.88) and a high correlation with the DRS (0.84). In a prospective cohort study, with repeated patient assessments at multiple points (admission, 8 weeks after discharge, at 6 and 12 months after admission), patients aged over 65 with delirium and dementia ($n = 165$), with delirium only ($n = 57$), with dementia only (n=55), and with neither ($n = 41$) were administered, among other measures, the DI, the CAM, and the MMSE. The DI was shown to be a reliable, valid, and responsive measure of the severity of delirium in patients with delirium, with or without dementia (McCusker et al. 2004).

Delirium Symptom Interview

Among structured interviews, the Delirium Symptom Interview (DSI; Albert et al. 1992) has been designed for diagnosing the presence of symptoms of delirium. It consists of seven domains in a present–absent format according to the DSM-III criteria for delirium: disorientation, perceptual disturbances, disturbance of consciousness during the past 24 hours, disturbance of sleep, incoherent speech, level of psychomotor activity, and fluctuation of symptoms. Each item is evaluated through direct questions to the patients or judged by the interviewer. By consensus, it has been indicated that the diagnosis of delirium can be made if at least one of three critical items (i.e. disorientation, perceptual disturbances, disturbance of consciousness during the past 24 hours) scores positive. When compared with clinical-rated interviews, however, sensitivity was high (90%), while specificity was lower (80%). Inter-rater reliability showed kappa-levels ranging from 0.90 to 0.93 for detecting one critical item. Although the DSI may be useful in epidemiological circumstances as trained lay interviewers can administer it, it is not easy to administer to severely ill patients who are unable to respond to questions (Trzepacz 1994b).

Delirium Writing Test

The Delirium Writing Test (DWT; Aakerlund and Rosenberg 1994), has been used in a study of patients who underwent thoracotomy for lung cancer, with the rationale that writing ability was impaired in patients who developed delirium in comparison with patients who did not develop delirium. It consists in examining certain features, namely reluctance to write, motor impairment because of tremor, clumsiness, and migrographia, and spatial disorders in writing, syntactical disorders, and spelling disorders, which were impaired in delirious patients (see Chapter 4 for more clinical detail). The authors indicate a high specificity/sensitivity of the instrument in detecting delirium in postoperative patients.

The usefulness of methods that assess dysgraphia in delirious patients has been confirmed in palliative care (Macleod and Whitehead 1997), while a recent study in psychiatry indicated the role of dysgraphia and constructional apraxia as having predictive diagnostic value (Baranowski and Patten 2000), and although sensitivity was low (33%), specificity was quite high (98%); see also Chapter 4.

Delirium Observation Screening

The Delirium Observation Screening (DOS) is a 25-item scale rated on a 5-point Likert scale developed to facilitate early recognition of delirium, according to the DSM-IV and based on nurses' observations during regular care. Internal consistency, predictive validity, and concurrent and construct validity were tested in two prospective studies with geriatric medicine patients and elderly hip fracture patients. The DOS showed high internal consistency (Cronbach's alpha = 0.93–0.96) with a good predictive validity against the DSM-IV. Concurrent validity, as tested by comparing the DOS with the CAM, was 0.63 ($p \leq 0.001$). The overall conclusion of these studies is that the DOS scale shows satisfactory validity and reliability, to guide early recognition of delirium by nurses' observation. The scale can be reduced to 13 items that can be rated as present or absent in less than 5 minutes. A score of 0 is defined as 'normal behaviour', meaning absence of behavioural alterations. Three items (3, 8, and 9) are reverse-scored, i.e. 'normal behaviour' is rated as 'always'. The highest total score is 13 with a cut-off point of 3, indicating delirium.

NEECHAM Confusion Scale

The NEECHAM Confusion Scale (Neelon et al. 1996) is a 9-item scale divided into three subscales investigating information processing (score range 0–14 points; attention and alertness, verbal and motor response, and memory and orientation), behaviour (score range 0–10 points; general appearance and posture, sensory-motor performance, and verbal responses), and performance (score range 0–16 points; vital signs, oxygen saturation level, and urinary incontinence). The total score is the sum of the scores on the three levels. The scale can be rated in 10 minutes on the basis of observations and measurements of vital signs. The scores may range from 0 (minimal function) to 30 (normal function) with a cut-off point of 24 (range from 0–24 indicates delirium). Several studies have examined the usefulness of the NEECHAM Confusion Scale, showing its ability to identify delirium in different contexts (Gemrt and Schuurmans 2007; Hattori et al. 2009; Immers et al. 2005; Matsushita et al. 2004). Recently, a study comparing the scale with the CAM-ICU indicated good levels of sensitivity (87%) and specificity (95%) with positive and negative predictive values of 79 and 97%, respectively (Van Rompaey et al. 2008).

Nursing Delirium Screening Scale (Appendix 5)

The Nursing Delirium Screening Scale (Nu-DESC; Gaudreau et al. 2005b) is a 5-item scale consisting of the 4 items of the Confusion Rating Scale (CRS) and one item rating unusual psychomotor retardation, taking into account medical condition (delayed responsiveness and few or no spontaneous actions/words; for example, when the patient is prodded, reaction is deferred and/or the patient is unarousable). Each items is rated from 0 to 2 based on the presence and intensity of each symptom, and the individual ratings are added to obtain a total score (maximum score = 10). In a study of 146 consecutive hospitalized patients assessed for delirium symptoms by bedside nurses, the Nu-DESC was found to be a valid instrument in comparison with the CAM and the MDAS in patients receiving a DSM-IV diagnosis of delirium ($n = 59$), with a sensitivity and specificity of 85.7 and 86.8%, respectively.

Communication Capacity Scale and Agitation Distress Scale

The Communication Capacity Scale (CS) and the Agitation Distress Scale (ASD) are two operational observer-rating scales that have been recently developed by

Morita et al. (2001) specifically for evaluating terminal delirium. The authors have conducted a study in a palliative care setting in order to quantify patients' communication capacity and agitated behaviour in terminal delirium. They used, along with the CS and the ASD, the DRS and the MDAS on 30 terminally ill cancer patients with delirium. Both the CS and the ASD achieved high internal consistency (Cronbach's alpha = 0.91 and 0.96, respectively) and inter-rater reliability (Cohen's kappa values on each item ranged 0.72–1.00). The principal components analysis resulted in the emergence of only one component for each scale. The CS total score was associated with the MDAS ($r = 0.78$), and cognitive items from the MDAS and DRS ($r = 0.83$). The ADS total score was significantly correlated with the DRS ($r = 0.61$) and agitation items from the MDAS and DRS ($r = 0.61$).

Intensive Care Delirium Screening Checklist

The Intensive Care Delirium Screening Checklist (ICDSC) is another instrument (Bergeron et al. 2001; Dubois et al. 2001) for assessing delirium in patients admitted to ICUs. The scale is completed by using information collected from the previous 24 hours. It consists of 8 items evaluating the following parameters: altered level of consciousness, inattention, disorientation, hallucination, psychomotor agitation or retardation, inappropriate speech or mood, sleep–wake cycle disturbance, and symptom fluctuation. For each abnormal item a score of 1 is given. The authors showed a sensitivity of 99% by using a cut-off score of 4 on the ICDSC. A recent study carried out on 71 patients with delirium showed that the kappa coefficient of agreement determined over 7 days of ICU stay was high (0.80; $p < 0.001$) between CAM-ICU and the ICDSC (Plaschke et al. 2008).

Other instruments

Other instruments have focused on assessing delirium severity to be able to repeat assessments in the short time and therefore to follow the clinical course of the syndrome. One of them is the Delirium Assessment Scale, which is based on observation of the patient, interview of staff or relatives, and the DSM III criteria (O'Keeffe 1994). Another tool is the Delirium Severity Scale, which is more focused on cognitive function assessment and consists of a modified version of cognitive tests such as the forward digit span and the similarities test from the Wechsler Adult Intelligence Scale and Wechsler Adult Memory Scale (Bettin et al. 1998). This scale showed sensitivity to change over a short period of time and in the authors' opinion has the advantage of not valuing anamnestic data for scoring as in the case of the DRS or MDAS (Bettin et al. 1998).

8.3 **Conclusions**

The diagnosis of delirium can be based on a variety of clinical procedures and of instruments, and can be aided by the use of different assessment tools. These tools respond in part to the desirable characteristics of instruments aimed at diagnosing and evaluating delirium (Roth-Romer et al. 1997), but in general, it is not advisable to use just one of them for both purposes at this time. Some instruments are clearly specifically designed for diagnosing the presence of delirium, whereas other instruments are used to describe symptoms and rate their severity. This distinction is not always so clear for some of the instruments described. For instance (see also appendices), it is clear that the assessment of delirium severity and clinical features is feasible with the DRS and the MDAS, and that others, such as the CAM and the DSI, are operational systems for making a diagnosis; others are screening instruments (ICDSC, NuDesc). Attempts to combine these two characteristics by using cut-off points over the severity scores provided by DRS and MDAS have been made but, in general, results were less than completely satisfactory (Breitbart et al. 1997; Grassi et al. 2001b; Rockwood et al. 1996). The NEECHAM confusion scale provided better results than the CAM-ICU (van Rompaey et al. 2008). Other authors have observed that, for instance, including the presence of a possible or definite precipitating physical disorder in a scale aimed at rating delirium severity may be inappropriate, if severity must be assessed on the basis of symptoms and signs (O'Keeffe 1994). In our opinion the diagnosis of delirium can be improved by a continual perfection of the application of diagnostic criteria but that clinical experience and decision should, however, be valued and incorporated in any diagnostic system. Severity scores will have fundamental importance in evaluation and screening procedures, if they are of a high enough sensitivity, but should not be a substitute for clinical diagnosis. The recent new version of the DRS is an attempt to combine in a single instrument a method for diagnosis and assessment. It is important to use this instrument to confirm the potential improvement that it represents.

The availability of different instruments is important to help clinicians and researchers to choose a method that is adequate for their specific requirements. However, the continuous proliferation of instruments for the diagnosis and assessment of delirium is not per se serving the purpose of perfecting homogeneous guidelines and of producing reproducible and comparable results across different international settings of care.

Chapter 9

Management[1]

9.1 Guidelines

The cornerstone of delirium management has varied little over the centuries, being identified with aetiological, environmental, nursing, and pharmacological interventions (Lipowski 1990b; Trzepacz and Meagher 2005). The area that has received most attention from modern medicine is drug therapy with the introduction in the fifties of major and minor tranquillizers (see below).

Quite interestingly pharmacological sedation has been considered helpful and necessary since the second century AD, when Areteus suggested the use of boiled poppy for this purpose (Adams 1861), whereas opium has been the most popular drug for this indication since the nineteenth century (Lipowski 1990b). Indeed the current use of opioids in critical care and anaesthesia confirms their fortunate historical background. Some authors still recently recommended opioid-based regimens as first-line therapy for agitated deliria (Adams 1988; Fernandez et al. 1989). This use is obsolete and more recently delirium has become regarded also as one of the potential toxic reactions to opioid pharmacotherapy.

With respect to some years ago, however, when management was largely empirical, attempts have been made by several agencies and institutions to produce guidelines for delirium. The American Psychiatric Association (APA) published the first guidelines in 1999 (American Psychiatric Association 1999), with few recent indications summarizing the important elements of the incremental progress in this area (Cook 2004) (Table 9.1 reports their general terms). The European Delirium Association (EDA) (http://www.europeandeliriumassociation.com) also created a training programme on delirium and delirium management, with clinical vignettes and aetiological, pharmacological, and non-pharmacological intervention, under the campaign Stop Delirium. The Royal College of Physicians and the British Geriatric Association published in 2006 national guidelines on delirium in older patients and in the same year the Royal College of Psychiatrists updated the Guidelines for the prevention, diagnosis, and management of delirium in older people in hospital. The same thing happened in Australia, under the commission of the Australian Health Ministers' Advisory Council (2006).

Specific recommendations for the management of patients with delirium at the end of their life were released by a consensus panel of the American Society of Internal

---

[1] Maria Giulia Nanni, MD, Section of Psychiatry, Department of Medical Disciplines of Communication and Behaviour, University of Ferrara, Italy, has contributed to the writing of this chapter.

Table 9.1 Coordinate with other physicians caring for the patient

Identify the aetiology

Initiate intervention for acute conditions

Provide other disorder-specific treatment

Monitor and ensure safety

Assess and monitor psychiatric status

Assess individual and family psychological and social characteristics

Establish and maintain alliances

Educate patient and family regarding the illness

Provide post-delirium management

Medicine (Casarett and Inouye 2001) and useful guidelines were published by the Canadian Coalition for Senior Mental Health in 2006 (Canadian Coalition 2006). It is possible that some guidelines are, however, not recognized by the health system, as indicated in the survey carried out by Leentjens and Diefenbacher (2006). In fact, the authors found that among the European Association for Consultation-Liaison Psychiatry and Psychosomatics in twelve European countries only two (i.e. the Dutch Psychiatric Association and the German Association of Scientific Medical Societies) seemed to report having national delirium guidelines. Specific guidelines exist for delirium tremens (DT; Mayo-Smith et al. 1997, 2004). In this indication the use of benzodiazepines alone or in combination with other drugs is first choice.

Some systematic reviews on the use of antipsychotics (Lacasse et al. 2006; Lonergan et al. 2007; Seitz et al. 2007) and specifically on the management of advanced patients (Jackson and Lipman 2004) are also available. Controlled clinical trials, are, however, lacking and most recommendations are clinical-experience-based rather than evidence-based (Britton and Russell 2000; Cole et al. 1998; Meagher 2001). In the cases with an underlying acute event that may allow for at least temporary recovery, management should consider supportive therapies for maintaining vital functions and treat complications.

Ethical aspects are also raised in the field of management of delirium. A potentially difficult question may arise when informed consent or patient competence is required for any reason (Auerswald et al. 1997). The response for these types of requests has been discussed only to a limited extent in the literature and may deserve more attention on ethical or medico-legal grounds.

9.2 Identify the cause and other aetiologically oriented interventions

9.2.1 Aetiological and general interventions

As already iterated in Chapters 6–8 the identification of a relevant aetiology should be part of any rational approach, even when potentially no action can be considered appropriate for removing the cause. Reversible causes, on the other hand, can be found in any population and can be potentially corrected (de Stoutz et al. 1995; Fainsinger et al. 1993; Grassi et al. 2001a; Lawlor et al. 2000b, Leonard et al. 2008).

General principles of management in emergency medicine suggest providing treatment for potential acute biochemical abnormality (such as hypoglicaemia), drug intoxication, and vitamin B1 deficiency, factors that may be relatively rare in the palliative care setting or difficult to correct, as in the case of the toxicity of an opioid drug otherwise needed for pain control.

9.2.2 Hydration and opioid toxicity

Recommendations based on the clinical experience of palliative medicine specialists and on systematic observation, but not on totally satisfying scientific evidence criteria, suggest that, besides all other procedures already reviewed in several parts of this book, moderate hydration is beneficial in dehydrated palliative care patients with complex pharmacological regimes for reducing the likelihood of accumulation of toxic drug or metabolites levels (Bruera et al. 1995, 2005).

In case of opioid toxicity several observations support the use of switching from one opioid to another one to obtain a more favourable balance between analgesia and side effects. The practice of switching (or 'rotating') opioids seemed useful in solving opioid-related delirium in several case series. It is our opinion that the most useful switching attempts imply changing from morphine or hydromorphone to methadone, fentanyl, or oxycodone (Cherny et al. 2001; Gagnon et al. 1999; Maddocks et al. 1996). Only one study prospectively described a series of 20 cases for whom switching from morphine to fentanyl was systematically used to try to reverse opioid-induced delirium (Morita et al. 2005). Although the dosages of oral morphine inducing delirium were unusually low in this study (64 ± 45 mg/day) the authors found an improvement in delirium severity in almost all patients after switching to transdermal or parenteral fentanyl.

9.3 Pharmacological management

Agitated delirium can be dangerous for the patient and the caregivers, and is a difficult experience for the family. A pharmacological symptomatic intervention is certainly justified. To implement an efficacious treatment regimen, continuous monitoring and frequent assessment are necessary as an integral part of treatment. Systematic recording of the patient mental status can be facilitated by using one of the assessment tools described in Chapter 8 and is needed to account for fluctuations, partial recovery, and to reduce the impact of differing views among staff members and family, which may jeopardize therapeutic outcome. The aim of pharmacological management is to calm the patient, avoid dangerous behaviours, and control hallucinations and delusions that can have subjective negative contents, while allowing for aetiological and supportive therapies that can contribute to delirium resolution in the reversible cases. At times this aim can be obtained by relatively simple drug regimens, but more intensive approaches, such as sedation or physical restraint in cases unresponsive to therapy, may be required.

Keeping in mind that better outcomes are related to pre-morbid general conditions (Cole et al. 1998), in the cases associated with multiple medical problems and unfavourable prognosis, the aims of therapy are at least in part the same. In the palliative care of this particular condition special attention should be paid to the assessment of symptoms unrelated to the altered mental state but concurrent with it (Bruera et al. 1992a), and to the benefit of improving the level of consciousness and awareness, which is always based on a case-by-case individual decision, where knowledge of the patient's wishes should have an important role (Morita et al. 2000). Another related, but complicated issue is whether quiet somnolent patients suffering from hypoactive deliria would need or benefit from treatment at all (Platt et al. 1994; Stiefel and Bruera 1991). Conversely, the therapeutic recourse to sedation to control delirium and related suffering is often specific to the clinical situation of the terminal patient although the frequency of this need varies across the experiences of different palliative care specialists (Fainsinger et al. 2000a, b). For the treatment of delirium the published guidelines indicate the necessary steps and drugs to use, of which neuroleptics, or antipsychotics, have a major role (Lonergan et al. 2007; Seitz et al. 2007). Other drugs have also been proposed as adjuvant pharmacological treatment both for the possible side effects of neuroleptics for rapid tranquillization and for the need for other options of treatment in specific forms of delirium (e.g. DT; Bourne et al. 2008; Grace and Holmes 2006; Grassi and Antonelli 2009; McAllister-Williams and Ferrier 2002).

9.3.1 Classic Neuroleptics or Conventional Antipsychotics

Neuroleptics are a broad class of different drugs discovered almost fifty years ago (chlorpromazine in 1950 and haloperidol in the following years), which are characterized by a potent antipsychotic action and, for that reason, routinely used in psychiatry and in medicine to treat psychotic symptoms present in several disorders (schizophrenia, affective disorders with psychotic features, and psychotic symptoms in organic mental disorders, such as dementia and delirium; Marder 1998). This class of drugs consists of several subclasses, namely phenothiazines (e.g. chlorpromazine, thioridazine, fluphenazine), tioxanthenes (e.g. tiothixene, flupentixol), butyrophenones (e.g. haloperidol, droperidol) and dibenzoxazepines (e.g. loxapine). Known as conventional or typical antipsychotics (to be distinguished from the most recent atypical antipsychotics–see next paragraph), all these drugs share the property of blocking dopaminergic D_2 activity in different areas of the central nervous system (CNS). This action exerted in the mesolimbic pathway results in a block of positive psychotic symptoms (hallucinations, delusions), while the same action in other areas are responsible for significant side effects. More specifically, blockade of dopamine receptors in the nigrostriatal pathway results in extrapyramidal symptoms (EPS; Parkinsonism after pure block, or dyskinesia as a consequent up-regulation of the system); blockade in the mesocortical pathway produces blunting of emotions and cognitive symptoms (known as negative symptoms); blockade in the tuberoinfundibular pathway determines increase in prolactin secretion. Conventional antipsychotics have also blockade properties of muscarinic receptors, resulting in generalized anticholinergic symptoms (e.g. blurred vision, dry mouth, constipation) of histamine H_1 receptors, with the onset of drowsiness and weight gain, and of noradrenergic α_1 receptors, which are responsible for orthostatic hypotension, drowsiness, and dizziness.

The use of antipsychotics in delirium is well established and constantly reported in all the guidelines mentioned, with the aim of both reducing psychotic symptoms, ameliorating the cognitive filter, and improving sleep. Sedation in case of aggressive behaviour or agitation can also be an important effect of the use of antipsychotics. However, sedation is more appropriately described as a side effect of neuroleptics and can be avoided, when not necessary, by an accurate individualization of drug choice and dosage. It is not always the case, however, and the tranquillization or control of some cases of delirium and suffering can only be achieved through significant sedation.

Haloperidol

Haloperidol is pharmacologically a butyrophenone with etherocyclic structure. The use of haloperidol and neuroleptics in general to control delirium is supported by pharmacological rationale and by clinical experience. One controlled clinical trial (Breitbart et al. 1996) confirmed these empirical and theoretical assumptions by demonstrating that while haloperidol and chlorpromazine were associated with the improvement of delirium symptoms, lorazepam worsened clinical symptoms. In a randomized controlled trial on the prophylaxis of postoperative delirium it was demonstrated that haloperidol reduced severity and duration of delirium in comparison with placebo; this is the only available, albeit indirect, evidence of the efficacy of haloperidol against placebo for delirium (Kalisvaart et al. 2005).

Haloperidol has long been considered the first-line drug for this indication with the exception of alcohol and benzodiazepine withdrawal delirium, because of its fewer vasomotor, cardiac, and central side effects in respect to all the other potentially useful drugs (see Table 9.2). It is worth noting that haloperidol has been considered the drug of choice even in liver transplant patients for its favourable profile of side effects (Trzepacz et al. 1993). It is still one of the most frequently used antipsychotics in delirium, even though risperidone seems to be replacing haloperidol as the drug of choice (Briskman et al. 2010) (see the later section on risperidone).

Table 9.2 Different profile of side effects among several neuroleptics

Drug	Sedative	Hypotensive	Extrapyramidal	Anticholinergic
Haloperidol	+	+	+ + + +	+
Droperidol	+ +	+ +	+ + + +	+ +
Methotrimeprazine	+ + + +	+ + +	+ +	+ + +
Promazine	+ +	+ +	+	+ +
Chlorpromazine	+ + +	+ + +	+ +	+ + +
Clozapine	+ + + +	+	-	+ + +
Olanzapine	+ +	-	-	+ +
Risperidone	+ +	+ + +	+	+

Haloperidol has 60% bioavailability after oral administration and is metabolized by liver oxidative dealkylation. Absorption via the oral route is slow with plasma levels detectable after 60 to 90 minutes and peak levels not earlier than 4 hours. Intramuscular administration leads to peak plasma levels in 20–40 minutes, while, after IV injection, the action is rapid–within minutes–and concentration decay is rapid as well–within 1 hour in the distribution phase (Forsman and Ohman 1977; Settle and Ayd 1983). Its half-life ranges from 12 to 36 hours, leading to sustained plasma levels long after repeated administration is discontinued.

Guidelines on haloperidol dosing in cases of agitated delirium are variable. Lipowski (1990b) suggests the use of oral administrations of 5–10 mg in the morning and at bedtime in mild to moderate cases, and IM injections of 5–10 mg every 30–60 minutes until tranquillization is achieved in severe cases. IM injections should be followed by oral maintenance doses equal to 1.5–2 times the parenteral dose. These guidelines apply to young patients without liver disease; in the elderly, aged 60 or older, dosing for rapid tranquillization should start with 0.5 mg IM every hour.

APA guidelines are not very detailed about dosing. For acute parenteral treatment, it is suggested to administer 1–2 mg, for younger patients, and 0.25–0.5 mg, for elderly patients, repeated every 2–4 hours as needed. Usual doses, independent of route of administration, are 0.5–1 mg for mild, 2–5 mg for moderate, and 5–10 mg for severe delirium with agitation. The dose should not be repeated before 30 minutes has elapsed, until the clinical effect is achieved (Wise et al. 1999; Wise and Trzepacz 1996).

While the intravenous use of haloperidol is not approved in the UK and USA, consensus exists on the usefulness and safety (e.g. lower incidence of EPS) of this type of administration for the severe cases and in critically ill patients (Ayd 1987; Gelfand et al. 1992; Shapiro et al. 1995). Typical doses are reported to be 2–5 mg every 20–30 minutes until the clinical effect is reached (Gelfand et al. 1992).

Published experiences can help in choosing the initial dose and titration regimen. One study on the emergency control of agitated disruptive behaviour due mostly to alcohol intoxication and head trauma found that mean doses of 8.2 ± 4.5 mg given as 1.4 ± 0.75 IM doses per patient controlled agitation in 113 over 136 patients (Clinton et al. 1987).

In critical patients, very high doses of IV haloperidol have been used successfully to control agitation, from more than 100 to 1000 mg in 24 hours (Levenson 1995; Riker et al. 1994; Wilt et al. 1993).

Lower doses have been reported in two other cases of hyperactive delirium treated with IV infusion, one starting off with 6 mg/h, lowered after a few hours to 3 mg/h and the second with 2 mg/h infusion (Dixon and Craven 1993).

A retrospective case series of delirious patients seen at a comprehensive cancer centre found that in 54 cases of hyperactive delirium, haloperidol doses employed were low in 61% of cases (mean = 2.5 mg/24 h), intermediate in 32% (mean = 15 mg/24 h), and high in 7% (mean = 30 mg/24 h) (Olofson et al. 1996).

Another study in the cancer patient population applied prospectively a 6-hour every-half-hour titration schedule (Table 9.3) using IM, IV, or oral haloperidol in 10 consecutive patients. The mean ± SD dose of haloperidol on the first day was 6 ± 4.0 mg (range 0.5–11 mg) and the mean daily dose over the whole follow-up

Table 9.3 Haloperidol 30-minute titration schedule

Time	Haloperidol IV or IM dose (mg)
1	0.5
2	0.5
3	0.5
4	1
5	1
6	1
7	2
8	2
9	2
10	5
11	5
12	5

This schedule is given as a published example of titration, understanding that it should be applied with specific judgement to individual cases. Doses are repeated every 30 minutes according to clinical effects and increased every three doses if clinical effect requires it.
Modified from Akechi et al. (1996) with kind permission from Springer Science+Business Media

period until recovery was 5.4 ± 3.4 mg (range 0.5–10.5 mg). The dose needed on the first day of treatment was significantly related to the following average daily dose (Akechi et al. 1996). The most important general rule is that without dose titration and individualization to patient response, many cases are going to result in therapy failures.

These doses are profoundly different from the doses reached in another report on terminally ill AIDS patients, using a combined protocol of IV haloperidol and lorazepam with an average daily dose of haloperidol of 42 mg and lorazepam 7.5 mg (Fernandez et al. 1989).

It is important to recall that haloperidol may be insufficient for controlling symptoms of delirium. In one case series of consecutive patients with delirium and advanced cancer, only 60% could be managed by haloperidol alone–the others required various combinations of other neuroleptics (chlorpromazine, methotrimeprazine) or benzodiazepines (lorazepam, midazolam). In 26% of cases symptom control could be achieved only by sedation, which was implemented with midazolam (Stiefel et al. 1992), confirming the experience of several case reports (Fainsinger and Bruera 1992).

In a retrospective series of 99 cancer inpatients with reversible delirium haloperidol was given in 72% of cases and the daily haloperidol equivalent dose for all patients was 2.5 mg (Q1-Q3 = 1–4.7) (Hui et al. 2010). As already mentioned in Chapter 6, haloperidol is also classified as a drug with high potential for metabolic interaction with many other drugs commonly used in palliative care (Bernard and Bruera 2000).

Droperidol

Droperidol is related to haloperidol but it is available only for IM or IV use, and usually limited to hospital use. It has a short half-life (2–3 hours) and is usually reserved for anaesthesiological or intensive care use. It differs from haloperidol in its more rapid, potent, and sedative effects. It also has strong α_1-adrenergic blocking activity that justifies significant hypotensive effects. Dosages of 5 to 15 mg can be used and repeated every 4 to 6 hours if necessary (van Leeuwen et al. 1977), but bolus injections are often followed by hypotension especially in critically ill patients (Frye et al. 1995). Two controlled clinical trials compared haloperidol with droperidol for the treatment of agitation. One study compared 5 mg IM double-blind injections of haloperidol or droperidol in 27 agitated patients and found that after 30 minutes 81% of the patients treated with haloperidol needed another injection compared to only 36% of the patients treated with droperidol (Resnick and Burton 1984). In another study 5 mg of IM or IV droperidol were compared with the same dosage of haloperidol to control agitation and combativeness in patients admitted to an emergency room and requiring physical restraint (Thomas et al. 1992). Droperidol was more rapid in controlling agitation within 30 minutes from administration. There are no official results available on the use of droperidol in patients with a diagnosis of delirium in palliative care. In a report of three intensive care unit cases, a continuous IV infusion of 1, 8, and 20 mg/h caused a mean increase of QTc interval of 17% (Frye et al. 1995).

For these reasons and the risk of possible death (Haines et al. 2001) droperidol has been withdrawn from some countries and caution has been recommended in its use.

Chlorpromazine

The prototypical phenothiazine and the first neuroleptic medication to be discovered, available for oral and parenteral administration subcutaneous (SC) use, is not recommended because it is an irritant. It has a half-life ranging from 16 to 30 hours. An oral dose of 100 mg is equivalent to 25–50 mg parenterally (oral bioavailability is 32 ± 19% and decreases after repeated administrations, mean half-life is 30 hours) and to 2–5 mg of parenteral haloperidol. As well as thioridazine it has strong α_1-adrenergic blocking activity, which justifies the frequency of orthostatic hypotension and cardiovascular effects; for this reasons its use is not recommended, especially in the elderly, frail and medically ill patients. Chlorpromazine has been used at times in advanced cancer patients for its more potent sedative effects (Stiefel et al. 1992). Phenothiazines have been implicated in exacerbating symptoms of restlessness and myoclonus in dying patients treated with high-dose opioids (Dunlop 1989; Potter et al. 1989). Phenothiazines indeed lower the threshold for epileptic discharges. Chlorpromazine is sometimes indicated in this setting to control dyspnoea or other more rare symptoms such as hiccup (De Conno et al. 1991b).

Methotrimeprazine

This drug gained some popularity in palliative care because of its analgesic (Beaver et al. 1966; Green B et al. 2004; Lasagna and DeKornfeld 1961) and potent antiemetic properties, suggesting its use in situations such as pain unrelieved by opioids or bowel obstruction (Baines 1993). Half-life is 16 to 78 hours. It is available as a parenteral preparation in the US and UK (the oral preparation is available in Italy only). It has a powerful sedating effect and can be used for this purpose in treating otherwise unresponsive agitation or severely insomniac patients (Stiefel et al. 1992). In a review it was the preferred drug for sedation together with chlorpromazine after midazolam (Cowan and Walsh 2001).

9.3.2 Atypical Antipsychotics

Atypical antipsychotics represent a class of new drugs characterized by a specific pharmacological property of serotonin$_{2A}$-dopamine$_2$ ($5HT_{2A}/D_2$) antagonism, which is absent among conventional antipsychotics. This property has significant clinical effects, mainly little or no propensity to cause EPS, reduced capacity to elevate prolactin levels, and reduction of negative symptoms of schizophrenia (Owens and Riscj 1998; Stahl 2000). However, the receptor binding profiles of the atypical antipsychotics vary consistently, with some (e.g. clozapine, olanzapine) interacting with multiple receptors, including noradrenergic (α_1 blockade), cholinergic (muscarinic blockade), histaminergic (antihistamine property), and serotoninergic ($5HT_{2C}$, $5HT_3$, $5HT_6$, besides $5HT_{2A}$), and others (e.g. risperidone, ziprasidone), with a predominant $5HT_{2A}$ selectivity (Goldstein 2000). The use of atypical antipsychotics in palliative care is now supported by a series of studies, including those carried out on delirious patients (Boettger and Breitbart 2005).

Clozapine

Clozapine is the first atypical antipsychotic drug synthesized in the mid-1960s and used from the early 1970s. Its use was discontinued in many countries because of its side effects (i.e. agranulocytosis), then re-evaluated and used in clinical practice. Its property of $5HT_{2A}/D_2$ antagonism at limbic than at striatal dopamine receptors explains the relative freedom from EPS. Clozapine is also an antagonist at adrenergic, cholinergic, histaminergic, and serotonergic receptors. Following a dosage of 100 mg b.i.d., the average steady-state peak plasma concentration occurs after about 2.5 hours (range: 1–6 hours). Clozapine is almost completely metabolized prior to excretion to inactive components or desmethyl metabolite, which has only limited activity. The mean elimination half-life of clozapine after a single 75mg dose is 8 hours (range: 4–12 hours). It is used mainly in psychiatry for the treatment of refractory schizophrenia. It has significant sedative properties that justify its use in treating aggressive and agitated patients and as a sleep adjuvant drug in patients with Parkinson's disease manifesting agitation, insomnia, or symptoms of delirium. Available in doses of 25 and 100 mg oral tablets in the elderly it is better to start with the initial dose of a quarter of the 25 mg tablet. Its adverse cardiovascular effects (orthostatic hypotension, tachycardia, ECG repolarization changes), the possible onset of seizures, and, especially, the occurrence of clozapine-induced agranulocytosis (1–2%) limit the use of clozapine in patients with severe medical illness, especially if concomitant drugs are employed (e.g. chemotherapy). Furthermore, the relevant anticholinergic effects justify the observation of delirium favoured by clozapine administration (van der Molen-Eijgenraam et al. 2001; Wilkins-Ho and Hollander 1997).

Olanzapine

Olanzapine is related structurally to clozapine with high affinity binding to the serotonin $5HT_{2A/2C}$, dopamine D_{1-4}, muscarinic M_{1-5}, histamine H_1, and α_1-adrenergic receptors. Antagonism of M_{1-5} receptors may explain its anticholinergic effects; antagonism of H_1 and α_1 receptors may explain the somnolence and orthostatic hypotension, respectively, observed with this drug. Olanzapine is well absorbed after oral administration and reaches peak concentrations in about 6 hours. It is eliminated extensively by first-pass metabolism, with approximately 40% of the dose metabolized before reaching the systemic circulation. Its half-life ranges from 21 to54 hours.

Olanzapine has been reported to be useful in delirium in a series of anecdotal cases (Passik and Cooper 1999; Sipahimalani and Masand 1998). Its mean half-life is 30 hours. Also devoid of EPS, it is much less likely than clozapine to decrease white blood cell counts. In a non-randomized comparison study of 22 patients, 11 treated with olanzapine and 11 with haloperidol for delirium of several aetiologies, the mean oral haloperidol dose was 5.1 ± 3.5 (SD) mg/day and the mean daily olanzapine dose was 8.2 ± 3.4 mg. Olanzapine was started at 5 mg qhs (*quaque hora somni*, before going to sleep) and titrated upwards as needed, the highest dose used being 15 mg/day. Patients tolerated olanzapine better than haloperidol; no side effect were seen with olanzapine while three patients had EPS and two had excessive sedation with haloperidol (Sipahimalani and Masand 1998). Efficacy was assessed with the Delirium Rating Scale (DRS) and was similar between the two treatments. Olanzapine was also useful for treating a complicated case of delirium due to the combined toxicity of many drugs including opioids and prochloperazine, in a patient with non-Hodgkin's lymphoma and secondary leukaemia. Delirium was not controlled with haloperidol and lorazepam and extrapyramidal symptoms were relevant. Olanzapine was given at 5 mg qhs in the early evening and increased to 10 mg with 2.5 mg as needed doses available during the day (Passik and Cooper 1999).

In an open, prospective trial of olanzapine for the treatment of delirium, Breitbart et al. (2002b) showed that out of 79 delirious patients, 57 (76%) had complete resolution of their delirium, with no patients experiencing EPS. A series of factors, including age >70 years, history of dementia, CNS spread of cancer and hypoxia as delirium aetiologies, 'hypoactive' delirium, and delirium of 'severe' intensity (i.e. Memorial Delirium Assessment Scale (MDAS) > 23), were associated with poorer response to olanzapine treatment for delirium.

Olanzapine is also available as a parenteral preparation and gave good results in the management of agitated demented patients when compared with lorazepam (Karena et al. 2002). It could be an interesting alternative for rapid tranquillization in case its efficacy and safety profile compared favourably with the standard treatment with haloperidol. In a randomized study of delirious critical care patients (Skrobik et al. 2004) the enteral use of olanzapine showed to be as efficacious as haloperidol, with less EPS.

Risperidone

Risperidone is an atypical antipsychotic ($5HT_{2A}/D_2$ antagonism) with high affinity for α_1- and α_2-adrenergic, and H_1 histaminergic receptors and a low-to-moderate affinity for the $5HT_{1C}$, $5HT_{1D}$, and $5HT_{1A}$ receptors, weak affinity for the D_1 receptor, and no affinity for cholinergic muscarinic or β_1-and β_2-adrenergic receptors. Risperidone is well absorbed after oral administration and it is extensively metabolized in the liver to a major active metabolite (9-hydroxy-risperidone), which is equi-effective with risperidone with respect to receptor-binding activity. Mean peak plasma concentrations occur at about 1 hour, while a peak of 9-hydroxyrisperidone occurs at about 3 hours (17 hours in poor metabolizers). The apparent half-life of risperidone is 3 hours in extensive metabolizers and 20 hours in poor metabolizers, while half-life of 9-hydroxyrisperidone is about 21 hours in extensive metabolizers and 30 hours in poor metabolizers. In clinical practice, it is widely accepted for treatment of agitation and aggression in elderly demented patients in doses ranging from 0.5 to 1.5–2 mg/day, and at low doses for a few cases of delirium (Ravona-Springer et al. 1998; Sipahimalani and Masand 1997). Doses of 3–4 mg/day can be reached. The existence of liquid formulation is important in clinical practice when the use of tablets is difficult. A pharmaco-epidemiological study estimated that risperidone can be associated with delirium in 1.6% of the cases (Zarate et al. 1997). In a double-blind comparative study of 28 patients with delirium, no difference was shown between haloperidol and risperidone over a 7-day period (Han and Kim, 2004). Similar results were reported by Mittal et al. (2004) and Parellada et al. (2004), who used low doses of risperidone (0.75–2.5 mg/day) to obtain a good response in almost all patients treated for delirium.

Quetiapine

Quetiapine is a new atypical antipsychotic with serotonin $5HT_{1A}$, $5HT_{2A}$, $5HT_6$, $5HT_7$, dopamine D_2, histamine H_1, and α_1 and α_2 noradrenergic blocker activity, without muscarinic properties. The antagonism of H_1 receptors may explain the somnolence observed with quetiapine, while antagonism of α_1-adrenergic receptors may explain the orthostatic hypotension secondary to its use. Rapidly and completely absorbed after oral administration, quetiapine reaches peak plasma concentrations in 1.5 hours and it is extensively metabolized by the liver, with metabolites that are pharmacologically inactive. Quetiapine's short half-life (3–6 hours) facilitates rapid discontinuation in case of adverse or negative effects. Attention should be paid to elderly patients in whom oral clearance is reduced by 40%. It is used in the treatment of delirium starting with low doses (e.g. 25 mg at night) and low increments according to clinical response (100–200 mg/day b.i.d. or t.i.d.). Recent preliminary clinical reports have indicated the efficacy and safety of quetiapine in treating delirium (Schwartz and Masand 2000; Torres et al. 2001). In a small open-label study, Sasaki et al. (2003) found that all patients with delirium treated with quetiapine ($n = 12$) achieved remission several days after starting quetiapine (4.8 ± 3.5 days) and that quetiapine was well tolerated, without onset of EPS. Similar results were reported by Kim et al. (2003) in 12 elderly patients with delirium treated with a dose of 93.75 ± 23.31 mg/day, and in a study of 24 inpatients with delirium (Pae et al. 2004).

More recently, in a randomized study of 36 intensive care unit (ICU) patients with delirium (Devlin et al. 2010), quetiapine (50 to 200 mg every 12 hours) was associated with a shorter time to first resolution of delirium, a reduced duration of delirium, and less agitation. Mortality (11% quetiapine vs 17% placebo) and ICU length of stay

(16 days quetiapine vs 16 days placebo) were similar, but subjects treated with quetiapine were more likely to be discharged home or to rehabilitation (89% quetiapine vs 56% placebo) and required fewer days of as-needed haloperidol.

Ziprasidone

Ziprasidone is a recent atypical antipsychotic with $5HT_{2A}/D_2$ blockade properties, associated with binding affinity for the D_3, $5HT2_A$, $5HT1_D$, and α_1-adrenergic receptors, and moderate affinity for the histamine H_1 receptor. It is also characterized by an agonism at the $5HT_{1A}$ receptor and a 5-HT and norepinephrine (noradrenaline) reuptake blockade, which justifies its anxiolytic and antidepressant properties. Antagonism at H_1 and α_1-adrenergic receptors is responsible for the somnolence and orthostatic hypotension side effects. Ziprasidone is rapidly absorbed by oral administration (peak plasma concentrations in 6 to 8 hours) and its bioavailability is increased up to twofold by food. Half-life of the drug is estimated to be 7 hours. The recent marketed IM formulation could be of help in several clinical situations, including palliative care, when oral administration is difficult or impossible. The dose for treatment of psychotic symptoms is in a range of 120–160 mg/day orally and 5–20 mg t.i.d. in IM injection. Ziprasidone has no EPS and little anticholinergic activity. A prolongation of QT interval has been reported, which suggests caution in its use in clinical practice, particularly in the elderly, patients using other drugs, and severely physically ill patients. Somnolence and dizziness are further side effects of ziprasidone. There are some case reports regarding the use of this drug in treating delirium. An oral dose of 100 mg/day (40 mg/20 mg/40 mg) was considered effective in a patient with cryptococcal meningitis and electrolytes abnormalities for whom risperidone was stopped due to EPS (Leso and Schwartz 2002). A further report showed the efficacy in the treatment of delirium in ICU by using IV ziprasidone (Young and Lujan 2004).

Amisulpride

Amisulpride is also considered an antipsychotic with atypical properties, showing antagonism at D_2 and D_3 receptor level at standard doses (200–1200 mg), while at low doses (40–200 mg) the drug blocks the inhibitory pre-synaptic autoreceptors, facilitating the dopaminergic transmission. A further action is represented by the activation of the gamma-hydroxybutyrate receptor and consequently the inhibition of dopamine release. In patients with delirium, Lee KU et al. (2005) provided preliminary data on the effectiveness and tolerability of amisulpride (16 subjects) versus quetiapine (15 subjects). The mean daily dose was 156.4 mg/day for amisulpride and 113 mg/day for quetiapine. After treatment, DRS-R-98 scores were significantly decreased from the baseline in both treatment groups ($p < 0.001$) without group difference. The mean duration of stabilization were 6.3 ± 4.4 days for the amisulpride group and 7.4 ± 4.1 days for the quetiapine group without group differences. There was no group difference in the mean quality of sleep score and the mean total sleep time. Both atypical antipsychotics were generally well tolerated. More recently, Pintor et al. (2009) showed significant improvement in the DRS score by using amisulpride (100-300 mg/day) in medically ill patients with delirium. Psychotic symptoms also improved from first day and cognitive status showed a significant improvement from day 2.

Aripiprazole

Aripiprazole is also a new drug that, unlike other atypical antipsychotics, has D_2 and 5-HT_{1A} partial agonist properties and like other atypical antipsychotics shows an antagonist profile at the 5-HT_{2A} receptor. In two case studies Alao et al. (2005) and Alao and Moskowitz (2006) used aripiprazole 15–30 g to treat delirium, showing an improvement of delirium in both the MMSE and DRS scores. In a report on 14 patients with delirium treated with aripiprazole, Straker et al. (2006) showed that 12 patients had a 50% reduction in DRS-R-98 scores, and 13 showed improvement on Clinical Global Impression Scale scores. The rate of adverse side effect was low, leading the authors to suggest that aripiprazole may be an appropriate first-line agent for the treatment of delirium because of its minimal effect on QTc interval, weight, lipids, and glucose levels.

Perospirone

Perospirone is an antipsychotic drug, developed in Japan, with dopamine D_2 antagonist and serotonin 5-HT_2 antagonist effects. It has been found to be significantly more effective against negative symptoms, and tended to be more effective against general symptoms and most positive symptoms at a dose of 8–48 mg/day compared with haloperidol 2–12 mg/day, and as affective as risperidone (De Paulis 2002). A recent study indicated that perospirone and risperidone are equally effective in the treatment of positive and negative symptoms of schizophrenia (Okugawa et al. 2009). Besides schizophrenia it is also used to treat psychotic and behavioural symptoms in dementia (Sato et al. 2006).

The effectiveness and safety of perospirone in patients with delirium was shown in a study carried out by Takeuchi et al. (2007) on a group of 38 patients with DSM-IV diagnosis of delirium. Perospirone was effective in 86.8% (33/38) of the cases, with the effect appearing within several days (5.1 ± 4.9 days). The initial dose was 6.5 ± 3.7 mg/day and maximum dosage of perospirone was 10.0 ± 5.3 mg/day. No serious adverse effects were reported, although increased fatigue (15.2%), sleepiness (6.1%), akathisia (3.0%), and a decline in blood pressure (3.0%) were observed.

9.3.3 Side effects of Neuroleptics

Interaction with other drugs and disease conditions are relevant in some cases (Bernard and Bruera 2000). Drug interactions are briefly described in Section 6.3 reviewing opioid toxicity. Potentially significant interactions can be envisaged, for instance, when using haloperidol, which inhibits the CYP 2D6 isoenzyme, in combination with codeine or oxycodone, which are metabolized to active compounds by CYP 2D6. This interaction may explain the case of patients not achieving significant analgesia notwithstanding incremental doses of oxycodone or codeine administered in combination with haloperidol (Gagnon et al. 1999). Also serotonin reuptake inhibitors and tricyclic antidepressants can interact with the metabolism of haloperidol. The role of drug interaction in modifying individual patient response increases as the number of drugs co-administered increases and is certainly complex. It is useful to remind that antidepressants (both TCAs and SSRIs), haloperidol, midazolam, opioids, steroids, anticonvulsants, some antibiotics and antifungals can have significant interactions (Bernard and Bruera 2000).

Side effects of neuroleptics are very similar. Differences between one drug and the next are more quantitative than qualitative and can be distinguished as having neurological side effect and non-neurological and toxic effects.

Neurological side effects

Involvement of the extrapyramidal system is the most significant problem with the use of conventional antipsychotics, especially high-potency ones (e.g. haloperidol). These effects are directly due to the primary antidopaminergic action at the nigrostriatal pathway. Acute dyskinesia or dystonic reaction can manifest as spasm of the buccofacial, neck, and back muscles, oculogyric crisis, and possible laryngeal spasm and can be relieved by benztropine mesylate or biperiden.

Akathisia is also an early and quite common reaction characterized by subjective need to move and often mistakenly interpreted as exacerbation of psychotic symptoms or anxiety. Lowering the dose of antipsychotics or using β-adreneric blocking drugs (e.g. propranolol) reduces the phenomenon. Parkinsonism is a gradual side effect that mimics Parkinson disease and is treated by re-equilibrating the acetylcholine–dopamine balance by administering anticholinergic drugs. However, both akathisia and parkinsonism are less problematic in short- to medium-term management of an acute episode of delirium and are less pronounced after parenteral haloperidol administration than after oral administration (Blitzstein and Brandt 1997; Menza et al. 1987). Other EPS, such as perioral tremor or 'rabbit syndrome' and tardive dyskinesias, are long-term consequences of antipsychotics that rarely apply to the palliative care patient.

The neuroleptic malignant syndrome (NMS) is a rare and life-threatening complication of antipsychotic drugs. It is characterized by catatonia, stupor, fever, autonomic instability, elevated levels of white cell count and creatinine phosphokinase, myoglobinuria, and delirium. It requires intensive care treatment. Administration of danthrolene and bromocriptine are considered beneficial.

Sedation is probably due to the anticholinergic effects of neuroleptics on muscarinic receptors. Phenothiazines are more sedating than haloperidol and also more often associated with paradoxical effects such as delirium itself. This is particularly true of thioridazine, clozapine (Szymanski et al. 1991; Wilkins-Ho and Hollander 1997), and olanzapine, but no drug is totally devoid of this risk (Tavcar and Dernovsek 1998).

The risk of seizures is more commonly associated with phenothiazines and is relevant especially in patients with other risks for seizure disorders, since the antipsychotics may lower the threshold for seizures. The use of phenothiazines in combination with opioids has been considered to explain the agitated delirious states with myoclonus seen by some palliative care specialists (Burke 1997).

Non-neurological side effects

Adrenergic side effects consist mainly of orthostatic hypotension and dizziness, due to α-adrenergic blockade. The least hypotensive drug is haloperidol (see Table 9.2). This effect is particularly important in cases with already compromised regulation of baroceptive reflexes, such as in the elderly and patients already on most antihypertensive medications.

Peripheral anticholinergic effects are a significant problem with many neuroleptics, especially low-potency conventional antipsychotics (e.g. chlorpromazine, thiori-dazine). Blockade of muscarinic activity causes blurred vision, dry mouth, constipation, decreased bronchial secretion, decreased sweating, difficulty in urination, and tachycardia. Dry mouth, which is often very bothersome in the presence of multiple symptoms and polypharmacy often characterizing palliative care, can at times be counteracted by the use of pilocarpine in sublingual drops (Mercadante 1998). Central side effects of anticholinergic properties of antipsychotics are represented by impairment in concentration attention and memory and, in the case of delirium, worsening of the symptoms of confusion. Anticholinergic delirium can be a consequence of excessive doses of neuroleptics with anti-muscarinic properties.

Apart from tachycardia, other cardiac effects should be considered. Arrhythmias and prolongation of the QT interval have been observed with oral and parenteral use of haloperidol with both high- and low-dose regimens (DiSalvo and O'Gara 1995; Jackson et al. 1997; Sharma et al. 1998; Wilt et al. 1993). Torsades des pointes have been seen in 4/1000 (Wilt et al. 1993) to 3.8% of patients receiving IV haloperidol and the relative risk increases with haloperidol doses ≥ 35 mg/day and with a QT interval ≥ 500 ms (Sharma et al. 1998). This should discourage the concurrent use of haloperidol with other drugs with similar effects of cardiac conductance and in patients with atrioventricular conduction blocks.

Sudden unexpected deaths have been reported with the use of other antipsychotics. However, torsade de pointes (TdP) and prolongation of the QTc interval have been related to death and sudden death in patients treated with these drugs, and extreme caution has been suggested when using haloperidol, droperidol, thioridazine, pimozide, and sertindole, which seem to be more frequently associated with possible cardiac toxicity and death (Glassman and Bigger 2001; Haddad and Anderson 2002).

Liver toxicity has been described frequently as an asymptomatic increase of liver enzymes. Severe toxicity has been associated mainly with phenothiazines. For this reason several authors would not recommend the use of haloperidol in hepatic encephalopathy delirium.

Ocular disorders can consist of pigmentary changes in the lens and retina, and in pigmentary retinopathy, especially after long-term treatment, which is not the case in the treatment of delirium.

Endocrine side effects deserve to be examined. Increased prolactine levels are related to dopamine receptor blockade at the tuberoinfundibolar pathway. Symptoms of hyperprolactinaemia (dysmenorrhoea, galactorrhoea, gynaecomastia, impotence) are quite frequent with conventional antipsychotics and risperidone, as well. The combination of endocrine, anticholinergic, and anti-adrenergic effects may also determine sexuality problems.

At the haematological level, blood dyscrasia and transient leukopenia have been reported while using antipsychotics, while the risk of agranulocytosis seems to be especially linked to clozapine use.

Dermatological side effects, consisting of rash and photosensitization, are possible consequences of antipsychotic use, mainly phenothiazines. If this is the case, the drug should be stopped and substituted with a structurally different antipsychotic.

Summarizing the studies relative to the use of conventional and atypical antipsychotics in delirium is, however, not an easy task. Although the literature regarding the side effects of conventional antipsychotics seems to favour atypical antipsychotics, recent reviews (Lacasse et al. 2006; Lonergan et al. 2007; Peritogiannnis et al. 2009; Rea et al. 2007) have indicated no difference between haloperidol in low dosage and atypical antipsychotics (e.g. olanzapine and risperidone) in terms of both efficacy and frequency of adverse drug effects in the treatment of delirium. Only high-dose haloperidol has been associated with a greater incidence of side effects, mainly parkinsonism, in comparison to atypical antipsychotics. More double-blind, randomized, placebo-controlled trials, however, are necessary in order to better evaluate the profile (efficacy and safety) of antipsychotic medication in the management of delirium (Boettger and Breitbart 2005; Campbell et al. 2009; Seitz et al. 2007).

9.3.4 Benzodiazepines and other drugs

Benzodiazepines

The role of benzodiazepine (BZD) in the management of delirium must be clearly defined. The idea that BZD would be beneficial in patients with delirium and severe physical illness with anxiety, insomnia, agitation, or excitement associated with hyperactive deliria is still frequent in medical settings. In contrast benzodiazepines are likely to impair cognition, can cause delirium (Pandharipande et al. 2006), especially in the elderly, and therefore are not recommended for delirium not due to alcohol withdrawal or similar clinical conditions. As already mentioned, BZD worsened the symptoms of delirium in the only randomized controlled study on this syndrome (Breitbart et al. 1996). They should therefore be considered second-line treatment when antipsychotics fail and when consciousness sedation is the aim of the therapy.

Important exceptions are delirium due to alcohol and benzodiazepine withdrawal, where BZD is the first-line treatment (Daeppen et al. 2002; Lonergan et al. 2009; Mayo-Smith et al. 1997, 2004; Newman et al. 1995). Usually lorazepam and chlordiazepoxide are the most commonly used in alcohol withdrawal delirium, although lorazepam seems to be safer (Kumar et al. 2009) and more efficacious if used according to clinical protocols (e.g. initial intermittent IV doses, progressing to a continuous IV infusion according to specific symptom scale) (De Carolis et al. 2007). Severe alcohol withdrawal syndrome, including DT (see Section 6.1), is considered an emergency and treatment has been based on old trials of paraldeide and diazepam (Mayo-Smith 1997, 2004). As reported recently drugs such as lorazepam, clonidine, and dexmedetomidine have become popular for treating severe delirium and adrenergic hyperactivity, and preventing seizures in DT. The doses of BZDs needed in these cases can be very high (from hundreds to thousands of diazepam milligrams per day) and treatment is usually given in ICU. Initial and less severe symptoms of alcohol withdrawal can be treated with lorazepam (8 mg/day) or chlordiazepoxide (80 mg/day) (Kumar et al. 2009).

Some authors would recommend BZD for patients with hepatic encephalopathy because of the risk of liver toxicity associated with the use of neuroleptics.

When BZDs are needed it is better to use those with a short half-life and no active metabolites. Lorazepam is our preferred drug. Half life is = 14 ± 5 hours. It has a very high oral availability and reaches peak concentrations 1 hour after oral and sublingual administration. Low doses can be used sublingually (1 mg) or orally (1–2.5 mg) and higher doses IV starting with 1 to 2 mg.

Midazolam has been employed mainly in the palliative care of advanced patients. It has the advantage of being well absorbed after SC administration. It has very fast onset of action and short elimination half-life 1.9 ± 0.6 hours and can be use also for short-term reversible sedation. Single IV doses can be used for induction of sedation and can be repeated after a short time. Prolonged sedation can be more difficult, requiring frequent dose adjustment after starting the infusion with 1 mg/h. Daily doses can range from 40 to 60 mg but higher doses are often administered as well (see below; Bottomley and Hanks 1990; Burke 1997; Burke et al. 1991; Stiefel et al. 1992).

Antihistamines

Antihistamine have sedative properties and for this reason, especially in the past, some authors would prefer hydroxyzine to aid sleep in patients with delirium (Lipowski 1990b) because of the lower potential of this drug for toxic reactions compared with BZD. Antihistamines all have anticholinergic effects and their use has been associated with delirium (Agostini et al. 2001; Garza et al. 2000). Therefore in our experience we limit their indication to cases for whom we want to emphasize sedation over other therapeutic options (see below).

Physostigmine

In anticholinergic delirium physostigmine can be used if anticholinergic toxicity is well proven and only with careful monitoring for the occurrence of side effect due to cholinergic hyperstimulation (Brown et al. 2004). Physostigmine salicylate (1 to 2 mg) should be given slowly IV or IM and repeated after 15 minutes. Contraindications to its use include a history of heart disease, asthma, diabetes, peptic ulcer, and bladder or bowel obstructions. It needs to be given cautiously to avoid seizures and cardiac arrhythmia. In a study on the treatment of proven anticholinergic intoxications physostigmine was superior to control agitation and to reverse delirium in comparison with BZD (Burns et al. 2000). Interestingly in this study BZDs were effective in controlling agitation in only 24% of cases (Burns et al. 2000).

Other drugs and miscellaneous case reports

The introduction of *cholinesterase inhibitors* for the treatment of dementia suggested their potential usefulness to ameliorate symptoms of delirium. Some clinical observations on the use of *donepezil* are interesting but preliminary (Fischer 2001; Kaufer et al. 1998; Slatkin et al. 2001; Wengel et al. 1998). These drugs act by making acetylcholine more available at CNS level. These observations therefore concur to suggest the relevance of acetylcholine transmission failure as one hypothesis in the pathogenesis of delirium. Their generalizability in the management of the syndrome is unknown and, as stated by Overshott et al. (2008), there is currently no specific evidence from controlled trials that donepezil is effective in the treatment of delirium. Two controlled trials evaluating rivastigmine and donepezil in the prevention of postoperative delirium gave negative results (Gamberini et al. 2009; Liptzin et al. 2005).

Mianserin, a second-generation antidepressant with antagonism to α_2-adrenergic presynaptic receptors (increase of noradrenergic activity), serotoninergic 5-HT$_{2A/2C}$ receptors (anxiolytic properties), and histaminic H$_1$ (sedative properties), has been reported to be effective in the treatment of symptoms of delirium in 62 consecutive elderly patients, 40% of whom suffered from pre-existing dementia. Mianserin at doses of 10 to 30 mg q.h.s. at night was effective for controlling behavioural symptom and, improving night-time sleep and hallucinations as measured by the DRS, but did not improve cognition (Uchiyama et al. 1996). The authors speculate that mianserin could exert a beneficial effect in delirious elderly patients by means of antihistamine (anti-H$_1$) and antiserotonergic (anti-5-HT$_2$) actions while devoid of the anticholinergic potential of traditional antihistamine drugs (Uchiyama et al. 1996).

Trazodone, an antidepressant drug blocking the postsynaptic serotonin (5-HT) receptors 5-HT$_{2A}$ and 5-HT$_{2C}$ and weakly inhibiting presynaptic 5-HT transporters, has been suggested as a possible drug for the further treatment of delirium not responding to neuroleptics (Okamoto et al. 1999). Because of the block of 5-HT$_2$ receptors, as with other atypical antipsychotics, the risk of extrapyramidal reactions present with conventional neuroleptics could be also an advantage for trazodone (Davis 2007).

Ondansetron (8 mg IV) has been used to treat postcardiotomy delirium in an open trial on 35 consecutive patients admitted to an ICU. As much as 80% of the patients are reported to have improved after treated with ondansentron (Bayindir et al. 2000). This observation may combine with studies advocating a role of the serotonergic system and amino acid metabolisms in postoperative delirium, but more controlled observations are needed (van der Mast et al. 2000).

One case report supported the use of *pimozide* in delirium due to hypercalcaemia not responding to conventional neuroleptic therapy (Mark et al. 1993), because of its high potency in blocking T-type Ca channels (Santamauro et al. 1994).

Carbamazepine was combined with buspirone in treating agitation associated with head trauma in a case report (Pourcher et al. 1994).

Dexmedetomidine, an α_2 receptors agonist, is a drug with sedative, analgesic, sympatholytic, and anxiolytic effects, without causing respiratory depression (Gerlach et al. 2009). In a pilot study, Raede et al. (2009) randomized 20 delirious patients to receive an infusion of either haloperidol 0.5–2 mg/h or dexmedetomidine 0.2–0.7 μg/kg/h, with or without loading doses of 2.5 mg haloperidol or 1 μg/kg dexmedetomidine, according to clinician preference. They found that dexmedetomidine significantly shortened median time to extubation and decreased ICU length of stay. Of patients who required ongoing propofol sedation, the proportion of time propofol required was halved in those who received dexmedetomidine. In contrast, three patients receiving haloperidol could not be successfully extubated and underwent tracheostomy and one prematurely discontinued haloperidol due to QTc interval prolongation. A reduced rate of delirium was found by using dexmedetomidine (3%) in comparison with propofol (50%) and midazolam (50%) in patients who underwent cardiac surgery (Maldonado et al. 2009).

Drugs used in hypoactive deliria

As already mentioned the pharmacological treatment of hypoactive deliria in palliative care has no straightforward answer. Some cases with clouded sensorium and somnolence, which may partially overlap with excessive sedation as a pharmacological side effect, may benefit from psychostimulant therapy (Gagnon et al 2005; Levenson 1992; Morita et al. 2000; Stiefel and Bruera 1991). Neuroleptic medication has been shown to improve delirium also in hypoactive cases (Platt et al. 1994). In our experience the patient with a moderate, quiet delirium who can still assume oral medication should have a trial with oral haloperidol. Advanced cases with irreversible causes of delirium and/or actively dying would suggest abstention from treatment. In some cases, as presented in Section 7.4, such as substance-induced delirium (namely fluoroquinolones), the possible mechanisms of inhibition of the binding of gamma-aminobutyric acid to its receptor sites suggest the use of BDZ as treatment of choice (Farrington et al. 1995; Unseld et al. 1990).

A relatively new drug *modafinil* with the primary indication for narcolepsy has been shown to improve vigilance in several other conditions (Holder et al. 2002; Nieves and Lang 2002). The mechanism of action of modafinil is different from the amphetamines' aspecifc activation of noradrenergic pathways. Modafinil should act at the level of the hypothalamic cells containing hypocretin implicated in the promotion of normal wakefulness (Scammell et al. 2000; see also Section 2.6). The potential use of modafinil in palliative care has been recently underlined (Cox and Pappagallo 2001). We used it successfully in two cases of encephalopathy with hypersomnia due to antineoplastic treatment toxicity and a randomized controlled trial confirmed its efficacy in improving cognitive performance in patients with advanced cancer (Lundorff et al. 2009).

9.4 Sedation

9.4.1 Definition

Palliative sedation is a term that appeared recently in the medical literature. There is now consensus (Cherny et al. 2009; de Graeff and Dean 2007) in using it in substitution of the older term, terminal delirium (Cowan and Walsh 2001; Fainsinger et al. 1998; Morita et al. 2001a).

9.4.2 Controversies—frequency and indications

A heated controversy took place years ago on the role of palliative sedation to control specific symptoms or complications characterizing the terminal phases of advanced illnesses, mainly focusing on the frequency of cases needing this type of intervention. One initial report by Ventafridda et al. (1990a) evaluated that in a home care programme, 52% of patients had symptoms that were controllable only by means of sedation in the last weeks of life (median survival 23 days). A total of 80 different symptom episodes (a patient could have more than one difficult symptom at a time) were treated with sedation; 11 episodes were due to delirium. The controversy was fuelled by a subsequent report by Fainsinger et al. (1991), who showed that, in a study conducted at a palliative care unit, in over 100 consecutive admissions the need to sedate patients with uncontrollable symptoms was reduced to 16%. The leading symptom requiring palliative sedation was delirium (10 patients out of 16). Several authors reported frequencies in between these extremes (16–52%; see Fainsinger et al. 1998 for a review), until a multicentre trial also failed to give a homogenous answer. In four geographically and culturally diverse centres of palliative care (three hospices and one hospital palliative care unit) the intent to sedate varied from 15 to 36%. Delirium was the main indication for sedation in 29% (Israel), 15% (Durban), 32% (Cape Town), and 60% (Madrid) of cases, respectively (Fainsinger et al. 2000b).

One prospective analysis of the home care programme from the same centre that produced the highest rate of recourse to palliative sedation showed that only 21% of patients needed sedation, at the end of life, in over 299 consecutive cases (De Conno et al. 1996; Groff 1993). Similar data were recently reported in a US experience; 12% of patients were sedated at home in the terminal phase and in 62% of them the cause for sedation was delirium (Alonso-Babarro et al. 2010).

A literature review found that over 328 cases of palliative sedation indications included agitation/restlessness in 26% of cases, confusion in 14%, and muscle twitching or myoclonus in 11% (Cowan and Walsh 2001).

In our experience the use of sedation in patients with very short prognosis was primarily indicated by the occurrence of agitated deliria in 19% of the cases that were sedated (Caraceni et al. 2002). The quality of the literature about palliative sedation has been improving in recent years; the cohort control study conducted by Maltoni and co-workers (2009) in Italy in a multicenter national setting showed in more than 500 patients that palliative sedation does not shorten life expectancy. In this study delirium was an indication for sedation in 78% of cases but the authors did not state when delirium was the only indication for sedation.

Guidelines for implementing sedation for 'refractory' symptoms have also been published with a specific definition of what should be considered a refractory symptom (Cherny 1994; Cherny et al. 2009; de Graeff and Dean 2007; Verkerk et al. 2007). This definition can be useful as an example of the complexities that we are facing when we would like to investigate the presence of refractory symptoms and potential therapeutic response to them in a way that is valid and reproducible (Cherny et al. 2009).

9.4.3 Drugs used in sedation

Midazolam

Midazolam is the most popular drug used, at the moment, for sedation in palliative care, as reported by Cowan and Walsh (2001). Midazolam is a benzodiazepine with high solubility that allows SC administration and a short elimination half-life of about 3 hours. It is highly bound to plasma proteins (>90%). After IM administration its bioavailability varies from 40 to 100% and plasma peak concentrations are achieved in 20–30 minutes. It is metabolized by the liver P450 cytochrome system (isoenzyme CYP3A4) to an active metabolite (hydroxyl-1-midazolam), which is responsible for 60–80% of the clinical effects. This metabolite is readily cleared from bloodstream after glucuronization and renal excretion, and therefore does not prolong the clinical effects of the drug. In long-term sedation in the ICU a high individual variability of effects has been seen. Clearance is dependent on hepatic function, hepatic blood flow, and interaction with other drugs with hepatic metabolism. A more pronounced sedative effect is seen in the elderly and accumulation may occur in hepatic and renal failure. A reduction of midazolam concentrations and effects has been documented by co-administration of carbamazepine, phenytoin, and rifampicin. Prolonged sedative effects were seen when midazolam was administered in combination with macrolid antibiotics, ketoconazole, and itroconazole (Bolon et al. 2002).

Indications for the use of midazolam in palliative care, however, would greatly benefit from studies documenting, specifically, clinical end-points and effective doses. It has been reported that in 23 patients requiring treatment for restlessness and agitation who were mostly (18 patients) already on diamorphine infusion for pain, SC midazolam was effective for resolving these symptoms in 22 cases by using a starting dose of 10–20 mg/24 h, followed by dose titration. The mean maximum dose achieved was 69 mg/24 h, but doses ranged from 5 to 200 mg/day (Bottomley and Hanks 1990). In one patient 120 mg/day midazolam infusion was not effective, and also methotrimeprazine 80 to 300 mg SC daily infusion failed to control the symptoms. No information is given as to the level of consciousness. General guidelines on the use of sedation included recommendations to use 2.5–10 mg SC midazolam injections 2 to 4 hourly to obtain rapid symptom control and 10-30 mg over 24 hour infusion thereafter (Burke 1997).

While it is likely that the use of SC midazolam is effective in offering adequate sedation in a number of patients (Bottomley and Hanks 1990), in agreement also with our experience, comparative studies giving specific indications to this practice are lacking. In our experience often the SC route of infusion is less effective than the IV route to keep control of the level of consciousness. This is true, in particular, when confronting very difficult acute situations such as dyspnoea or haemorrhage, when rapidity of clinical effect is fundamental. We also found that the IV route facilitated the need to monitor the level of consciousness and adapting pharmacological treatments to it.

Indications on the doses needed to obtain prolonged sedation with midazolam come from the experience of ICUs, where it is also common practice to administer it together with opioids. If rapid sedation is needed, midazolam should be used at a starting dose of 0.07 mg/kg IV (minimal dose). In one case series of patients requiring mechanical ventilation the mean dose for inducing sedation was 0.22 ± 0.07 mg/kg (Chamorro et al. 1996). Midazolam requires frequent dose adjustment after inducing sedation and its clinical effect may be prolonged after withdrawing it. In the same study maintenance doses varied (mean 0.14 ± 0.10 mg/kg/h). After discontinuing continuous infusion, reversibility was achieved after 13.6 ± 16.4 h in patients without renal failure and after 44.6 ± 42.5 h in patients with renal failure. Two patients with combined hepatic and renal failure took 124 and 140 h, respectively, to awaken (Shelly et al. 1991).

The sedative effect of midazolam is obtained at plasma concentration above 150 ng/mL, moderate sedation has been associated with concentrations of 346 ± 208 ng/mL, and deep sedation required mean concentrations of 661 ± 477 ng/ml, confirming a very high individual variability (Bolon et al. 2002).

Midazolam can fail even at high doses. In this case it is suggested to add a barbiturate, propofol, or, according to our experience, an antihistamine or α_2 agonist (see Cheng et al. 2002).

Lorazepam

Lorazepam is an effective alternative to midazolam with the only drawback of requiring the use of the IV route for administration. Lorazepam has a longer half-life than midazolam (8–24 hours). It is independent of liver cytochrome oxidative metabolism as it is glucoroconjugated and inactivated by liver enzymes and excreted by renal glomerular filtration. For this reason less variability of its sedative properties could be expected from metabolic changes or drug interactions. Lorazepam was compared with midazolam in achieving sedation in the ICU. The average half-life of lorazepam was 13.8 hours and that of midazolam 8.9 hours but lorazepam showed less variability than midazolam. The average dose of lorazepam was 1 mg/h compared with 15.5 mg/h of midazolam for an average sedation period of about 7 days (Swart et al. 1999). In another study sedation was conducted over a much shorter time period (Barr et al. 2001) and lorazepam's average dose was 0.91 mg/h (mean), compared with 2.54 mg/h of midazolam.

Propofol

Propofol, a potent IV hypnotic agent, is also a drug commonly used in anaesthesia and intensive care (Marik 2004) that has been occasionally used in palliative care. Propofol is not related to the other general anaesthetic agents used for IV sedation. It is an oil and is manufactured as a 1% emulsion that can only be used via IV administration. Its effect is very fast, distribution occurring with a half-life of 2–8 minutes. Elimination half-life is 1–3 hours. Propofol is metabolized by the liver by glucuronization and excreted in urine. Its clearance is higher than liver blood flow suggesting an extrahepatic metabolism. A dose of 2 mg/kg is used to induce anaesthesia. Blood pressure is reduced by 30% during propofol anaesthesia due to peripheral vasodilatation. No direct cardiac effects are known. Apnoea and pain at the site of injection also occur. Only four cases of sedation in terminal phases with propofol are reported in the literature (Cowan and Walsh 2001; McWilliams et al. 2010).

Propofol has been proposed as the treatment of DT in the intensive care management of cases refractory to benzodiazepines. In a case series of 4 patients, doses of 90, 80, 45, and 40 mg/kg/h were used at the highest rates of infusion to control agitation. These patients are, of course all mechanically ventilated (McCowan and Marik 2000).

One case report of a patient with agitated delirium due to terminal hepatic failure was managed with propofol infusion, by giving a 20 mg loading bolus IV followed by 50 mg/h infusion that needed to be increased to 70 mg/h after 2 hours because of insufficient sedation. Overall infusion lasted 8 hours (Mercadante et al. 1995). Our opinion is that its use should seldom be considered appropriate in palliative care.

Alpha-2-adrenergic agonists

Alpha-2-adrenergic agonists are used mainly in critical care and postoperative sedation protocols but also in managing DT for their central sedative activity, produced via inhibition of the activation of the cortical mantle by noradrenergic projections from the locus coeruleus. They are, therefore, more useful in cases of adrenergic hyperactivity. Clonidine and, more recently, dexmedetomidine can be administered parenterally (clonidine IV infusion 0.1–2 µg/kg/h, dexmedetomidine 1 µg/kg in 10 loading doses, followed by an infusion of 0.2–0.7 µg/kg/h). In our experience, doses of clonidine up to 0.6 mg/day have been used in hospices with good sedative effects and no significant side effects. These agents have no respiratory depressant action but can cause orthostatic hypotension. The experience from ICUs seems in any case to indicate no difference between dexmedetomidine and midazolam or propofol in inducing deep sedation (Riker et al. 2009; Ruokonen et al. 2009).

Antihistamines

Antihistamines are useful sedative drugs without respiratory depressant effects, and although they have anticholinergic effects, their primary sedative activity can be important for improving night-time sleep or reducing agitation in hyperactive deliria. Promethazine (hydroxyzine is a possible alternatives) is, in our clinical experience, the drug with the most favourable profile in this indication (25–50 mg IM or IV can be repeated up to t.i.d. q8h). Its use proved efficacious in controlling agitated behaviour and reducing the risk of acute dystonias in psychiatric patients treated with high-dose (5–10 mg) injections of haloperidol (Huf et al. 2007).

Other drugs or drug combination

As clarified by reviewing the literature, a number of different drugs are used for sedation that are more or less appropriate for this task. In particular the combination of opioids with BZDs is potentially useful and we would favour at this stage a more consistent use of midazolam for this indication. The combination of opioids and neuroleptics is also common as a result of trying to control delirium with increasing doses of haloperidol or of the more sedative phenothiazines (Fainsinger and Bruera 1992; Stiefel et al. 1992).

The addition of an antihistamine to opioids and neuroleptics when sedation is required and not easily achieved is suggested by anaesthesiological experience (Laborit's cocktail). In the absence of clearly defined guidelines our suggestions,

Table 9.4 Stepwise approach for the treatment of refractory delirium

1) Haloperidol IV infusion can be titrated to effect within hours; the full effect can be appreciated after about 24 hour of infusion.

2) Switch to more sedative neuroleptics such as chlorpromazine 50 mg IV or IM every 8 h.

3) Add antihistamine to an opioid and neuroleptic combination: promethazine 50 mg IV or IM every 8 h.

4) If immediate effect is needed, start midazolam 0.07 mg/kg IV and titrate to effect. Continuous IV or SC infusion can be planned depending on indication and context of care starting with 1 mg/h.

Drugs and doses are indicative and should be adapted case by case.

summarized in Table 9.4, rely on clinical experience. They are, therefore, general and cannot be applied to single cases without specific considerations. In our experience delirium is not the most frequent indication for palliative sedation nor the most difficult if we consider that patients with delirium in very advanced phases of disease already have, by definition, significant failure of consciousness and cognition. On the other hand, patients with dyspnoea or haemorrhage can present with a preserved state of awareness. One significant case example is reported in Chapter 7.

9.4.4 **Key issues in palliative sedation** (Cherny et al. 2009)

Key issues of palliative sedation may explain the differences between cases that can be easily managed at home with SC infusion or and cases that need more aggressive interventions and intensive monitoring:

- Patient level of consciousness before sedation, performance status, and age;
- Indication to sedation;
- Level of suffering associated with the indication;
- Rapidity of effect required;
- Duration of sedation before death (very short interventions may last hours and just require the acute administration of a sedative drug); and
- Monitoring of the level of consciousness (particularly important when sedation is prolonged over hours and days).

9.5 **Non-pharmacological management**

Behavioural and educational interventions represent a further important part of the treatment of delirium. Although aetiologic and psychopharmacological interventions are the hallmark of the treatment of delirium, a more integrated, non-pharmacological approach should be available and routinely utilized in clinical settings (Cole 1999; Jacobson and Schreibman 1997; Maldonado 2008; Miller 2008; Rabins 1991). Current research has provided data about the importance and the efficacy of multicomponent intervention in delirious patients in terms of both prevention and efficacy. A first aspect regards the need to improve the education of nurses in delirium features, cognitive assessment, and factors associated with risk of delirium in order to facilitate its recognition (Inouye et al. 2001). Then, training the staff, particularly nurses, on educational and behavioural interventions seems to be pivotal for a more appropriate management of delirious patients (Milisen et al. 2005; Rockwood 1999; Young et al. 2008).

With regard to this, Meagher et al. (1996) have studied the use of eight basic nursing strategies in managing delirious patients. More specifically the authors evaluated the following strategies: frequent observation (four hourly or more), efforts by staff to re-orientate the patient to his surroundings, efforts made to avoid excessive staff changes, efforts to keep the patient in a single room, use of an individual night light, efforts to minimize environmental noise levels, relatives or friend specifically requested to visit the patient regularly as a way to re-orientate him, and uncluttered nursing environment (no more than two non-orienting, non-vital objects in vicinity of the bed, beds spaced an adequate distance apart). The authors found also that use of behavioural strategies were not routinely used, with only four strategies implemented for fewer than half of the patients. Furthermore, nursing strategies were more frequently employed for patients with hyperactive delirium and more severe symptoms (agitation, mood lability, and disturbances of the sleep–wake cycle), but were associated more with difficulties in ward management than the severity of the patients' cognitive disturbances.

Other studies carried out on elderly patients with delirium indicated that focusing attention on the environmental factors and supportive elements within the interpersonal relationships with the patients themselves are relevant factors of treatment (Cole et al. 1994; Simon et al. 1997). Likewise, studies on elderly hip fracture patients indicated that integrated intervention can in part favour prevention and, to a further extent, the treatment of delirium (Brännström 1999).

A study on delirious patients with hip fracture showed that certain factors, such as education of nursing staff; systematic cognitive screening; consultative services by a delirium resource nurse, a geriatric nurse specialist, or a psychogeriatrician; and use of a scheduled pain protocol, improved the patients' cognitive functioning, decreased the duration of delirium and decreased the postoperative length of hospital stay (Milisen et al. 2001). In line with these results, Marcantonio et al. (2001) indicated that proactive geriatric consultations using a targeted recommendations protocol, to be followed by orthopaedics and repeated symptom evaluation, can reduce delirium by over one-third, and severe delirium by over a half in comparison with usual care patients. Likewise, Inouye et al. (2003) examined the impact of level of adherence on effectiveness of the intervention strategy to prevent delirium. In a study of 422 consecutive in-patients 70 years or older admitted to the medicine service at a university hospital, the authors found that complete adherence rates for individual intervention protocols ranged from 10% for the sleep protocol to 86% for the orientation protocol, with a rate of complete adherence with all protocols of 57%. Higher levels of adherence resulted in lower delirium rates, with a significant graded effect, for orientation, mobility, and therapeutic activities protocols, and for the composite adherence measure. After controlling for potential confounding variables, such as illness severity, co-morbidity, baseline delirium risk, and functional status, adherence continued to demonstrate a consistently strong and significant protective effect against delirium, with patients in the highest adherence group showing an 89% reduction in delirium risk compared with patients in the lowest group. More recently, Vidán et al. (2009) in a consecutive series of 542 inpatients aged 70 years and older with any of the risk criteria for delirium (cognitive impairment, visual impairment, acute disease severity, dehydration) found that an intervention based on educational measures and specific actions in seven risk areas (orientation, sensory impairment, sleep, mobilization, hydration, nutrition, drug use) was associated with lower incidence of delirium, with an adherence to the intervention protocols of 75.7%. The intervention also reduced the rate of functional decline and improved other quality indicators (e.g. mobilization and physical restraints reduction).

According to these data, it is clear that awareness of the importance of delirium in palliative care and training of the staff in multicomponent, non-pharmacological interventions integrated into routine practice are key elements for both prevention and treatment of the syndrome (Siddiqi et al. 2007). A correct knowledge of the risk factors for delirium, the regular assessment of cognitive status, and the application of standardized protocols have a significant role. Once delirium has developed, the application of standardized procedures of behavioural and educational interventions is necessary to reduce the many consequences of the disorder and to help the family in dealing with the situation. According to what has been described in the literature and our own experience (Borreani et al. 1997), we will briefly present the most useful strategies to take into account in palliative care settings, by examining environmental and supportive strategies for the patient and for the family members (Tables 9.5 and 9.6).

9.5.1 Intervention for the patient

The role of environmental and social factors in precipitating or maintaining delirium has not been extensively examined, although it has been clear that their contribution is important in clinical practice (Eriksson 1999) as now conformed in clinical trial (McCusker et al. 2001a).

As mentioned, there is now evidence deriving from well-conducted randomized trials that an integrated pre-emptive environmental, nursing, and cognitive intervention can reduce the number of incident cases among elderly hospitalized patients (Inouye et al. 1999a, Vidan et al. 2009). Another large randomized clinical trial, on the other hand, failed to demonstrate that early detection and targeted multidisciplinary care has an impact on delirium duration and recovery (Cole et al. 2002).

In a recent study of more than 150 patients with delirium (Van Rompaey et al. 2009) it was shown that environmental risk factors such as isolation, absence of visit, absence of visible daylight, transfer from another ward, and use of physical restraints were significantly associated with the risk of delirium. Thus, integrated intervention for delirium should consider the meaningful significance of practical and relationship variables, which we will summarize.

Manipulation of the environment

When possible, the patient should be transferred to a single room, where contact with other patients, who are strangers to the patient and who are often themselves suffering from severe medical conditions, could represent a 'pathogenic' stimulus, increasing the

Table 9.5 Manipulation of the environmental

- Provide quiet, non-noisy environment
- Avoid over- and understimulation
- Provide light (including night)
- Provide clock and calendar
- Make the environment familial (photographs, personal objects, pictures)
- Allow patient to have family members and well-known persons available
- Allow patient to be familial with at least one staff member through proper shift

vulnerability of the patient as far as his perception and thought processes are concerned. Furthermore, the noises of the often overcrowded medical or oncology wards (e.g. nursing activity, beeps, alarms, ringing bells, respirators, monitors) may be reduced if the patient is in his own room. Keeping the room quiet and well lit, with adequate light during the night-time, is useful to improve the patient's confusion and decrease frightening illusions. Availability of objects familiar to the patient (e.g. photographs, pictures, personal objects) is also of great help in giving a sense of reassurance and safety. Also returning aids (e.g. eyeglasses, hearing aids) to patients that normally need them is helpful in ameliorating the quality of sensory input and, consequently, in decreasing misinterpretation of the surroundings.

Orientation

Reorienting the patients to time and space is a further helpful strategy. Reorientation to time can consist in frequently repeating the date and the time to the patient and in providing the room with a calendar and a big clock. Reorientation to space, context, and persons can consist in repeating where the patient is, why he is there, and the identity of the people assisting him, and reinforcing the sense of control and familiarity with those who are present.

Giving information

Regular explanation of the procedures the staff are applying (e.g. blood exams, pharmacological treatment and route, restraints when needed) and reassurance about what is happening is extremely important for increasing the patient's sense of safety. When the symptoms of confusion decrease or delirium is cleared, information about what happened (e.g. why the patient has restraints, what kind of symptoms the patient has had) and what can be expected in the following hours (e.g. fluctuations and possible returning of symptoms) is necessary to reduce the frequent distress condition which can follow delirium and to help the patient in understanding his bizarre experiences and the frightening memories of his symptoms. We have shown that experiences during ICU admission, including sensations, factual memories, and emotional memories, are remembered by at least two-thirds of the patients, irrespective of the treatment (no sedation, morphine, morphine plus other sedatives; Capuzzo et al. 2001). This seems to be a long-lasting phenomenon persisting up to 1 year after discharge (Löf et al. 2006).

Company

Family members and close relatives or friends should be permitted to visit the patient and stay with him. Their presence can in fact reduce the feeling of abandonment and strangeness determined by unknown persons (e.g. other patients, family members visiting their own relatives in overcrowded wards). Staying with the patient, speaking to him, and touching him are important in that vocal and visual stimuli can favour the patient's awareness of his environment. Family members can also help the staff in facilitating and correcting the patient's reinterpretation of the surroundings, in reorienting him to time and space and giving him positive feedbacks to what is happening. A balance between overstimulation (that could increase the patient's confusion) and understimulation (that could leave the patient in his poor conditions) should be found.

Table 9.6 Supportive intervention for the patient

- Maintain open communication channels
- Maintain active listening
- Give meaning to symptoms
- Evaluate the patient's emotions and the defences underlying the symptoms
- Explain to patient what the staff is doing (procedures, interventions)

Staff

When possible, staff members who care continually for the patient should be maintained in their rotation scheme, trying to avoid that the patient is attended by new, unknown, and unfamiliar professionals. Creating an atmosphere of trust is easier if the patient is allowed to be familiar with at least one nurse per shift. This reduces the sense of strangeness and reinforces alliance and interpersonal relationships.

For these reasons, communication is extremely significant in the care of delirious patient. Communication channels should be always open. It is important to remember that the content of the patient's utterances always has a meaning and should not be dismissed as strange, incomprehensible, or bizarre. Attention should be paid to the patient's fears and worries and to his possible illusions and hallucinations, reassuring him about the situation, his feelings, and his perceptions, and respecting his emotions. Challenging the patient about delusions is not helpful and can worsen the trust in the staff. Patients should also be allowed to respond in their own time and non-verbal skills can be used to fill sudden communication gaps. Table 9.6 presents some of the significant goals of communicating with a patient with delirium.

It also must be remembered that delirium does not happen in a vacuum, but it is a phase during a process of the illness of a patient with his own history and experience. Thus collecting data about the patient's life can be useful in interpreting the symptoms of delirium in a more comprehensive way, if and when it develops.

The following case is an example of significant life elements, not known by the staff, that appeared during a confusional state and that could have been useful in the management of the disorder.

Case report

Ms P. is a 49-year-old woman admitted to the oncology ward because of worsening of her physical conditions. She has been suffering from bone metastases secondary to breast cancer for several months. After a few days following admission the patient begins to show sleep–wake disorders and within the following day a full-blown hyperactive delirium is present. Along with confusion, disorientation, and agitation, prominent thought disorders, persecutory type, and perception disorders are also evident. The patient is convinced to be in hell and she screams about the devil threatening her from the top of her bed. The staff members are mistakenly perceived as enemies allied with the 'obscure forces of the hell'. The patient seemed to live in a nightmare where a fight between her, as an angel, and the devil is taking place. Fragments of her past, especially her father's death, appear during the short periods of awareness and return to a state of consciousness. The patient is referred to psychiatric consultation. Alcohol use and other possible causes of delirium are ruled out and a significant hypercalcaemia results to be the only possible cause of delirium. Her clinical situation improves in a few days, after treatment of the metabolic disorder and a course of haloperidol 3 mg/day. After a week the patient is discharged from the hospital and returns home. A home-care assistance programme is planned through the domiciliary oncology service. During a scheduled home visit by the psychiatrist who saw her in the hospital, many aspects linked to the content of her delirium become clear and understandable. The home is full of pictures of saints and holy images on all the walls of her bedroom. During a long and moving interview, the patient reveals dramatic experiences of her life, especially the death of her father, who committed suicide fifteen years earlier after a diagnosis of an inoperable stomach cancer. A few years later the patient's mother was diagnosed with breast cancer and the patient followed and assisted her during the course of the illness until her death, which happened five years later. The patient was profoundly shocked by this second death and gradually moved towards faith to give meaning to her destiny, including the sudden discovery of a malignant lump in her breast. 'It was like the ghosts of the past were returning with their bad forces in our home.' She joined a group of people called the Angels of Salvation, who met regularly and who used to sing together as a way to be in contact with God and the 'good' forces. Besides the clinical meaning of these thoughts and convictions, all these aspects of the patient's life were completely unknown to the doctors who had followed the patient in the two years she was seen for breast surgery, chemotherapy, and regular check-ups.

Other problems can be found when delirium develops. A home and the home staff can have the advantage of the help of the family and the disadvantage of carrying out intervention in a less safe context with respect to the hospital, the palliative care unit, or the hospice (Bond 2009).

9.5.2 Intervention for the family

The patient's family should also be involved in different ways in order to provide the best possible treatment of delirium. For this reason, specific intervention should be provided to family members, in order to reduce the frightening experience of caring for their loved one who, during fluctuations of delirium, is unable to communicate in a coherent and 'familial' way with his relatives (Fitzgerald and Parkes 1998; Gagnon et al. 2002). We will focus our attention in the next chapter on the complex problem of psychosocial impact of terminal illness on the family and on the needs that should be addressed in palliative care, limiting this section to the most important strategies to apply in the management of delirium, as summarized in Table 9.7.

Education and counselling

A number of factors that suggest a role for counselling and education for the family of the delirious patient can be recognized (Table 9.8). Education about the symptoms of delirium, especially disinhibition and agitation, hallucinations and delusions, is extremely important for the family. This can alleviate the profound sense of helplessness, incredulity, and anxiety that family members can feel during delirium

Table 9.7 Supportive intervention for the family

- Elicit and respond to the family's concerns, problems, and needs
- Identify and accept the family emotional reactions (e.g. fear, anger, guilt, helplessness)
- Understand the meanings underlying emotions and behaviour
- Give clear information about the patient's symptoms and the necessary interventions
- Involve family in the assistance plan
- Involve other professionals or helping figures, when needed (e.g. volunteers)
- Favour more adaptive strategies to cope with the situation
- Improve communication between the family (or the key family member) and the single members of the staff
- Reduce attrition
- Link the patient's 'bizarre' content of speech with possible previous experiences (e.g. work, interpersonal relationships)

('He doe not recognize me', 'He seems like another person, someone that I never knew', 'His personality has changed'). The fear of a psychological death that will prevent the relative from having any further contact with their loved one is extremely frustrating and source of desperation for not having had enough time to share. Furthermore, delirium can be interpreted as a sign of an impending death long anticipated but not yet accepted. Helping the family to find a possible sense in the patient's 'bizarre' behaviour, linking it with previous experiences (e.g. family life, social life, interpersonal relationships, work) can also be useful.

It is also important to explain the fluctuating nature of delirium, indicating that transitory phases of awareness, in which the patient is still in contact with reality, do not necessarily mean a recovery and that symptoms can recur.

The possible causes of delirium (e.g. metabolic imbalances, use of drugs), as well as treatment options, should also be clearly explained. The fact that control of symptoms, such as pain, is important even if the drugs (e.g. opioids) could favour the onset of

Table 9.8 Critical issues in counselling for the family of delirious patients

Communication barrier

Patient's awareness of physical and psychological suffering

Reversibility

Short-term prognosis

Fluctuations of cognitive functions

Role of opioid and other therapies in aetiology

Role and goal of sedation

Goals of care

Reproduced from Borreani et al. (1997) with permission.

delirium should be honestly communicated to the family. This is particularly important in home-care assistance programmes, where the family can feel abandoned by the team and can develop ambivalent emotions about the use of pain drugs. Likewise, information about the pharmacological treatment of delirium (e.g. haloperidol) and possible side effects should be given. Involvement of the family in the assistance plan is obviously in order, given the role of family members to stay with the patient, to reorient him and accept his confused speech.

In cases in which the patient's clinical conditions are rapidly deteriorating or the reversibility of physiological functions can be achieved at enormous costs in terms of suffering, the family should be informed and involved in decision-making process. The patient's wishes and the family opinion about deep sedation should be known and openly discussed; likewise the opposite situation in which the family requests that their relative be 'put to sleep' should be evaluated and discussed in a sincere and open way.

Attention to family emotions and needs

Identifying and accepting family emotional reactions is a basic intervention. Allowing the family to express their doubts and feelings is necessary to reduce their burden in caring for their relative. Fear about irreversibility of the clinical situation and death, anger towards the health care system or the staff, guilt about their inability to sustain the situation, and hopelessness and helplessness about the possible loss are common reactions that should be addressed and accepted in a non-judgmental way. It is possible that these emotional reactions are sustained by behaviours that, at first glance, can be seen as inadequate and inappropriate (e.g. reducing visiting to their relative, not asking the staff for the relative's clinical situation, isolation or intrusion). In any case the possible and multiple meanings underlying these behaviours should be scrutinized and understood. Attention and responses to practical needs can also help the family find more adaptive coping mechanisms towards the situation. If good communication channels between the family (or the key family member) and the single members of the staff are maintained, it is possible to identify and give priority to problems and concerns and to find possible solutions. Involving other figures and liaising with other professionals (e.g. hospital or community social workers, volunteer association) who may provide assistance can give the family a sense of non-abandonment and model strategies for a better management of their loved one's situation.

During the terminal phases of illness interventions that permit the family to express their feelings, to cry, and to grieve are the most significant part of assistance, as we will describe in the next chapter.

Chapter 10

Family Issues[1]

Your pallor
startled me.
One could read on your face
the abandonment of life
and like clear water
your look meant the departing
from things human.
You carried your pain inside
and did barely answer.
Then, with a brief nod,
you quickly slipped away.
Leaving me with my grief.
Speechless.

Eugenio Montale (translation by Jody Fitzhardinge and Lorenzo Matteoli)[2]

10.1 Introduction

The impact of the patient's disease on the family psychosocial equilibrium and the role of the family members merits special attention in palliative medicine (Liao and Arnold 2006) both for the role of the family in offering assistance in the management of delirium and for the consequences of the terminal phase of illness on family members.

In fact, cancer and life-threatening disease leading to palliative care intervention are events of the whole family, often indicated as 'family diseases' (Northouse 1988). For this reason family members are referred to as 'second order patients' (Lederberg 1998a) or 'hidden patients' (Kristjanson and Aoun 2004) with their own needs. At the same time they are also considered to be 'second order therapists' in that they provide the majority of assistance and work with the staff in the care of their relative (Emanuel et al. 1999).

---

[1] Maria Giulia Nanni, MD, Section of Psychiatry, Department of Medical Disciplines of Communication and Behaviour, University of Ferrara, Italy, has contributed to the writing of this chapter. The Authors are indebted to Lea Baider for her thoughtful comments and helpful suggestions.

[2] The authors are indebted to Lorenzo Matteoli for his work 'A Reading of the Life and Works of Eugenio Montale within the Context of Italian History from 1896 to 1981', for Department of Italian, School of European Languages, University of Western Australia.

It is especially in home-care palliative programmes that the active involvement of the family in providing continuous assistance to their relative may often cause problems, given the ambiguity and conflict in being caregivers and care-recipients (Schachter and Coyle 1998). The diffusion of home-care programmes, the shift from a patient-focused to a patient/family-focused approach in health organizational systems, and the development of health community-based palliative care services coordinated by family physicians represent further elements indicating the need for a holistic vision of terminal illness (Burge et al. 2001; Kutner and Kilbourn 2009; Robinson and Stacy 1994; Steinmetz et al. 1993).

The aspects concerning the family as a unit and the mixed emotional reactions during the palliative care process, before and after the loss of their loved one, should be an ethical and clinical consideration for health care professionals (Hudson et al. 2004; Kristjanson 1997; Kristjanson and Ashercraft 1994; McClement and Woodgate 1998).

It is apparent that the emotional aspects involving the family during palliative care vary greatly according to many significant variables, such as who is the dying person (e.g. child, adolescent, young wife, mother), his/her gender, his/her age, his/her role, the context of care (e.g. hospital ward, hospice or palliative units, or patient's own home), as well as the cultural background and rituals (Bosma et al. 2009; Kagawa-Singer and Blackhall 2001; Nyatanga 2002), which all influence the process of illness/death.

The focus of this chapter is on briefly reviewing the most significant psychological aspects evident in the family during the terminal phase of their relative's illness and after his/her death, and giving the reader elements that facilitate the analysis of delirium and terminal delirium in a broader and more integrated framework.

10.2 The psychological impact of delirium and terminal illness on the family

Families are profoundly influenced by the hopeless disease progression of their relative. It is the conclusion of a long and difficult journey in the domains of suffering, adjustment, reframing, expectations, illusions of recovery and fears of relapse, uncertainty, dilemmas, and, finally, inevitability of the terminality of one's own life. Understanding the continuity of this journey is paramount for a more precise awareness of the psychological impact of the terminal phase of illness on the family and, inextricably, on the patient and on the team caring for them (Cherny et al. 1994; Jo et al. 2007; Klagsbrun 1994; Leis et al. 1997).

10.2.1. General aspects on the role of the family in the advanced phases of illness

Several factors are to be considered in contributing to the family psychosocial distress during the terminal phase. Although these factors are intimately connected and entwined, they can be classified into (i) patient-related factors, (ii) family-related factors, and (iii) family/staff-related factors (Table 10.1).

Patient-related factors

Patient-related factors are mainly represented by the symptoms caused and by the problems determined by the progression of illness. Watching a loved one deteriorate and experience unbearable physical symptoms is a major source of suffering for the family.

Table 10.1 Sources of distress for the family during the terminal phase of illness

Patients's domain

◆ Physical issues (e.g. loss of mobility, pain, fatigue, constipation, nausea and vomiting, medication side effects)

◆ Psychological and psychiatric issues (e.g. fear of death, guilt, anger, requests for hastening death, psychiatric symptoms, e.g. cognitive deterioration, delirium, depression, anxiety)

◆ Existential and spiritual issues (e.g. meaning of one's own life, fear of nothingness)

Family domain

◆ Psychosocial issues (e.g. impending bereavement, fear of separation, loss and abandonment, anxiety, helplessness and hopelessness, guilt, role changes, interpersonal relationships, conflicts)

◆ Physical issues (e.g. fatigue, health behaviour, sleep–wake cycle disorders)

◆ Practical issues (e.g. need for acquiring technical skills, economic strain, need for reorganization, work-related problems, changes in daily-life rhythms, modifications of social relationships, dependency on others)

Healh-care team domain

◆ Psychosocial issues (e.g. communication with health staff members, ambiguity in the reciprocal roles, conflicts, burned-out staff)

◆ Practical issues (e.g. organizational problems, relationship with the health-system organization, availability of resources)

Speaking about delirium and the cognitive deterioration of their own loved one is a significant source of distress for the family (Breitbart et al. 2002a; Cohen et al. 2009; Susan 2003). The several symptoms of delirium, such as the patient's inability to recognize his relatives, the bizarre content of thoughts, the disturbance of perceptions and mood, the inability to control impulses, and the alterations in the sleep–wake cycle are extremely frightening for the family and can easily be interpreted as an anticipation of death (Lawlor et al. 2000a), with consequent intense feelings of impotence and the need to be helped by the health staff. In a study of the family perception of palliative care services, it has been shown that expectations of the family members tend to be higher than the perception of the actual palliative care they receive in the families of delirious or unconscious patients, as compared with the families of conscious patients (Kristjanson et al. 1996). Furthermore, in certain circumstances delirium and terminal delirium are considered part of a process, in other circumstances as a terrible and distressing phenomenon. Namba et al. (2007), for example, qualitatively analysed the reports of the experience of the family towards the terminal delirium of their loved ones. Family experiences varied (e.g. 'patients talked about events that actually occurred in the past', 'patients were distressed as they noticed that they were talking strangely', 'patients talked about uncompleted life tasks', 'patients expressed physiologic desires such as excretion and thirst') and family emotions were positive, neutral, or negative (e.g. distress, guilt, anxiety and worry, difficulty coping with delirium, helplessness, exhaustion, and feeling a burden on others). Families perceived the delirium to have different meanings, including positive meanings (e.g. relief from real suffering), a part of the dying process, and misunderstanding of the causes of delirium (e.g. effects of drugs, mental weakness, and pain).

Confronting with the patient's concerns and emotional symptoms is also a very difficult task for the family. The patient's fears of physical deterioration and dependency; feelings of anger, hopelessness, and despair; existential and spiritual concerns (e.g. knowing that life had had a meaning, finding comfort in one's faith); and preoccupation with their own family (e.g. perceiving appreciation from the family, saying good-bye, knowing that the family will survive without them) are all sources of suffering that affect the family too (Greisinger et al. 1997). In fact, it has been shown that the patient's poor adjustment to illness is a factor favouring the increase of levels of distress in the family (Wellisch et al. 1989). Furthermore, the patient's level of depression, determined in large part by physical suffering and loss of mobility, has been related with high levels of depression in the family (Given et al. 1993; Kurtz et al. 1995). Family requests for help to the health care system tend to exponentially increase at the worsening of the patient's clinical conditions (Hileman et al. 1992; Lewis 1990).

Family-related factors

The quality of interpersonal relationships within the family, the level of communication between family members, adjustment to role changes, possible intrafamily conflicts, physical exhaustion or health problems, existential concerns (e.g. unfulfilled aspirations, unresolved guilt, searching for a meaning), lack of support from close or diffuse social resources (e.g. other relatives, friends, neighbours, associations), economical problems, and cultural variables represent further factors that intervene in determining family distress (Cherny et al. 1994; Sales et al. 1992).

It is apparent that within the family context, the nature of the relationships between the members is an important variable in moulding the emotional response during the terminal phase of illness. As we will discuss (see section on anticipatory grief), these are major issues in influencing the impact of terminal illness on the family.

A significant area regarding the level of communication between the family and the patient can become problematic in the advanced phases of illness. Hinton (1981) indicated that restricted communication among couples during the terminal phase of illness of one of the members may be related to previous family patterns of communication antedating the illness or to the attempt to prevent emotional distress and to facilitate coping with the problems caused by the disease. The family tendency to hide the patient from the truth or to minimize the severity of his/her clinical situation is often an act made in order to protect their loved one from hopelessness and desperation. Even if it is understandable, it may cause problems in the relationship between the family and the patient as it becomes a major trap for the family (Fallowfield et al. 2002; Hancock et al. 2007; Maguire 2000; Parker et al. 2007). In fact, the 'conspiracy of silence' and 'collusion', as so it is sometimes seen, is a problem when the patient becomes aware of what is happening. At this time, the patient can feel a sense of betrayal and abandonment, with consequent distrust towards their family, which in turn, can experience feelings of guilt, remorse, and futility. In other cases, the family and the patient know what is happening but they prefer not to openly discuss it, with the intention of not concerning each other. However, the game of 'I know that you know that I know' can influence the family relationships in a negative way, since the effort of not expressing one's own emotions has a high psychological cost, causing feelings of dishonesty, preventing the family from feeling really cohesive, and reducing the possibilities of discussing 'unfinished business'. In other cases, again, open communication is simply not possible because the patient has chosen to remain unaware of the situation, leaving every decision to the family or the health staff.

Family–staff related factors

All the aspects described in the previous sections are evidently entwined with the factors regarding the relationship between the family and the health care team. This is a de facto 'second family', in touch with the 'primary (or true) family' at both a technical and a psychological level (Rolland 1994). In fact, being part of the treatment team requires the family to acquire complex technical skills (e.g. tube feeding, wound and skin care, use of oxygen, bowel and bladder management, use of drugs), and to share responsibilities with the health care providers with regard to the medical conditions of the patients (e.g. evaluating and 'objectively' reporting symptoms, such as pain, administering p.r.n.—*pro re nata* 'as circumstances may require—therapy; Grobe et al. 1981). Thus, significant sources of stress between family members and the team may emerge as a consequence of the overwhelming pressure and complexity of caring (Siegel et al. 1991). On the other hand, the staff itself, as a part of the caregiver system, have to deal with repeated confrontation with death and dying, with their own existential and emotional concerns (e.g. feelings of anxiety, anger, abandonment, hopelessness, or guilt), with overwhelming requests from the patient and the family, and with possible conflicts between the single team members or between the team and the health care organization (Feldstein and Buschman Gemma 1995; Graham et al. 1996; Lederberg 1998b; Ramirez et al. 1998; Vachon 1998; Yancik 1984a, b). This can in turn reverberate onto the family increasing its level of distress. With regard to this, Shinjo et al. (2010) evaluated family members and the perceived necessity for improvement in the care for imminently dying patients in 670 families, of whom 76% responded. Families reported their experiences as very distressing in 45% of cases. Determinants of high-level distress were a younger patient age, being a spouse, and, interestingly, overhearing conversations between the medical staff outside the room at the time of the patient's death. Furthermore, those reporting high-level necessity of improvement were less likely to have encountered attempts to ensure the patient's comfort, received less family coaching on how to care for the patient, and felt that insufficient time was allowed for the family to grieve after the patient's death.

The same authors (Morita et al. 2007) identified also some aspects of care which were perceived as important by family members witnessing their relatives' delirium, including respect for the patient's subjective perceptions and experiences, coordination of care to enhance communication, and improvement in communication to explain the reasons for delirium and its course. It also emerged that a caregiver's being with the patient was associated with lower family emotional distress, emphasizing one of the oldest palliative care tenets: 'to be there' (Saunders 1965).

Meetings with the family are thus a basic resource for health care professionals in palliative medicine both for prevention and treatment reasons when necessary and for planning and continuing care, as also demonstrated by recent research (Dumont and Kissane 2009; Guegen et al. 2009).

10.2.2 Family psychosocial morbidity

For all these reasons, it is not surprising that a number of studies have tried to examine the extent and characteristics of psychosocial morbidity in the family of terminally ill patients, both as a consequence of delirium and, more in general, as a consequence of the situation involving the pending loss of their loved one. More data are necessary in this area, however (Swore et al. 2008). In a quantitative study of 212 family caregivers (Dumont et al. 2006), a high level of psychological distress was shown in 41–62% caregivers (vs 19.2% in the general population). Family caregivers' psychosocial distress was strongly associated with the patients' terminal disease progress and declined functioning, along with the caregiver's burden, the patient's young age, the patient's symptoms, the caregiver's young age and gender, a poor perception of his/her health, and dissatisfaction with emotional and tangible support. Buss et al. (2007) assessed the frequency of caregiver-perceived delirium among 200 caregivers of patients with advanced cancer, by using the Stressful Caregiving Response to Experiences of Dying (SCARED). The authors found that 38 (19.0%) reported seeing the patient 'confused, delirious' at least once per week in the month prior to study enrollment and 7 (3.5%) met criteria for generalized anxiety. Caregivers of patients with caregiver-perceived delirium were 12 times more likely to have general anxiety ($p < 0.01$), with a relationship persisting after adjusting for caregiver burden and exposure to other stressful patient experiences. In a study carried out by Bruera et al. (2009) on 99 patients who had completely recovered from an acute delirium episode and paired 99 family caregivers 73 patients (74%) remembered the episode of being delirious, with 59 of them (81%) reporting the experience as distressing. However, the median overall delirium distress score was higher in family caregivers than in patients ($p = 0.0004$). Similar data has also been published by Breitbart and co-workers (2002a).

In a multicentre Japanese experience, 50% of family members reported being very emotionally distressed about the experience of terminal delirium (Morita et al. 2004). These data are in line with the literature regarding psychiatric morbidity in the family of terminally ill patients. In a preliminary study of 102 families taking care of patients with cancer, for example, Kissane et al. (1994a) have found that 35% of spouses and 28% of offspring showed symptoms of clinical depression ('cases') on the Beck Depression Inventory. About one-quarter of the family members were also 'cases' as far as anxiety, phobia, and obsessive-compulsiveness were concerned. Harrison et al. (1995), by studying 198 key relatives of cancer patients, found that 48% scored as possible cases on the General Health Questionnaire (GHQ), especially within the domain of anxiety/insomnia and somatic symptoms. In this study it was also shown that female family members were at a higher risk than males (63 vs 39%).

Thus, although the trajectory of caregiving during the terminal phase of illness is not a rigid process, but changes and fluctuates according to changes and ongoing of the situation (Nijboer et al. 1998), being actively supported throughout the palliative care process is a major need for the family. Giving honest information about the patient's disease, including the prognosis, the way to control symptoms, the correct use of medications (dose, use, schedule time, side effects) and technical devices, and providing emotional support are all important elements of palliative care that help the family to handle the difficult situation of their loved one's terminal illness (Cherny et al. 1994; Hinds 1985; Houts et al. 1991; Northouse 1988; Tulsky 2005; Weiner and Roth 2006).

Although some studies carried out in home settings have indicated that emotional support seemed less effective than the staff's active intervention aimed at reducing the patients' physical discomfort (De Conno et al. 1996; Peruselli et al. 1997), variations are possible according to the family structure and wishes. It has been shown, for instance, that some families express preference for home-palliative programs, which permits the family to be better connected with other relatives and friends, to search for and receive support (Beck-Friis and Strang 1993; Brown et al. 1990), while other families tend to gradually reduce their praising of home-care assistance as the disease progresses (Hinton 1994).

In any case, as we will also discuss later, all the multiple dimensions of physical, psychosocial, existential, and spiritual dimensions of the human experience should be incorporated into the care of terminally ill patients and their family (Breitbart et al. 2004; De Haes and Teunissen 2005).

10.3 The assessment of family functioning

Assessment of the family needs and evaluation of the main characteristics of family functioning are thus extremely important in palliative care (Hickey 1990; Osse et al. 2000; Zaider and Kissane 2009). Although during the process of illness/death, families switch their modes of functioning many times in order to adapt to the modifications imposed by the progression of illness, some central elements that characterize the family functioning should be considered and understood (Lipsitt and Lipsitt 1991; Rolland 1994; Wellisch 2000).

The number of the family members present during the palliative care process and their respective roles are a first significant element to take into account. Some families consist only of two members (e.g. a couple of elderly persons); other are multigenerational families with many members. The capacity of the family to maintain its internal stability and, at the same time, to be flexible in front of events that need new adaptations is another significant element to assess. The degree of closeness between members with respect, at the same time, to separateness and autonomy of each member is a key factor. Families in which the members are extremely dependent each other or completely disengaged about family life are two opposite extremes of possible family functioning. The boundaries between the family members are also important. The rules, the roles, the rights, and obligations are points from which one can interpret how the members relate to each other (e.g. the relationship between the spouses, between parents and children, between grandparents and grandsons). Likewise the family–community boundaries are important in describing to what degree the family

Table 10.2 Assessing family functioning

Family history

1. Has the family already coped with difficult health situations, including life-threatening disease or death events?

2. Has the family had psychological or psychiatric needs in the past and what has been done for that? (Specify who, when, and in what situation of family life.)

History of the disease

1. To what extent and in which way have the diagnosis and treatment modified the family roles?

2. What were the main crises during the 'journey' determined by the disease (diagnosis to treatment; recurrence to treatment; advanced phase to palliation)?

Communication and coping patterns

1. Is it possible for family members to speak openly about the illness and therapy among themselves and for the ill relative to speak openly with family members about the illness and therapy?

2. Are there members who are excluded from discussions about relevant aspect of emotional or physical problems the patient has? Who are they? For what reasons?

3. What are the main coping mechanisms of the family (or some members) with regard to the situation?

   • Minimization or, less often, denial of the reality of the disease as a way of reducing the devastating anxiety implicated in anticipated loss

   • Overprotection, with the often-marked tendency to protect their loved one from information about his condition (collusion)

   • Overinvolvement and -identification, causing both depression and anxiety in the family and search for miracle cures

   • Distancing, with delegation of every responsibility to the health system (hospital, staff)

4. What are the main family emotional reactions (e.g. anger, sadness, guilt, anxiety, hopelessness, coldness, detachment)

Relationship with the staff

1. What is the relationship with the staff? Are the staff accepted into the family system? Does it cause conflicts, competitions, distrust?

2. Is there a sharing of viewpoints in regards to health staff recommendations and family expectations?

has a clear sense of unit and, at the same time, is permeable to community systems (e.g. other families, neighbourhood, social or religious associations).

The time in which the illness develops and progresses must also be considered in order to understand the family reactions. The development of the family (life cycle) is, in fact, characterized by different phases and the impact of illness is different according to these phases (e.g. a terminal illness in a spouse of a newly developed family, rather than in a family consisting of two elderly people who have already experienced many losses, including retirement, or departure of sons). According to Rolland (1994), the dimensions of time is extremely important, since illness, individuals, and family development have in common the notion of periods or phases marked by different developmental tasks. Thus, the personal history of single members, the history of the family, and the history of the illness (its onset, its course and outcome) are all factors intervening in moulding the emotional reactions of the whole family (and of their single members) to the terminal phase of illness.

Having a broad picture of what is the family perception of the crisis imposed by the advanced phase of illness ('What is your understanding of what is happening?', 'How is this situation affecting you?') and the main concerns ('What are your main concerns about your loved one's condition'?, 'What would help you to deal with these concerns?') can favour the relationship with the staff and a gradual deepening of investigation about the family as a unit (Welch-McCaffrey 1988; Table 10.2). Hudson et al. (2006a), by studying caregiver preparedness, competence, mastery, social support, anxiety, and self-efficacy, found that self-reported 'anxiety' and 'competence' subscale total scores at the time of commencement of home-based palliative care services were associated with caregivers at risk of lower levels of psychosocial functioning five weeks later.

Examination of these elements provides helpful information that can guide the staff along the process of palliative care. With respect to this, Davies et al. (1994), by transcribing individual and group interviews with families in a palliative care programme, have identified eight major themes that can still be used as indicators of the functioning of the family as a unit. More specifically the authors considered the following elements:

1) How the family integrates the past (e.g. remembering positive and negative events of the past, linking painful past experience to the present, and learning from the past rather than dwelling on the past, without integrating it with the present or learning from previous experiences);

2) How the family deals with feelings (e.g. ability to express a variety of feelings, including fear, vulnerability rather than the tendency to express a few feelings, especially the negative ones, such as anger, hurt, bitterness);

3) How the family solves its problems (e.g. identifying problems, considering multiple options, being open to suggestions, reaching consensus on a common plan of action rather than focusing on fault and guilt without finding solutions, withholding or inaccurately passing information onto the other members, and feeling powerless in dealing with the problem);

4) How the family uses the resources (e.g. taking initiative in searching for resources, utilizing them, and expressing satisfaction rather than not searching or finding or utilizing resources or expressing dissatisfaction with them);

5) How the family consider others (e.g. focusing attention on other family members and their needs rather than being focused on their own emotional needs);

6) How the family portrays the family identity (e.g. capacity to identify typical coping styles of the family as a unit, to consider present situation as an opportunity for growth rather than describing one's own characteristics, giving a portrait of a fragmented family);

7) How the family fulfils roles (e.g. demonstrating flexibility in adapting to role change, sharing extra responsibilities willingly rather than showing rigidity in adaptation, feeling caregiving as a duty or obligation, criticizing caregiving provided by others); and

8) How the family tolerates the differences among their members (e.g. tolerating different views from members of the family and persons outside the family, willing to examine own belief and value system rather than showing intolerance for different opinions, adhering rigidly to beliefs and value systems).

Starting from a different perspective and using their consolidated experience in both consultation psychiatry and palliative care, Kissane et al. (1994b) assessed the functioning of a group of 102 families (patients, spouses, and offspring) referred to a palliative care programme. According to the parameters of family cohesion, levels of conflict, and expressiveness of thoughts and feelings, the authors described five possible typologies of families. Of these, two were well functioning (*supportive* and *conflict-resolving*), two were dysfunctional (*sullen* and *hostile*), and one was intermediate between the two groups (*ordinary*). Supportive families were characterized by high levels of intimacy between members and capacity to share their distress and provide mutual support. These families were able to deal with the difficult process of caregiving, working together with the palliative care staff in a straightforward way. A conflict-resolving pattern was typical of families where the conflict, even if present, was faced and solved through the high level of cohesiveness between members and moderate, but significant, expressiveness. The most significant dysfunctional pattern was represented by *hostile* families. They showed the highest rate of conflict between the members and the lowest levels of cohesion and expressiveness. Furthermore, psychiatric morbidity was the highest and social adjustment the poorest among this typology. Working with these families was problematic since their distress reverberated throughout the treatment system, creating conflicts and emotional burden to the staff. Another dysfunctional pattern was represented by *sullen* families, in which members showed moderate levels of conflict, but tended to demonstrate poor cohesion and expressiveness and reported high levels of psychological morbidity, especially depression. The *ordinary* pattern had intermediate levels of conflicts, cohesion, and expressiveness but presented levels of psychological morbidity needing clinical attention. Identification of severe family conflicts is, however, not always helpful in resolving the situation, as indicated in the following example.

Case report

The patient is a 65-year-old man affected by prostate cancer with diffuse bone metastases. He has been bed-ridden for 3 months. He lives with his wife and a 24-year-old daughter, while an older son got married some years earlier and lives in another town, but not far away from his father's town. A palliative home-care programme planned to assist the patient is rapidly challenged by the increasing demands and requests from the family, especially the patient's wife. She complains about the unavailability of the home-care service as far as practical ('My husband is too heavy and I cannot move him for a proper washing'), and emotional needs are concerned ('He is depressed and has a lot of trouble with pain, since pain killers do not work at all'). Dissatisfaction has caused the sudden admission of the patient to different hospital wards, especially on the weekends, followed by equally sudden discharges for 'improper admission'. The tension between the family and the staff progressively increases with reciprocal accusations. The patient, caught in between, tries to negotiate, asking the staff to forgive his wife 'who is very anxious and depressed'. On the other hand, the tension between the daughter and her mother increases also to very high levels, with accusation of the former to 'have always been hated by you, mum. You are envious of the relationship I had with dad, who was the only one who protected me when you interfered with all my relationships with my boyfriends, by following me, ruining my love affairs and never allowing my boyfriends to come home.' The intervention of the son to mediate the fight, which has extremely negative consequences on the patient, miserably fails. The inability to adjust with the role reversal in the family, the economical problems determined by the patient's disease, the unresolved mother–daughter conflicts, and the impossibility for the patient, a strong man now stuck in a bed and completely dependent on his wife, to conduct his family seem to be major problems for the family. Offers by C-L Psychiatric Service to regularly meet the family and help the wife and the daughter in clarifying the sense of what is happening also fails. In one of the biggest arguments between the two women, with open physical violence, the daughter, screaming, leaves the house, saying 'I am sorry, Dad, your wife won,' and slams the door. She lives away from home for many months, while the wife concludes her relationship with the home-care programme, admitting her husband to a hospice unit. In this case, the problems of previous family relationships emerge in all their force during the crisis determined by progression of the illness. The inability of two family members (mother and daughter) to adapt to the change in their roles and to face the pending loss of their relative is shown by the emphasis given to the old rivalry between them. The high level of criticism between the members was also projected onto the staff and only served to exacerbate the situation.

For these reasons, a continuous assessment of the levels of family functioning and adjustment in palliative care is always important. First, as already mentioned, it gives vital information about the family system as a unit and about the best way to deal with the numerous and special tasks the palliative care staff must deal with when assisting the patient, from both the medical and the psychological point of view. Secondly, it allows a better tailoring of the supportive and educational interventions directed to the family during the difficult or critical phases of terminal illness (e.g. pain management, onset of delirium, or other psychiatric disorders). Thirdly, it can demonstrate the need for referral of dysfunctional families to more specific psychiatric or psychological interventions, as a way of reforming alliances with the staff and coping with the anticipation of loss. As a direct consequence of which, it represents a way to work through the subsequent phases, namely bereavement, promoting early intervention when needed.

Given the importance for the family of these last two issues in palliative care, namely anticipatory grief, on the one hand, and bereavement and grief, on the other, we will

Table 10.3 Definitions of the terminology regarding bereavement and grief

Bereavement–the loss of a person to whom one is attached

Grief–the cognitive, emotional, and behavioural reactions to bereavement

Grief work (or *grieving process*)–the psychological process of working through the loss over time

Mourning–the social expression of grief, which varies according to religion and culture

Anticipatory grief–the psychological and emotional experiences that precede bereavement

Complicated grief–the possible psychological complications of grief and the grieving process

give a short framework of this clinical area (Kissane and Bloch 1994). The definitions of the terminology used in this field are reported in Table 10.3.

10.4 **Anticipatory grief**

Anticipatory grief or anticipatory mourning is commonly described as the experience (in the broad Latin meaning of *experiri*, 'to feel', but also 'to know through', 'to learn through', 'to try') that the family, but also the patient (Hottenson 2010), goes through before the death, involving the expectations of emotional pain and the life changes that the loss will determine (Skinner Cook and Dworkin 1992; Clukey 2008).

Regarding specifically the family, it represents a way for the members to rehearse or imagine in advance the loss of their loved one and prepare themselves for working through the trauma of actual death, facilitating the adjustment to bereavement (Sweeting and Gilhooly 1990). The profound fears of the patient about his own pending death (e.g. fear of not having completed his plans, of abandoning his family to an unknown future, of being alone at the very moment of death, fears of nothingness) are intertwined with the family fears (e.g. fear of being left alone, desire for more intimacy, and at the same time for letting their loved one go).

10.4.1 **The concept and the determinants of anticipatory grief**

With regard to the literature, it must be said that different terms have been used to indicate the series of emotional events relating to the impending death of a loved one. Forewarning of loss, anticipatory loss, family emotional responses to terminal illness (or terminal response), anticipatory grief, and 'pre-mourning' phase (Evans 1994) are the most common terms used, which indicate different theories and conceptualizations in this area. In fact, some authors tend to confirm the existence of the anticipatory grief (Rando 1988), others tend to rejected this concept, rather considering a continuum between pre- and post-loss reactions (Bourke 1984), and others, complaining about the lack of data in this field, tend to criticize oversimplification of terms and point out that a vast number of variables involved should be taken into consideration (Fulton and Gottesman 1989).

Several aspects regarding this problem deserve discussion. First, the family psychological reactions during anticipatory grief are different with respect to grief, which, by definition, represents the psychological and emotional response to the actual death of a loved one (Parkes 1998c). The complex interplay of family emotional responses during anticipatory grief occurs, in fact, in a context in which the patient is not dead and still has a role, although different from the past. Intensification of attachment is shown by a strong tendency to stay close to the loved one, and overprotection may be evident in the family during anticipatory grief, but not during grief (Parkes 1998a, b, c). In contrast with these data, Hays et al. (1994) found that the family's psychological symptoms in the weeks and months before their loved one's death were undistinguishable from the early emotional reactions after his/her death. More research is needed to clarify these aspects.

A second issue concerns the concept of death itself. It has been indicated that death has multiple meanings and that, when linked to the concept of loss, it should be considered from different perspectives (Evans 1994). One perspective regards social death (thus, a form of loss), which is largely anticipated during the process of the patient's illness, as represented by the changes in and/or irreversibility of social roles, loss of identity, loss of temporal boundaries (e.g. uncertainty about the future, disillusions, regrets with lost opportunities and with plans still to be achieved). Another perspective refers to clinical and psychological deaths, which are also evident in the palliative care process, as represented by the worsening of both the patient's physical (e.g. disfigurement, pain, fatigue, debilitation, cachexia) and psychological conditions (e.g. modification of the patient's personality and onset of severe psychiatric disorders, including delirium and depression). Finally, biological death concerns the actual event of death, as a transitional point from which grief begins.

A third topic regards the nature of the interpersonal relationships between the family members and the individual psychological traits and coping abilities of the each family member, including the patient. As we have seen in the different possible styles of family functioning, it should be expected that the dynamics within the family influence the ways in which the loss of the relative is perceived and anticipated, making evident that anticipatory grief is not an 'all or nothing' phenomenon. In this respect, Zisook (2000) considers the difficult tasks for palliative care teams in dealing with possible distortions in the family anticipation of loss, such as 'premature' grief. In this situation, withdrawal from the patient, as if he had died, before the actual event can provoke in him/her feelings of abandonment and loneliness, with evident negative consequences on the terminal phase of his/her life.

A fourth problem regards sociocultural and context variables that should not be dismissed in analysing the phenomenon of anticipatory grief. The belonging culture both in broad (e.g. the values, norms, and rites of one's own culture) and in narrow terms (e.g. the values, norms, and rites of a single family) is an important variable to take into account. The interpersonal and practical resources available in the social milieu (e.g. social support systems, volunteer association, neighbourhood characteristics, church facilities) and their utilization should also be considered. Last, the context itself in which palliative care is provided (e.g. hospice, hospital palliative care units, home) makes a difference in moulding the emotional reactions of the family, as we have already discussed.

Failure to consider these multiple aspects is in large part the origin of contradictory data in the literature as far as the role of anticipatory grief in working through the process of grief after the patient's death (Fulton et al. 1996; Fulton and Gottesman 1989).

10.4.2 **The approach to anticipatory grief**

Despite all the problems we have discussed, the delicate phase of transition anticipating the loss of the patient should be approached by the health care staff with extreme attention. The specific needs of the family and their difficulties and problems should be taken into consideration and addressed in a proper way (Bates and the-Psychological-Work-Group-of-the-International-Work-Group-on-Death-Dying-and-Bereavement 1993; McMillan 2005). It has been pointed out that maintaining an honest and open communication with the family about the patient's clinical situation, giving information about the evolution of the disease, responding to questions and doubts the family can have, and reassuring them about the patient's symptom control and physical comfort and encouraging family members to express their feelings are important objectives the health staff should pursue (Ferrell 1998). Guilty feelings (e.g. 'We should have tried other options and therapies', 'We had not done all we could for him', 'I have horrible thoughts, hoping that all this can finish soon and wishing he can die'), fears (e.g. 'We are not able to see him worsening and deteriorating day after day', 'We are too weak and emotionally engulfed to help him'; 'Will we be able to meet his expectancies?'), anger (e.g. 'What have we done to deserve this?', 'How is possible that medicine cannot do anything?', 'The health system is servant of the power and does not care for real people with real problems'), or denial (e.g. 'We don't think the situation is so severe', 'There should have been some mistake, it is not possible that everything is going in a bad way') should be acknowledged, listened to, and understood (Faulkner and Maguire 1994; Maguire 2000). It is suggested that communication between family members should be favoured (Twycross and Lichter 1998), although the modality must follow the family and the patient's own needs, wishes, values, religion, and culture. Staying close to their relative and sharing with him feelings, affection, and love may help to address unresolved conflicts, to forgive and be forgiven, to reciprocally thank, and to say good-bye in the most proper way. It has been recently found that family caregivers who have the opportunity to express their love through care of a close member with terminal cancer can experience strong positive emotions (Grbich et al. 2001).

In the most advanced phases of illness, if the patient is delirious or unconscious, the family presence is important and communication, even if the patient seems unable to show any response, should be maintained. The family should feel helpful and adequate in what they are doing and every effort and action reinforced and complimented, as a tangible sign of their personal and unique way to comfort their loved one. Through constant support it is possible that the family is able to transcend and find meaning in their caregiving experience. In connection with this, it has been shown that, among family members of terminally ill patients, finding meaning involved 'being with' or 'doing for' their loved one, as death approached, and that this search for a meaning had positive consequences for the caregivers in the long run (Enyert and Burman 1999).

Attention to the family's own wishes and needs is also necessary. Family members should be encouraged to take into consideration their needs, correcting the misconception about being judged selfish or detached if they take some rest and reassuring them about the importance of recuperating energy in order to reduce the risk of their own psychological or physical breakdown. The family should also be respectfully encouraged to receive professional help if conflicts and emotional disruption emerge.

With respect to this, Kissane et al. (1998) developed a 6- to 8-session family intervention plan with the aim of reducing the level of distress in dysfunctional families during a palliative care programme. All the themes that emerged during the sessions (e.g. previous experiences with loss and bereavement, existential themes of suffering and death, difficulties in sharing intimacy and saying good-bye to their loved one, problems in receiving or utilizing care, conflicts within the members) were reviewed and analysed. The aim of the intervention is to facilitate cohesiveness among members and their communication and problem-solving skills, and to decrease, at the same time, family conflicts, in order to improve the functioning of the family as a unit in caring for their relative. More recently the same authors (Kissane et al. 2003, 2006) screened 257 families of patients dying from cancer by using the Family Relationship Inventory and identified 183 (71%) as dysfunctional and at risk for psychosocial morbidity. Those who participated in family-focused grief therapy (53 families, 233 individuals) and had high baseline scores on the Brief Symptom Inventory and Beck Depression Inventory reported significant improvements in distress and depression in comparison with controls, even if global family functioning did not change. The data indicated that family-focused grief therapy has the potential of preventing pathological grief. Benefit is clear for intermediate and sullen families.

In a different study, McMillan et al. (2006) used a coping skills training to help families to adjust to the different difficult situations to be dealt with in palliative care in hospice among 354 family caregivers of advanced cancer patients. By randomly dividing the sample into standard hospice care, standard hospice care plus three supportive visits, and standard care plus three visits to teach a coping skills intervention, they found that the coping skills intervention led to significantly greater improvement in caregiver quality of life ($p = 0.03$), burden of patient symptoms ($p < 0.001$), and caregiving task burden ($p = 0.038$) than did the other two conditions.

More recently, Hudson et al. (2008) tested the efficacy of a group education programme delivered in three consecutive weekly sessions and conducted at six home-based palliative care services. Among 44 caregivers completing the program, the authors found a significant positive effect for preparedness for the caring role, caregiving competence, caregiving rewards and having information needs met from commencement of the programme (T1) and upon completion (T2).

Further data regarding the role of early intervention in palliative care derive from the studies carried out by Chochinov and his group in Canada. Dignity therapy is a novel therapeutic intervention designed to address psychosocial and existential distress among the terminally ill that allows patients to discuss things most important to them and to articulate things they would most want remembered as they neared death, eventually recording and transcribing these discussions into a 'generativity document' to be given to the family (Chochinov et al. 2004, 2005), McClement et al. (2007) showed that 78% of the family members reported that the therapy helped them during their time of grief; 77% reported that the generativity document would continue to be a source of comfort for their families and themselves; and 95% reported they would recommend dignity therapy to other patients of family members confronting a terminal illlness, considering it as a therapeutic intervention that moderates their bereavement experiences and lessens suffering and distress in terminally ill relatives.

Thus attention to the psychological reactions of the family during anticipatory grief is a specific component of the palliative care programme, in order to provide support and recognize both dysfunctional patterns and the possible onset of psychiatric symptoms as early as possible (Zeitlin 2001), as illustrated in the following situation that we had to deal with in our practice.

Case report

The home palliative-care staff are having difficulties dealing with the family problems emerging in the care of Mrs A, a 65-year-old woman affected by diffuse bone metastasis, secondary to breast cancer, and who has been bed-ridden for 3 months. In fact, the relationship between the staff and Mrs A's husband, Mr P., a 68-year-old man, has gradually worsened because of his increasing requests for home intervention ('my wife needs a home visit twice a day'), his dissatisfaction of and complains about whatever the staff are doing, his inability to help his wife, and a diffuse sense of impotence and despair that prevents the man from leaving the home, since he wants to be with his wife 'every minute of the day and night'. The couple live alone and there is no other support from relatives or friends. After a few weeks, the situation seems unmanageable, and the sense of failure and anger in the staff is increasing, with negative consequences on the quality of the care provided to the patient. After discussing the situation in a meeting with the C-L psychiatric service, a domiciliary psychiatric visit is programmed. Mrs A. seems to be well adjusted to her situation and satisfied of the care she is receiving, but worried for the deterioration of her husband's psychological status. Mr P., seated at his wife's bedside, shows high levels of anxiety and only after several attempts is he convinced to move to another room to speak more openly about his perception of the situation. At mental status examination, Mr P. appears hypervigilant and anxiously attentive, and, with a low tone of voice, begins to speak about his problems. He describes the difficult situation at home, rapidly shifting his attention to his own physical conditions, specifically his diabetes that he has been affected by for ten years and has caused several hospital admissions and medical complications, such as sight problems and difficulty in deambulation. He is markedly preoccupied about the deterioration of his diabetes, his mood is depressed, he feels desperate, worthless, and guilty for his inability to help his wife ('I am too tired and weak that I cannot do anything at home') and hopeless about the future ('My wife will die and I also will die soon from my own disease'). Assessment of his personal history shows two previous episodes of major depression in the past ten years. During the first one (concomitant with the diagnosis of diabetes), Mr P. was followed by the Community Mental Health Service for a while through psychopharmacological intervention and supportive counselling. A diagnosis of a major depressive disorder, recurrent type, is made, antidepressant therapy is prescribed, and a joint home-care programme with the Mental Health Service is planned for the following day.

In this case, the history of the family, its previous and current functioning, and the impact of the present illness would have been of remarkable help to the palliative care team in order for them to be able to respond in the correct manner. The fact that the husband was affected by an important physical illness, such as diabetes, may have determined a significant impact on the couple, with a sense of vulnerability in the husband, need for readjustment as far as the roles in the family are concerned, and maybe economic problems. The onset of depressive episode in concomitance with the diagnosis of diabetes and of a recurrent one some years later indicate in fact the high psychological vulnerability of the husband, which caused the need for psychiatric help. Thus it would have been predictable that, given these antecedents, the onset and progression of cancer in the wife might have had a severe impact on the husband himself, creating the basis for a new depressive episode.

10.5 Bereavement

At the death of the patient, the family begins the process of grieving. Grief is a human, universal, and healthy psychological response to the loss of a loved one. It has important aims, specifically that of gradually accepting the reality of the death, accommodating to the absence of the loved one, coming to terms with the changes of that the

Table 10.4 Common symptoms and phenomenology of normal grief

Feelings	Cognitive and perceptual symptoms
Shock	Disbelief
Numbness	Confusion
Yearning	Preoccupation
Anxiety	Sense of presence
Anger	Perceptual alterations (illusions, misinterpretations, possible hallucinations)
Sadness	
Guilt and self-reproach	**Behavioural symptoms**
Loneliness	Restless overactivity
Apathy	Searching and calling out
Helplessness	Sleep disturbances
Emancipation	Appetite disturbances
Relief	Social withdrawal
	Sighing and crying
Physical symptoms	Visiting places or carrying objects that remind the survivor of the deceased
Hollowness in the stomach	
Tightness in the chest and throat	Treasuring objects that belonged to the deceased
Breathlessness	
Lack of energy	Avoiding reminders of the deceased
Weakness	
Pain and muscle tension	

loss has determined in the life of the bereaved, and reorganizing one's own internal models. The main symptoms that emerge during grief are presented in Table 10.4.

These symptoms do not occur contemporarily, but follow the grief trajectory, which, although it is non-linear and tends to vary from person to person, it is usually conceptualized as a series of stages or phases. Over time, several authors, such as Kübler-Ross (1969), Worden (2009), Parkes (1998b), Maciejewski et al. (2007), and Prigerson and Maciejewski (2008) have proposed theoretical models that can be used as a way for understanding the process of grief, as synthetically described in Table 10.5.

Although grief is a normal reaction to a human event, i.e. the loss of a loved one, this does not mean that support during the grieving is unnecessary. Usually bereaved persons are helped by other family members, close friends, and interpersonal and social resources, including religious affiliation systems, associations, or self-help groups, where they exist. However, the importance for clinicians and health professionals to be trained in helping persons who are experiencing grief after the death of a loved one has been pointed out as a necessity in palliative care (Katz and Chochinov 1998; Grassi 2007).

As far as palliative care settings are concerned, data from the hospice experience indicate the importance of maintaining a relationship with the bereaved family and providing them with different kinds of support (e.g. practical, educational, counseling; Sheldon 1998). Parkes (1998b) warns us to avoid simplistic and schematic approaches to a complex, but at the same time natural phenomenon, like grief. Medicalization of what is part of life is not useful, whereas humanity, empathy, and compassion in the relationship with the bereaved is welcomed. Basically, active listening to the person, allowing expression of the feelings that family members can or want to express (e.g. anger, guilt, anxiety, sadness, hopelessness, helplessness, fear of not being able to carry on one's life), reassuring about the normality of these reactions, offering support, and maintaining follow-up is important for the bereaved family in being accepted and not left alone in their suffering (Gregory 1994).

For these reasons, it has been strongly suggested that community palliative care teams improve their skills in evaluating the specific needs and in providing proper care during the bereavement follow-ups for families of deceased patients (Broomberg and Higginson 1996; Kutner and Kilbourn 2009; Payne and Relf 1990). This seems well worth considering in order to provide the family with a continuity of care that involves community health care systems, including general practitioners (GPs). In fact, although some studies have indicated that the family does not expect special action from their GP (Dangler et al. 1996), others have shown that almost 50% of the families consider their GP's intervention as helpful (Siegel et al. 1991). In a more recent evaluation of bereaved families, the majority would have appreciated a letter of sympathy form their GPs, and over half expressed some form of dissatisfaction either with their GP or with the hospital (Main 2000).

Given the significant change in the health care organization in palliative care services in many countries and the significant role of GPs in providing home care for patients with advanced illness (Robinson and Stacy 1994; Steinmetz et al. 1993), more effort and research are necessary to address the training needs of primary care physicians in assessing bereavement and in counselling families (Farber et al. 1999; Hermann et al. 1999). In this respect, it has been shown that most GPs tend to be worried about

Table 10.5 Models of normal grief

Stages of grief (Kübler-Ross 1969)	
Denial	Shock and numbness about death, scanning the environment for sights or sounds of the deceased one
Bargaining	Hoping for the return of the loved one and making promises if it would happen
Anger	Frustration, anger towards the fate and/or the doctors
Depression	Deep sadness and pain for the reality and irrimediability of the death
Acceptance	Reorganization and return to live, retaining the memories without prolonged pain
Phases of grief (Parkes 1998b)	
Numbness and blunting	Shock, denial, feelings of unreality that can last hours or days
Pining and yearning	Intense pining, cry, separation anxiety, anger, irritability, self-reproach, loss of security and self-esteem
Disorganization and despair	Apathy and despair, isolation and disengagement from social life, feelings of mutilation
Reorganization and recovery	Gradual return to life, resurgence of interests, willingness to plan for the future
Tasks of grief (Worden 2009)	
To accept the reality of the loss	Confront the reality of loss and overcome normal tendency to deny the event of death
To work through the pain of grief	Experience pain and feelings of depression, isolation, emptiness due to the loss of the loved one
To adjust to an environment in which the deceased is missing	Develop new skills to adjust to new roles, to a new sense of self, to a new sense of the world
To emotionally relocate the deceased and move on with life	Find a place for the deceased in one's emotional life, think of the loved one with sadness, but not with overwhelming feelings of despair

States Theory of Grief (Maciejewski et al. 2007; Prigerson and Maciejewski 2008)

Based on 5 indicators: disbelief, yearning, anger, depression, and acceptance

Disbelief is high in the first period then decreases;

Yearning is high in a second period then decreases while anger increases;

Then anger decreases while depression increases;

Then depression decreases;

Acceptance gradually increases throughout the period.

a) Between 1 and 6 months post-loss and 6 and 12 months post-loss, disbelief and yearning decline and acceptance increases

b) From 6 to 12 months post-loss and 12 to 24 months post-loss, disbelief, yearning, anger, and depression decline and acceptance increases.

making clinical or diagnostic mistakes and report feelings of guilt about the death of their patients. However, they feel, at the same time, that it is their responsibility to make contacts with the bereaved patients, complaining of a lack of specific bereavement strategies to help the family (Saunderson and Ridsdale 1999). Likewise, other studies have indicated that family physicians acknowledge that bereavement presented significant health risks to their patients and that the identification and treatment of bereaved patients is an important part of their role (Lemkau et al. 2000). Over the past few years attention to this area has increased enormously, with literature clearly indicating that GPs, and clinicians in general, need more specific training about the clinical and intervention implications necessary for both palliative care intervention (Ewing et al. 2006; Mitchell, 2002) and bereavement (Casarett et al. 2001; Charlton and Dolman 1995; Hermann et al. 1999; Woof and Carter 1997a, b).

Providing continuity of care during bereavement can also facilitate the evaluation of the grieving process over time and the referral of maladaptive situations that need intervention by specialist services. In fact, although literature is lacking about this area, it has been found that almost half of bereaved people meet the criteria for a psychiatric disorder during the first year of bereavement or show forms of maladaptive grief (Jacobs et al. 1990; Middleton et al. 1996), as we will describe in the next section.

10.6 **Complicated grief**

The problem of psychiatric morbidity and maladaptive reactions following bereavement has been, in fact, the focus of intense research for a long time. Different definitions for describing the possible psychiatric complications during bereavement, such as *abnormal grief, complicated bereavement, atypical grief, unresolved grief,* and *pathological grief* have been proposed (Katz and Chochinov 1998; Stroebe et al. 2000; Zeitlin 2001). Even if it is clear that structural distinctions are possible between normal and complicated grief (Dillen et al. 2008), the different terminology used, in part, reflects disagreement about the different clinical characteristics of complicated grief. For some authors, in line with the current psychiatric nosological systems, depressive disorders should be considered the most frequent and significant pathological evolution of grief (Bonanno and Kaltman 2001), while other authors sustain the need to describe and classify complicated grief in a more detailed way (Jacobs et al. 2000) . As far as the former hypothesis, the DSM-IV (American Psychiatric Association 1994) and its Text Revision (DSM-IV-TR; American Psychiatric Association 2000) dedicate a short paragraph to bereavement, which is included in the chapter 'Other Conditions That May Focus Clinical Attention'. The DSM-IV-TR states that

> [the] duration and expression of normal bereavement vary considerably among different cultural groups. The diagnosis of Major Depressive Disorder (MDD) is generally not given unless the symptoms are still present two months after the loss. However, the presence of certain symptoms that are not characteristics of normal grief reaction may be helpful in differentiating bereavement from Major Depressive Episode [MDE]. These include: (1) guilt about things other than actions taken or not taken by the survivor at the time of the death; (2) thoughts of death other than the survivor feeling that he or she

would be better off dead or should have died with the deceased person; (3) morbid preoccupation with worthlessness; (4) marked psychomotor retardation; (5) prolonged and marked functional impairment; and (6) hallucinatory experiences other than thinking that he or she hears the voice, or transiently sees the image of the deceased person.

Uncomplicated bereavement as well as uncomplicated depressive reactions secondary to other losses are in this sense different from major depression (Wakefield et al. 2007), whereas complicated grief with depressed features is subsumed under the diagnosis of MDD. However, clinical experience and research data indicate that the problems of bereavement-related depression are not solved and that the exclusion criterion of bereavement from the diagnosis of MDD should be revised. In a study of more 300 subjects, Kendler et al. (2008) evaluated whether cases of bereavement-related depression that also met DSM criteria for 'normal grief' were qualitatively distinct from other depressive cases related to stressful events. The authors found that the similarities between bereavement-related depression and depression related to other stressful life events substantially outweigh their differences and, thus, questioned the validity of the bereavement exclusion for the diagnosis of MDD. Similar results were reported in a large study of 685 subjects (Karam et al. 2009) in which the multiple features of bereavement related to non-bereavement-related MDD were compared without showing specific differences between the two conditions. Likewise, Corruble et al. (2009), in a large population of patients with MDD without bereavement and bereavement-excluded subjects showing depressive symptoms, found that bereavement-excluded subjects were more severely depressed than MDE controls without bereavement and similar to MDD controls with bereavement. The authors concluded that symptom cues of the DSM-IV MDD bereavement exclusion criterion should be modified since they could result in patients failing to be correctly diagnosed and treated.

Besides the problem of depression, other clinical conditions that go unresolved should be considered in grief. In fact, symptoms and/or behaviours, other than depression, can develop and clearly indicate a poor grieving response that has significant interference of or impairment in the individual functioning.

Classification of complicated grief is not homogeneous. Worden (2009) and Skinner Cook and Dworkin (1992) described four possible pathological forms: chronic grief, delayed grief, masked grief, and exaggerated grief (with psychiatric features). The latter authors added also avoidance of grief. Jacobs (1993) and Parkes (1998b) generally agree to consider three forms: traumatic loss, conflicted grief, and chronic grief. Zisook (2000) suggested separating the forms that exacerbate or favour the onset of a medical or psychiatric condition (e.g. major depression, anxiety disorder) from specific complications of grief, namely absent, delayed, or inhibited grief; hypertrophied grief; and chronic grief. The characteristics of these disorders are indicated in Table 10.6.

By using a more specific methodological approach, over the past few years, psychiatric literature has confirmed that, within the realm of complicated grief, depressive disorders secondary to bereavement should be separated from other clinical disturbances, which have their own phenomenological expression. By starting from the concept of the traumatic nature that a death of loved one can have for the bereaved person, Horowitz et al. (1997) conducted a 14-month follow-up study of 70 bereaved spouses. They showed that symptoms of complicated grief did not overlap with those presented

Table 10.6 Possible forms of complicated grief

Psychiatric disorders following bereavement (exaggerated grief)

Major depression

Anxiety disorders

Eating disorders

Substance abuse disorders

Brief psychotic reactions

Avoidance of grief

Mummification with prolonged treasuring objects and tendency to leave everything (e.g. the person's room, personal objects, wearing) as immediately before death

Idealization of the quality of the deceased person and magnification of the loss

Persistent anger or guilt response rather than acceptance of death

Chronic grief (or prolonged grief)

Excessive duration of grief response, with difficulty to speak about the death without intense overwhelming after several years from loss

Themes of loss coming out during daily conversation

Inability to resume one's own life and adjust to new roles

Delayed grief

Re-experience of excessive grief reactions secondary to new stressful events or losses and re-emergence of symptoms linked to the past loss

Inhibited grief (or masked grief)

Onset of physical complaints resembling the physical illness of the deceased ('facsimile illness')

Physical symptoms (e.g. pain)

Behavioural problems (e.g. impulsive decisions, poor health care, promiscuity, acting out)

by subjects who received a diagnosis of major depression and, on this basis, they proposed diagnostic criteria for complicated grief (Horowitz et al. 1993) as a syndrome characterized by a combination of sustained intrusion, avoidance, and maladaptation symptoms following the loss of a close person (Table 10.7).

In a study of bereaved persons, Langner and Maercker (2005) confirmed Horowitz's classification of symptoms into intrusion, avoidance, and failure-to-adapt categories, with high diagnostic accuracy of the symptom criteria and a meaningful correlational pattern to standard measures of divergent psychopathology and normal grief reactions. According to the study the application of a stress response operationalization of complicated grief is supported.

In a series of studies Prigerson and her group (1995, 1996) could distinguish between symptoms indicating complicated grief and those indicating bereavement-related depression. The authors, in a longitudinal study of subjects interviewed at the time of their spouse's hospital admission and at 6, 13, and 25 months after the loved one's

Table 10.7 Proposed criteria for complicated grief disorder (Horowitz et al. 1997)

Event criterion/prolonged response criterion

Bereavement (loss of a spouse, other relative, or intimate partner) at least 14 months ago (12 months is avoided because of possible intense turbulence from an anniversary reaction)

Signs and symptoms criteria

During the past month, any three of the following seven symptoms have occurred with a severity that interferes with daily functioning

Intrusive thoughts

1. Unbidden memories or intrusive fantasies related to the lost relationship

2. Strong spells or pangs of severe emotion related to the lost relationship

3. Distressingly strong yearnings or wishes that the deceased were there

Signs of avoidance and failure to adapt

4. Feelings of being far too much alone or personally empty

5. Excessively staying away from people, places, or activities that remind the subject of the deceased

6. Unusual levels of sleep interference

7. Loss of interest in work, social, caretaking, or recreational activities to a maladaptive degree

---

death, also found that traumatic grief at 6 months after the death predicted negative health outcomes (e.g. high blood pressure, suicidal ideation, changes in eating behaviour) in the survivor (Prigerson et al. 1997). At a first consensus conference, the possible criteria of traumatic grief have been proposed by the same group (Prigerson et al. 1999) as a guide to help clinicians recognize and treat bereaved individuals who do not adjust to the loss of their relative (Table 10.8).

On this basis, the authors have tried to validate the criteria for what has been called *complicated grief* (Lichtenthal et al. 2004) and, more recently, *prolonged grief disorder* (PGD) as a proposal for inclusion in DSM-V and ICD-11, considering the distinctive phenomenology, aetiology, course, response to treatment, and adverse outcomes associated with PGD symptoms (Prigerson et al. 2008, 2009). PGD is characterized by the following criteria:

A. Event: Bereavement (loss of a significant other);

B. Separation distress: The bereaved person experiences yearning (e.g. craving, pining, or longing for the deceased; physical or emotional suffering as a result of the desired, but unfulfilled, reunion with the deceased) daily or to a disabling degree;

C. Cognitive, emotional, and behavioral symptoms: The bereaved person must have 5 (or more) of the following symptoms experienced daily or to a disabling degree:

  1. Confusion about one's role in life or diminished sense of self (i.e. feeling that a part of oneself has died);

  2. Difficulty accepting the loss;

Table 10.8 Proposed criteria for traumatic grief (Prigerson et al. 1999)

Crtierion A

1) Person has experienced the death of a significant other

2) Response involves 3 of the following 4 symptoms experienced at least sometimes:

    a) Intrusive thoughts about the deceased

    b) Yearning for the deceased

    c) Searching for the deceased

    d) Loneliness as a result of death

Criterion B

In response to the death, 4 of the 8 following symptoms are experienced as mostly true:

1) Purposelessness or feeling of futility about the future

2) Subjective sense of numbness, detachment, or absence of emotional responsiveness

3) Difficulty acknowledging the death (e.g. disbelief)

4) Feeling that life is empty or meaningless

5) Feeling that part of oneself has died

6) Shattered world view (e.g. lost sense of security, trust, control)

7) Assumes symptoms or harmful behaviours of, or related to, the deceased person

8) Excessive irritability, bitterness, or anger related to the death

Criterion C

Duration of disturbance (symptom lasting at least 2 months)

Criterion D

The disturbance causes clinically significant impairment in social, occupational, or other important areas of functioning

---

    3. Avoidance of reminders of the reality of the loss;

    4. Inability to trust others since the loss;

    5. Bitterness or anger related to the loss;

    6. Difficulty moving on with life (e.g. making new friends, pursuing interests);

    7. Numbness (absence of emotion) since the loss;

    8. Feeling that life is unfulfilling, empty, or meaningless since the loss; and

    9. Feeling stunned, dazed, or shocked by the loss.

D. Timing: Diagnosis should not be made until at least 6 months have elapsed since the death.

E. Impairment: The disturbance causes clinically significant impairment in social, occupational, or other important areas of functioning (e.g. domestic responsibilities).

F. Relation to other mental disorders: The disturbance is not better accounted for by major depressive disorder, generalized anxiety disorder, or post-traumatic stress disorder.

Despite these efforts, when different classification systems of complicated grief (e.g. Horowitz et al. 1997; Prigerson et al. 1999) were compared in a representative sample of elderly population, Forstmeier and Maercker (2007) found a prevalence of 4.2% by using Horowitz et al.'s system and 0.9% by using Prigerson et al.'s system, with a poor agreement between the two methods ($\kappa = 0.13$). Furthermore, the conditional probabilities of developing complicated grief after experiencing a major bereavement were 22.2% (Horowitz et al.'s system) and 4.6% (Prigerson et al.'s system).

10.6.1 Risk factors and consequences of complicated grief

An important aspect related to complicated grief refers to the identification of its risk factors. From a research point of view, Kissane et al. (1996) carried out a study, the Melbourne Family Grief Study, involving 115 families who were followed for a year after bereavement. The authors showed that dysfunctional families, as described in the previous section (i.e. sullen and hostile families) presented the highest psychosocial morbidity during bereavement. In the palliative care setting, Robinson et al. (1995) have confirmed the value of using a bereavement risk index in the course of the palliative care process to predict complicated grief after bereavement, and Kissane et al. (1998) showed that family coping style (related to family functioning) was the most consistent correlate of bereavement outcome (grief, distress, depression, and social adjustment). Table 10.9 summarizes the most significant risk factors implicated in complicated grief that can be acknowledged in the assessment of the family during the palliative care process.

The importance of identifying risk factors for all the possible forms of pathological/complicated grief is evident by examining the negative consequences on the bereaved person not only at the psychological level (e.g. higher risk of suicide; Johnson et al. 2008), but also at the levels concerning physical health and quality of life. In fact, it has been shown that bereaved persons with pathological/complicated grief are more prone to physical illness, especially cardiovascular diseases, and at higher risk of death (Lannen et al. 2008; Prigerson et al. 1997; Schaefer et al. 1995; Silverman et al. 2000; Stroebe and Stroebe 1993). The mechanisms are related to both indirect (e.g. poor healthy behaviours) and direct causes (e.g. neuroendocrine alterations and increased of proinflammatory cytokines, reduction of the immunity system activity; Glaser 2005; Irwin and Miller 2007; Kemeny 2009; O'Connor 2005).

Taken together all these aspects indicate the need for more attention to evaluation of grief responses in palliative care settings in order to ascertain the onset of possible complications and to intervene with early and appropriate treatment (Stroebe et al. 2000; Zhang et al. 2006), as the following case clearly explicates.

Table 10.9 Risk factors for complicated grief

Historical variables

History of family dysfunction

History of multiple losses

Previous complicated grief

Previous psychiatric disturbances (e.g. depressive disorders, substance abuse)

Personality variables

Poor self-esteem and self-efficacy

Tendency to repress emotions

Tendency to physiological activation in facing stress rather than psychological activation

Relational variables

Ambivalent relationship with the deceased

Dependent relationship with the deceased

Conflicted relationship with the deceased

Circumstantial variables

Uncertainty of death (e.g. disappeared persons, catastrophes)

Sudden and unpredictable death

Untimely death of young person

Stigmatized deaths (e.g. AIDS, suicide)

Culpable deaths

Social variables

Poor or inadequate support from social ties

Social reinforcement for secondary gains

Adapted from Sheldon (1998); Skinner Cook and Dworkin (1992); and Worden (2009).

Case report

Ms G., a 32-year-old woman, was admitted to internal medicine for physical complications and a facial trauma occurred during alcohol intoxication. Her physical conditions were very poor. She was suffering from a hepatic pre-cirrhosis state secondary to alcohol abuse with laboratory and clinical testing indicating the need for intensive treatment. Nevertheless, Ms G. tended to refuse every kind of medical intervention, including blood transfusion, oral and IV therapy, and insistently asked to be discharged. She was referred to the C-L Psychiatric Service to evaluate the possibility of involuntary physical treatment for psychiatric reasons. She reluctantly accepted psychiatric evaluation 'only to be let to leave the hospital'. At the meeting with the psychiatrist, Ms G. was very upset, angry, and contradictive. She wanted to be discharged immediately or she would call the police to sue the hospital. She denied any problem, including drug use, and minimized her clinical conditions, including her three previous admissions to the general hospital within the past two months. Gently confronted with the real risk she could die and the reasons she was punishing herself so badly, a very sad scenario gradually emerged 'from the dark' ('I live only in the dark'). Ms G. belonged to a very disruptive family, where the father had separated from the mother, even though he continued to live in the same apartment. Her father never cared for the family nor his two sons (Ms G. had an older brother, who was also an alcohol-abuser). The only affectionate bond was with her mother, a good and hard-working woman, the 'victim of my father'. Unfortunately, Ms G.'s mother developed a uterine cancer, which, at the time of the diagnosis, had already spread and curative treatments were not possible. Ms G.'s mother was repeatedly admitted to the hospital, because of rapid worsening of physical conditions. During the last admission, Ms G. was the only family member constantly present nearby her mother. Ms G. was not ready to lose her mother. She did not believe that she should be alone by her mother's side, but no one else wanted to share 'this responsibility' with her. She did not accept that the only good bond could be destroyed like 'a broken dream over night'. During the last day of her mother's life, Ms G. assisted her all day long. Her mother's abdominal pain, marginally controlled by drugs, and breathing problems, marginally controlled by an oxygen mask, were unbearable burdens for Ms G. Her mother wanted to speak with her, but the oxygen mask prevented a clear communication and, when the mask was taken off, breathing problems immediately worsened. The old lady whispered to her daughter 'help me, take off this mask, it is unbearable.' Ms G. obeyed and in a few seconds her mother died.

All this happened six years ago and since then Ms G. had started to drink heavily, convinced that she killed her mother. She thought that life had no meaning and no redemption. She said that she had never told this story before because no psychiatrist or psychologist ever saw her after bereavement.

It is evident that palliative care professionals have the opportunity to observe some problematic areas of family functioning and possible risk factors for psychological disorders that can emerge in both the anticipatory grief and bereavement phases. As indicated by the End-of-life Care Consensus Panel (Casarett and Inouye 2001), correct and repeated assessments and early and proper intervention, including psychological or psychiatric referral in case of complications, are thus the necessary elements that characterize a holistic process of care before and after the death of the patient (Table 10.10).

Table 10.10 Steps in the care of the family during anticipatory grief and bereavement

Anticipatory grief

- Assess family history and functioning
- Assess social support and coping resources
- Encourage open discussion [a]
- Facilitate emotional expression [a]
- Clarify plans for the future

Acute grief

- Be present
- Provide time and permission to grieve [a]
- Assess need for assistance and immediate plan
- Offer support and follow-up appointments

Early bereavement (< 1 month)

- Elicit concerns about the symptoms of grief
- Evaluate the characteristics of grief symptoms
- Reassure about the normality of grief reactions
- Reassess social support resources
- Examine possible practical needs and problems

Late bereavement (> 1 month)

- Assess progress of mourning
- Identify symptoms indicating possible complicated grief
- Refer for counselling or specialist intervention when needed

[a] According to the family own culture and values.
Data adapted from Casarett et al. (2001).

10.7 **Conclusions**

In this short review we have tried to show how the difficult voyage within the domain of palliative care involves all the members (patient, family, and staff) who are together protagonists of the life–death mystery. The different aspects that emerge during this phase should be taken into consideration when assisting terminally ill patients and their families. With this respect, confusional states are an example of the way in which a disorder that the patients may present can be interpreted by using a holistic perspective. This perspective should take into account not only biological and clinical aspects (i.e. aetiology, symptoms, clinical subtypes, treatment), but the psychological and interpersonal as well. From this point of view, delirium seems to represent the extreme attempt to chaotically maintain a sense in a world that is collapsing and, at the same time, the expression of the loss of contact with a painful reality. Delirium is also the expression of something uncontrollable and terrible that transforms for the family the sense of coherence of their system. Giving a sense to this disorder, as a part of the trajectory of the advanced phase of illness, is a complex but important task, especially when suffering seems to be endless, pointless, and meaningless. Assisting the patient and the family (according to the Latin etymology of *adsistere*, 'to stay nearby', 'to stay still', but also 'to defend') in a clinical sense (according to the Greek etymology of κλινω, 'to stay' and 'to be towards') has thus a precise significance for the palliative care programmes. Among the different significances, it means to give the patient and the family the hope that it is possible to accept to be in a world of finitude and fallibility and to face our own mortality as the ultimate truth of our being-in-the-world.

It also provides a sense of authenticity in the relationship between the health professional and the patient/family systems, as has been repeatedly pointed out by philosophical and psychiatric existential traditions both in the past (e.g. Frankl 1984) and in more recent times (Van Deurzen and Arnold-Baker 2005). This deserves to be specifically considered nowadays in the field of palliative medicine, which shares so many aspects with the areas of mental health and psychiatry (Chochinov 2008). The recent interest in existential foundations of meaning and spirituality in light of terminal illness and palliative care (Breitbart et al. 2004; Chochinov and Cann 2005; Okon 2005; Sinclair et al. 2006) represents one of the most significant examples of the integration and need for an ample perspective that health care professionals should have in the care of the family and patients at the end of their life.

References

Aakerlund, L.P., and Rosenberg, J. (1994). Writing disturbances; an indicator for postoperative delirium, *Int J Psychiatry Med*, **24** 245–57.

Alao, A.O., and Moskowitz, L. (2006). Aripiprazole and delirium. *Ann Clin Psychiatry* **18**, 267–9.

Alao, A.O., Soderberg, M., Pohl, E.L., and Koss, M. (2005). Aripiprazole in the treatment of delirium. *Int J Psychiatry Med*.**35**(4), 429–33.

Alonso-Babarro, A., Varela-Cerdeira, M. A., Torres, I., Rodrí Guez-Barrientos, R., and Bruera, E. (2010). At-home palliative sedation for end-of-life cancer patients. *Palliat Med*. [Epub ahead of print]

Adams, F. (1861). The extant work of Aretaeus, The Cappadocian, Sydenham Society, London.

Adams, F. (1988). Neuropsychiatric evaluation and treatment of delirium in cancer patients, *Adv Psychosom Med*, **18**, 26–36.

Adams, R.D., and Foley, J.M., (1953). The neurological disorder associate with liver disease, *Res Publ Assoc Res Nerv Ment Dis*, **32**, 198–237.

Adamis, D., Morrison, C., Treloar, A., Macdonald, A.J., and Martin, F.C. (2005). The performance of the Clock Drawing Test in elderly medical inpatients: does it have utility in the identification of delirium? *J Geriatr Psychiatry Neurol*. **18**(3), 129–33.

Adamis, D., Van Munster, B.C., and Macdonald, A.J. (2009). The genetics of deliria. *Int Rev Psychiatry*.**21**, 20–29.

Agostini, J.V., Leo-Summers, L.S., and Inouye, S.K., (2001). Cognitive and other side adverse effects of diphenhydramine use in hospitalized older patients. *Arch. Intern. Med*. **161**, 2091–97.

Akechi, T., Uchitomi, Y., Okamura, H., Fukue, M., Kagaya, A., Nishida, A., Oomori, N. and Yamawaki, S., (1996). Usage of haloperidol for delirium in cancer patients. *Supp. Care Cancer* **4**, 390–2.

Akechi, T., Kugaya, A., Okamura, H., Nakano, T., Okuyama, T., Mikami, I., Sima, Y., Yamawaki, S. and Uchitomi, Y., (1999). Suicidal toughts in cancer patients: clinical experience in psycho-oncology. *Psychiatry Clin. Neurosci*. **53**, 569–73.

Akechi, T., Okuyama, T., Sugawara, Y., Nakano, T., Shima, Y., and Uchitomi, Y. (2004). Suicidality in terminally ill Japanese patients with cancer. *Cancer* **100**,183–91.

Albert, M.S., Levkoff, S.E., Reilly, C.R., Lipzin, B., Pilgrim, D., Cleary, P., Evans, D., and Rowe, J.W., (1992). The delirium symptom interview: an interview for the detection of delirium symtoms in hospitalized patients. *J. Geriatr. Psychiatry Neurol*. **5**, 14–21.

Alciati, A., Fusi, A., D'Arminio Monforte, A., Coen, M., Ferri, A. and Mellado, C.M.-. (2001). New-onset delusions and hallucinations in patients infected with HIV. *J. Psychiatry Neurosci*. **26**, 229–34.

Aldemir, M., Ozen, S., Kara, I.H., Sir, A. and Bac, B., (2001). Predisposing factors for delirium in the surgical intensive care unit. *Crit. Care Med*. **5**, 265–70.

American Psychiatric Association (1980). Diagnostic and Statistical Manual of Mental Disorders, 3rd edn [DSM-III]. American Psychiatric Press, Washington.

American Psychiatric Association (1987). Diagnostic and statistical manual of mental disorders. 3rd edn revised [DSM-III-R]. American Psychiatry Association, Washington, DC.

American Psychiatric Association (1994). Diagnostic and Statistical Manual of Mental Disorders, 4th edn [DSM-IV]. American Psychiatric Association, Washington DC.

American Psychiatric Association (1995). Diagnostic and Statistical Manual of Mental Disorders, 4th edn [DSM-IV-TM], Primary care version. American Psychiatric Press, Washington.

American Psychiatric Association (1999). Practice guideline for the treatment of patients with delirium. Am. J. Psychiatry **156**, 1–20.

American Psychiatric Association (2000). Diagnostic and Statistical Manual of Mental Disorders, 4th edn, Text revision [DSM IV-TR]. American Psychiatric Press, Washington.

Amodio, P., Marchetti, P., Del Piccolo, F., Beghi, A., Comacchio, F., Carraro, P., Campo, G., Baruzzo, L., Marchiori, L. and Gatta, A. (1997). The effect of flumazenil on subclinical psychometric or neurophysiological alterations in cirrhotic patients: a double-blind placebo-controlled study. Clin. Physiol. **17**, 533–9.

Amstrong, S.C., and Schweitzer, S.M. (1997), Delirium associated with paroxetine and benztropine combination. Am. J. Psychiatry **154**, 581–2.

Ancelin, M.L., Artero, S., Portet, F., Dupuy, A.M., Touchon, J., and Ritchie, K. (2006). Non-degenerative mild cognitive impairment in elderly people and use of anticholinergic drugs: longitudinal cohort study. BMJ **332**, 455–9.

Anderson, G., Jensen, N.H., Christup, L., Hansen, S.H., and Sjogren, P. (2002), Pain, sedation and morphine metaolism i cancer patients during long-term treatment with sustained-release morphine. Pall Med. **16**, 107–14.

Annese, M., Bacca, D., Francavilla, R., and Barbarini, G. (1998), Flumazenil for hepatic encephalopathy grade III and IVa in patients with cirrhosis: an Italian multicenter double-blind placebo-controlled, cross-over study. Hepatology **28**, 1338–9.

Andrews, G., Goldberg, D.P., Krueger, R.F., Carpenter, W.T., Hyman, S.E., Sachdev, P., Pine, D.S. (2009). Exploring the feasibility of a meta-structure for DSM-V and ICD-11: could it improve utility and validity? Psychol. Med. **39**, 1993–2000.

Ansaloni, L., Catena, F., Chattat, R., Fortuna, D., Franceschi, C., Mascitti, P., and Melotti, R.M. (2010). Risk factors and incidence of postoperative delirium in elderly patients after elective and emergency surgery. Br. J. Surg. **97**, 273–80.

Arieff, A.L., Llach, F., and Massry, S.G. (1976), Neurological manifestations and morbidity of hyponatremia: correlation with brain water and electrolytes. Medicine **55**, 121–9.

Ashworth, M., and Gerada, C. (1997), ABC of mental health. Addiction and dependence-II. Alcohol. BMJ **315**, 358–60.

Auerswald, K., Charpentier, P., and Inouye, S. (1997), The informed consent process in older patients who developed delirium: a clinical epidemiologic study. Am. J. Med. **103**, 410–18.

Australian Health Ministers' Advisory Council (2006). Clinical Practice Guidelines for the Management of Delirium in Older People. Victorian Government Department of Human Services, Melbourne, Victoria, Australia.

Ayd, P.J. (1987), Intravenous haloperidol therapy. Int. Drug Ther. Newsletter **13**, 20–3.

Azorin, J.M., Dassa, D., Tramoni, V., Peretti, P., and Donnet, A. (1992), Confusione mentale. In Encyclopedie Medico Chirurgicale Psichiatrie, 37124 A10, pp. 1–9. Elsevier, Paris.

Basinski, J.R., Alfano, C.M., Katon, W.J., Syrjala, K.L., and Fann, J.R. (2010).Impact of delirium on distress, health-related quality of life, and cognition 6 months and 1 year after hematopoietic cell transplant. Biol. Blood Marrow Transplant. [Epub ahead of print]

Bagri, S., and Reddy, G. (1998), Delirium with manic symptoms induced by diet pills. *J. Clin. Psychiatry*, **59**, 83.

Baines, M. (1993), The pathophysiology and management of maliganant intestinal obstruction. In: D. Doyle, G.W. Hanks and N. MacDonald (Eds.), Oxford Textbook of Palliative Medicine. Oxford University Press, Oxford, pp. 311–316.

Baranowski, S.L., and Patten, S.B. (2000), The predictive value of dysgraphia and constructional apraxia for delirium in psychiatric patients. *Can. J. Psychiatry* **45**, 75–8.

Barbaro, G., Di Lorenzo, G., Soldini, M., Marziali, M., Bellomo, G., Grisorio, B., Annese, M., Bacca, D. and Barbarini, G. (1998), Flumazenil for hepatic coma in patients with liver cirrhosis: an Italian multicentre double-blind, placebo-controlled, cross-over study. *Eur. J. Emerg. Med.* **5**, 213–18.

Barbato, M., and Rodriguez, P.J. (1994), Thiamine deficiency in patients admitted to a palliative care unit. *Pall Med.* **8**, 320–4.

Barr, J., Zomorodi, K., Bertaccini, E.J., Shafer, S.L., and Geller, E. (2001), A double-blind, randomized comparison of IV lorazepam versus midazolam for sedation of ICU patients via a pharmacologic model. *Anesthesiology* **95**, 286–98.

Barry, J., and Franklin, K. (1999), Amiodarone-induced delirium [letter]. *Am. J. Psychiatry* **156**, 1119.

Bates, T. and the Psychological-Work-Group-of-the-International-Work-Group-on-Death-Dying-and-Bereavement (1993). A statement of assumptions and principles concerning psychological care of dying persons and their families. *J. Pall. Care* **9**, 29–32.

Bayindir, O., Akpinar, B., Can, E., Guden, M., Sonmez, B. and Demiroglu, C. (2000), The use of 5-HT-receptor antagonist ondansetron for the treatment of postcardiotomy delirium. *J. Cardiothoracic Vasc. Anaesthesia* **14**, 288–92.

Beaver, W., Wallenstein, S., Houde, R. and Rogers, A. (1966), A comparison of the analgesic effects of methotrimeprazine and morphine in patients with cancer. *Clin. Pharmacol. Ther.* **7**, 436–46.

Beck-Friis, B., and Strang, P. (1993), The family in hospital-based home care with special reference to terminally ill cancer patients. *J. Pall. Care* **9**, 5–13.

Bergeron, N., Dubois, M.J., Dumont, M., Dial, S., and Skrobik, Y. (2001). Intensive care delirium screening checklist: evaluation of a new screening tool. *Intensive Care Med.* **27**(5), 859–64.

Berggren, D., Gustafson, Y., Erikson, B., Bucht, G., Hansson, L., Reiz, S. and Winblad, B. (1987). Postoperative confusion in elderly patients with femoral neck fratcures. *Anesth. Analg.* **66**, 497–504.

Berggren, U., Fahlke, C., Berglund, K.J., Blennow, K., Zetterberg, H., and Balldin, J. (2009). Thrombocytopenia in early alcohol withdrawal is associated with development of delirium tremens or seizures. *Alcohol Alcohol.* **44**, 382–6.

Bernard, S.A., and Bruera, E. (2000), Drug interactions in palliative care. *J. Clin. Oncol.* **18**, 1780–99.

Berrios, G.E. (1981). Delirium and confusion in the nineteenth century. A conceptual history. *Br. J. Psychiatry* **139**, 439–49.

Bettin, K., Maletta, G., Dysken, M., Jilk, K., Weldon, D., Kuskowski, M. and Mach, J.J. (1998), Measuring delirium severity in older general hospital inpatients without dementia. The Delirium Severity Scale. *Am. J. Geriatr. Psychiatry* **6**, 296–307.

Bhat, R., and Rockwood, K. (2007). Delirium as a disorder of consciousness. *J. Neurol. Neurosurg. Psychiatry* **78**, 1167–70.

Bialer, P.A., Wallack, J.J., Prenzlauer, S.L., Bogdonoff, L. and Wilets, I. (1996), Psychiatric comorbidity among hospitalized AIDS patients vs. non-AIDS patients referred for psychiatric consultation. *Psychosomatics* **37**, 469–75.

Bitondo Dyer, C., Ashton, C.M., and Teasdale, T.A. (1995). Postoperative delirium. A review of 80 primary data collection studies. *Arch/ Intern. Med.* **155**, 461–5.

Black, K., Shea, C., Dursun, S., and Kutcher, S. (2000), Selective serotonin reuptake inhibitor discontinuation syndrome: proposed diagnostic criteria. *J. Psychiatry Neurosci.* **25**, 255–61.

Blass, J.P., and Gibson, G.E. (1999), Cerebromeabolic aspects of delirium in relationship to dementia, *Dement. Geriatr. Cogn. Disord.* **10**, 335–8.

Blitzstein, S., and Brandt, G. (1997), Extrapyramidal symptoms from intravenous haloperidol in the treatment of delirium [letter]. *Am. J. Psychiatry* **154**, 1474–5.

Block, S.D (2001). Perspectives on care at the close of life. Psychological considerations, growth, and transcendence at the end of life: the art of the possible. *JAMA* **285**, 2898–905.

Blum, D., Maldonado, J., Meyer, E., and Lansberg, M. (2008). Delirium following abrupt discontinuation of fluoxetine. *Clin. Neurol. Neurosurg.* **110**, 69–70.

Bodner, R.A., Lynch, T., Lewis, L., and Kahn, D. (1995), Serotonin syndrome. *Neurology* **45**, 219–23.

Boettger, S., and Breitbart, W. (2005). Atypical antipsychotics in the management of delirium: a review of the empirical literature. *Palliat. Support. Care* **3**, 227–37.

Bolon, M., Boulieu, R., Flamens, C., Paulus, S., and Bastien, O. (2002). Sedation par le midazolam en reanimation: aspects pharmacologiques and pharmacocinetiques. *Ann. Fr. Anesth. Reanim.* **21**, 478–92.

Bonanno, G.A., and Kaltman, S. (2001), The varieties of grief experience. *Clin. Psychol. Rev.* **21**, 705–34.

Bond, S.M. (2009). Delirium at home: strategies for home health clinicians. *Home Healthc Nurse* **27**, 24–34.

Bond, S.M., Neelon, V.J., and Belyea, M.J.(2006). Delirium in hospitalized older patients with cancer. *Oncol. Nurs. Forum* **33**, 1075–83.

Bond, S.M., and Neelo V.J. (2008). Delirium resolution in hospitalized older patients with cancer. *Cancer Nursing* **31**, 444–51.

Bonin, B., Vandel, P., Vandel, S., Sechter, D. and Bizouard, P. (1999), Serotonin syndrome after sertraline, buspirone and loxapine? *Therapie* **54**, 269–71.

Bonne, O., Shalev, A.Y. and Bloch, M. (1995), Delirium associated with mianserin. *Eur. J. Neuropsychopharmacol.* **5**, 147–9.

Borreani, C., Caraceni, A. and Tamburini, M. (1997), The role of counselling for the confused patient and the family. In: R.K. Portenoy and E. Bruera (Eds.), *Topics in palliative care*, Oxford University Press, New York, pp. 45–54.

Bortolussi, R., Fabiani, F., Savron, F., Testa, V., Lazzarini, R., Sorio, R., De Conno, F. and Caraceni, A. (1994), Acute morphine intoxication during high-dose recombinant Interleukin-2 treatment for metastatic renal cell cancer. *Eur. J. Cancer* **30A**, 1905–7.

Bortone, E., Bettoni, L., Buzio, S., Giorgi, C., Melli, G., Mineo, F. and Mancia, D. (1998), Triphasic waves associated with acute naproxen overdose: a case report, *Clinical electroenceph*, **29** 142–5.

Bosisio M, Caraceni A, Grassi L; Italian Delirium Study Group (2006). Phenomenology of delirium in cancer patients, as described by the Memorial Delirium Assessment Scale (MDAS) and the Delirium Rating Scale (DRS). *Psychosomatics* **47**(6):471–8.

Bosisio, M., Caraceni, A., Grassi, L., Borreani, C., Mercadante, S., Luzzani, M., Maltoni, M. and Caraceni, A. (2002), Fenomenologia clinica del delirium nel paziente oncologico, *Rivista Italiana di Cure Palliative*, **4** 17–30.

Bosma H, Apland L, Kazanjian A. (2009). Cultural conceptualizations of hospice palliative care: More similarities than differences. *Palliat Med.* [Epub ahead of print]

Bottomley, D. and Hanks, G. (1990), Subcutaneous midazolam infusion in palliative care., *J Pain Symptom Manage*, **5** 259–61.

Bourke, M. (1984). The continuum of pre- and post-bereavement grieving, *Br H Med Psychol*, **57** 121.

Bourne RS, Tahir TA, Borthwick M, Sampson EL (2008). Drug treatment of delirium: past, present and future. *J Psychosom Res.* **65**:273–82.

Bowdle, T.A. and Rooke, G.A. (1994), Postoperative myoclonus and rigidity after anesthesia with opioids, *Anesth Analg*, **78** 783–6.

Boyle D. (2006). Delirium in older adults with cancer: implications for research and practice. *Oncol Nurs Forum.* **33**: 61–78

Brännström, B. (1999). Care of the delirious patient., *Dementia Ger Cogn Dis*, **10** 416–419.

Brauer, C., Morrison, R.S., Silberzweig, S.B. and Siu, A.L. (2000), The cause of delirium in patients with hip fracture, *Arch Intern Med*, **160** 1856–60.

Breitbart, W. (1987), Suicide in the cancer patient, *Oncology*, **1** 49–54.

Breitbart, W. (1990), Cancer pain and suicide. In: K.M. Foley, J.J. Bonica and V. Ventafridda (Eds.), Second International Congress on Cancer Pain, vol. **16**, Raven Press, New York, pp. 399–412.

Breitbart W, Gibson C, Poppito SR, Berg A. (2004). Psychotherapeutic interventions at the end of life: a focus on meaning and spirituality. *Can J Psychiatry.* **49**:366–72.

Breitbart W, Gibson C, Tremblay A. (2002a). The delirium experience: delirium recall and delirium-related distress in hospitalized patients with cancer, their spouses/caregivers, and their nurses. *Psychosomatics.* **43**:183–94.

Breitbart, W., Marotta, R., Platt, M.M., Weisman, H., Derevenco, M. and Grau, C. (1996), A double-blind trial of haloperidol, chlorpromazine and lorazepam in the treatment of delirium in hospitalized AIDS patients, *Am J Psychiatry*, **153** 231–37.

Breitbart, W., Rosenfeld, B., Roth, A., Smith, M.J., Cohen, K. and Passik, S. (1997), The Memorial Delirium Assessment Scale, *J Pain Symptom Manage*, **13** 128–37.

Breitbart, W., Stiefel, F., Kornblith, A.B. and Pannullo, S. (1993), Neuropsychiatric disturbance in cancer patients with epidural spinal cord compression receiving high dose corticosteroids: a prospective comparison study., *Psychooncology*, **2**, 233–45.

Breitbart W, Tremblay A, Gibson C. (2002b). An open trial of olanzapine for the treatment of delirium in hospitalized cancer patients. *Psychosomatics.* **43**:175–82.

Breitbart, W, Lawlor P, Friedlander M. (2009). *Delirium in the terminally ill. In: H.M. Chochinov and W. Breitbart (eds.), Handbook of Psychiatry in Palliative Medicine*, 2nd edn, Oxford University Press, New York, pp. 81-100.

Brenner, R.P. (1991), Utility of EEG in delirium: past views and current practice., *Int Psychogeriatr*, **3** 211–29.

Briskman I, Dubinski R, Barak Y. (2010). Treating delirium in a general hospital: a descriptive study of prescribing patterns and outcomes. *Int Psychogeriatr.* **22**(2):328–31.

Britton, A. and Russell, R. (2000). Multidisciplinary team interventions for delirium in patients with chronic cognitive impairment, *Cochrane Database of* Systematic Reviews (2): CD000395.

Britton A, Russell R. (2007) WITHDRAWN: Multidisciplinary team interventions for delirium in patients with chronic cognitive impairment. Cochrane Database *Syst Rev*. (2):CD000395.

Broadhurst, C. and Wilson, K.W. (2001), Immunology of delirium new opportunities for treatment and research, *Br J Psychiatry*, **174** 288–89.

Brodal, A. (1981), Neurological Anatomy, Oxford University Press, Oxford, 527–30, 756-8.

Brogan K, Lux J. (2009). Management of common psychiatric conditions in the HIV-positive population. *Curr HIV/AIDS Rep.* **6**:108–115.

Broomberg, M.H. and Higginson, I. (1996), Bereavement follow-up: what do palliative support teams actually do? *J Pal Care*, **12**, 12–17.

Brown, A.S. and Rosen, J. (1992), Lithium-induced delirium with therapeutic serum lithium levels: a case report, *J Geriatr Psychiatry Neurol*, **5**, 53–55.

Brown DV, Heller F, Barkin R. (2004). Anticholinergic syndrome after anesthesia: a case report and review. *Am J Ther.* **11**:144–53.

Brown LJ, McGrory S, McLaren L, Starr JM, Deary IJ, Maclullich AM. (2009). Cognitive visual perceptual deficits in patients with delirium. *J Neurol Neurosurg Psychiatry.* **80**:594–99.

Brown, P., Davies, B. and Martens, N. (1990), Families in supportive care—Part II: Palliative care at home: a viable care setting, *J Palliat Care*, **6**, 21–7.

Bruera, E., Chadwick, S., Weinlick, A. and MacDonald, N. (1987), Delirium and severe sedation in patient with terminal cancer, *Cancer Treat Rep*, **71**, 787–88.

Bruera, E., Macmillan, K., Hanson, J. and MacDonald, R.N. (1989), The cognitive effects of the administration of narcotic analgesics in patients with cancer pain, *Pain*, **39**, 13–16.

Bruera, E., Macmillan, K., Pither, J. and Mac, D.R. (1990), Effects of morphine on the dyspnea of terminal cancer patients, *J Pain* Symptom Manage, **5**, 341–4.

Bruera, E., Fainsinger, R.L., Miller, M.J. and Kuehn, N. (1992a), The assessment of pain intensity in patients with cognitive failure: a preliminary report, *J Pain Symptom Manage*, **7**, 267–70.

Bruera, E., Miller, L., McCallion, J., Macmillan, K., Krefting, L. and Hanson, J. (1992b), Cognitive failure in patients with terminal cancer: a prospective study., *J Pain Symptom Manage*, **7** 192–95.

Bruera, E., Miller, M.J., Macmillan, K. and Kuehn, N. (1992c), Neuropsychological effects of methylphenidate in patients receiving a continuous infusion of narcotics for cancer pain, *Pain*, **48**, 163–6.

Bruera, E., Schoeller, T. and Montejo, G. (1992d), Organic hallucinosis in patients receiving high doses of opiates for cancer pain, *Pain*, **48** 387–99.

Bruera, E., Franco, J.J., Maltoni, M., Watanabe, S. and Suarez-Almazor, M. (1995), Changing pattern of agitated impaired mental status in patients with advanced cancer: association with cognitive monitoring, hydration and opioid rotation, *J Pain Sympt Manage*, **10**, 287–91.

Bruera, E., Fainsinger, R.L., Schoeller, T. and Ripamonti, C. (1996), Rapid discontinuation of hypnotics in terminal cancer patients: a prospective study., *Ann Oncol.*, **7** 855–56.

Bruera, E. and Pereira, J. (1997), Acute neuropsychiatric findings in a patient receiving fentanym for cancer pain, *Pain*, **69** 199–201.

Bruera E, Sala R, Rico MA, Moyano J, Centeno C, Willey J, Palmer JL. (2005). Effects of parenteral hydration in terminally ill cancer patients. a preliminary study *J Clin Oncol*, **23** 2366–71.

Bruera E, Bush, SH, Willey J, Paraskevopoulos T, Li Z, Palmer JL, Cohen MZ, PhD, D Sivesind, MSN, Elsayem A (2009). The impact of delirium and recall on the level of distress in patients with advanced cancer and their family caregivers *Cancer* **115**, 2004–2012.

Buchman, N., Mendelsson, E., Lerner, V. and Kotler, M. (1999), Delirium associated with vitamin B12 deficiency after pneumonia., *Clin Neuropharmacol*, **22**, 356–8.

Burge, F., McIntyre, P., Twohig, P., Cummings, I., Kaufman, D., Frager, G. and Pollett, A. (2001), Palliative care by family physicians in the 1990s. Resilience amid reform., *Can Fam Physician*, **47** 1989–95.

Burke, A.L. (1997). Palliative care: an update on "terminal restlessness, *Med J Aust*, **166**, 39–42.

Burke, A.L., Diamond, P.L., Hulbert, J., Yeatman, J. and Farr, E.A. (1991), Terminal restlessness-its management and the role of midazolam, *Med J Aust*, **155**, 485–87.

Burns, M.J., Linden, C.H., Graudins, A., Brown, R.M. and Fletcher, K.E. (2000), A comparison of physostigmine and benzodiazepines for the treatment of anticholinergic poisoning, *Ann Emerg Med*, **35**, 374–81.

Buss MK, Vanderwerker LC, Inouye SK, Zhang B, Block SD, Prigerson HG. (2007). Associations between caregiver-perceived delirium in patients with cancer and generalized anxiety in their caregivers. *J Palliat Med*. **10**(5):1083–92.

Byelry, M.J., Christensen, R.C. and Evans, O.L. (1996), Delirium associated with a combination of sertraline, haloperidol, and benztropine, *Am J Psychiatry*, **153**, 965–66.

Caltagirone, C. and Carlesino, G.A. (1990), Lo stato confusionale acuto. In: G. Denes and L. Pizzamiglio (eds), *Manuale di neuropsicologia. Normalita' e patologia dei processi cognitivi.*, Zanichelli, Bologna, pp. 1245–61.

Campbell, K.M. and Schubert, D.S. (1991), Delirium after cessation of glucocorticoid therapy, *Gen Hosp Psychiatry*, **13**, 270–72.

Campbell N, Boustani MA, Ayub A, Fox GC, Munger SL, Ott C, Guzman O, Farber M, Ademuyiwa A, Singh R. (2009). Pharmacological management of delirium in hospitalized adults—a systematic evidence review. *J Gen Intern Med*. **24**(7):848–53.

Camus, V., Burtin, B., Simeone, I., Schwed, P., Gonthier, R. and Dubos, G. (2000), Factor analysis support the evidence of existing hyperactive and hypoactive subtypes of delirium, *Int J Geriatr Psychiatry*, **15**, 313–316.

Canadian Coalition for Seniors' Mental Health.(2006). National guidelines for seniors' mental health: the assessment and treatment of delirium. http://www.ccsmh.ca/en/guidelinesusers.cfm.

Capitani, E. (1985). *Alterazioni neurologiche della coscienza e del sonno*. In: P. Pinelli (Ed.), *Neurologia, Casa editrice ambrosiana.Milano*, pp. 79.

Capuzzo, M., Pinamonti, A., Cingolani, E., Grassi, L., Bianconi, M., Contu, P., Gritti, G. and Alvisi, R. (2001), Analgesia, sedation and memory ofintensive care, *J Crit Care*, **16**, 83–89.

Caraceni, A., Martini, C., Belli, F., Mascheroni, L., Rivoltini, L., Arienti, F. and Cascinelli, N. (1992), Neuropsychological and neurophysiological assessment of the central effects of interleuki-2 administration, *Eur J Cancer*, **29A**, 1266–69.

Caraceni, A., Martini, C., Gamba, A., Pugnetti, L., Cattaneo, A., Biserni, P., De Conno, F. and Ventafridda, V. (1993), Cognitive effects of oral morphine administration in cancer pain. A neurophysiological evaluation, *7th World Congress on Pain, Paris*.

Caraceni, A., Martini, C., De Conno, F. and Ventafridda, V. (1994), Organic brain syndromes and opioid administration for cancer pain, *J Pain Symptom Manage*, **9**, 527–33.

Caraceni, A., Scolari, S. and Simonetti, F. (1999), The role of the neurologist in oncology a prospective study, *J Neurology*, **246** (suppl I) I/68.

Caraceni, A., Nanni, O., Maltoni, M., Piva, L., Indelli, M., Arnoldi, E., Montanari, L., Amadori, D., De Conno, F. and an Italian multicenter study group on palliative care, (2000). The impact of delirium on the short-term prognosis of advanced cancer patients. *Cancer*, **89**: 1145–8.

Caraceni, A., Zecca, E., Martini, C., Gorni, G., Galbiati, A. and De Conno, F. (2002), Terminal sedation a retrospective survey of a three-year experience, 2nd Congres of the EAPC Research Network, Lyon (France).

Caraceni A, Andreola S, Simonetti F, Celio L. (2003). Acute confusional state with fatal outcome in a cancer patient. *Neurol Sci* **24** 424–25

Caraceni A, Simonetti F (2009). Palliating delirium in cancer patients. *Lancet Oncology* **10**: 164–72

Carlson, L.A., Gottfries, C.G., Winbland, B., Robertson, B. and (eds), (1999). Delirium in the elderly. Epidemiological, pathogenetic and treatment aspects, *Dement Geriatr Cog Disord*, **10** 306–429.

Cartwright, P.D., Hesse, C. and Jackson, O. (1993), Myoclonic spams following intrathecal diamorphine, *J Pain Symptom Manage*, **8** 492–5.

Casarett, D. and Inouye, S. (2001), Diagnosis and management of delirium near the end of life, *Ann Intern Med*, **135** 32–42.

Casarett, D., Kutner, J.S., Abrahm, J. and for the End-of-Life Care Consensus Panel (2001). Life after death: a practical approach to grief and bereavement., *Ann Intern Med*, **134**, 208–15.

Catalano, G., Catalano, M. and Alberts, V. (1996), Famotidine-associated delirium. A series of six cases., *Psychosomatics*, **37**, 349–55.

Chambost, M., Liron, L., Peillon, D. and Combe, C. (2000), Serotonin syndrome during fuoxetine poisoning in a patient taking moclobemide, *Can J Anesth*, **47**, 246–50.

Chamorro, C., de Latorre, F.J., Montero, A., Sanchez-Izquierdo, J.A., Jareno, A., Moreno, J.A., Gonzalez, E., Barrios, M., Carpintero, J.L., Martin-Santos, F., Otero, B. and Ginestal, R. (1996), Comparative study of propofol versus midazolam in the sedation of critically ill patients: results of a prospective, randomized, multicenter trial [see comments], *Crit Care Med*, **24**, 932–9.

Chang, P.H. and Steinberg, M.B. (2001), Alcohol withdrawal, *Med Clin North Am*, **85** 1191–1212.

Charlton, R. and Dolman, E. (1995), Bereavement: a protocol for primary care., *Br J Gen Pract*, **45** 427–30.

Chaslin, P. (1895), La confusione mentale primitive, Asselin et Houzeau, Paris.

Checkley, H., Sydenstricker, V. and Geeslin, L. (1939), Nicotinic acid in the treatment of atypical psychotic state., *JAMA*, **112**, 2107–10.

Chedru, F. and Geschwind, N. (1972a), Disorders of higher cortical functions in acute confusional states, *Cortex*, **8**, 395–411.

Chedru, F. and Geschwind, N. (1972b), Writing disturbances in acute confusional state, *Neuropsychologia*, **10**, 343–53.

Cheng, C., Roemer-Becuwe, C. and Pereira J. (2002), When midazolam fails. *J Pain Symptom Manage*, **23**, 256–65.

Cherny, N., Ripamonti, C., Pereira, J., Davis, C., Fallon, M., McQuay, H.J., Mercadante, S., Pasternak, G. and Ventafridda (2001). Strategies to manage the adverse effects of oral morphine: an evidence-based report, *J Clin Oncol*, **19**, 2542–54.

Cherny, N.I., Coyle, N. and Foley, K.M. (1994), Suffering in the advanced cancer patient: A definition and taxonomy, *J Palliative Care*, **10**, 57–70.

Cherny, N.I. and Portenoy, R.K. (1994). Sedation in the teatment of refractory symptoms: guidelines for evaluation and treatment., *J Palliat Care*, **10**, 31–8.

Cherny NI, Radbruch L; Board of the European Association for Palliative Care. European Association for Palliative Care (EAPC) (2009) recommended framework for the use of sedation in palliative care. *Palliat Med.* **23**:581–93

Chochinov HM. (2008). Psychiatry and palliative care: 2 sides of the same coin. *Can J Psychiatry.***53**:711–712

Chochinov HM, Cann BJ. (2005). Interventions to enhance the spiritual aspects of dying. *J Palliat Med.* Suppl 1:S103–111

Chochinov HM, Hack T, Hassard T, Kristjanson LJ, McClement S, Harlos M. (2004). Dignity and psychotherapeutic considerations in end-of-life care. *J Palliat Care.* **20**(3):134–42.

Chochinov HM, Hack T, Hassard T, Kristjanson LJ, McClement S, Harlos M. (2005). Dignity therapy: a novel psychotherapeutic intervention for patients near the end of life. *J Clin Oncol.* **23**:5520–5.

Chow, K.M., Wang, A.Y., Hui, A.C., Wong, T.Y. and Szeto, C.C. (2001), Nonconvulsive status epilepticus in peritoneal dialysis patients, *Am J Kydney Dis*, **38** 400–405.

Clark, D. (1999). 'Total pain', disciplinary power and the body in the work of Cicely Saunders, 1958-1967, *Soc Sci Med*, **49** 727–36.

Clinton, J.E., Sterner, S., Stelmachers, Z. and Ruiz, E. (1987). Haloperidol for sedation of disruptive emergency patients, *Ann Emerg Med*, **16**, 319–22.

Clouston, P.D., De Angelis, L. and Posner, J.B. (1992). The spectrum of neurological disease in patients with systemic cancer., *Ann Neurol*, **31**, 268–73.

Clukey L. (2008). Anticipatory mourning: processes of expected loss in palliative care. *Int J Palliat Nurs.* **14**(7):316, 318–25.

Cohen MA, Gorman JM, (eds) (2008). Comprehensive Textbook of AIDS Psychiatry. New York: Oxford University Press.

Cohen MZ, Pace EA, Kaur G, Bruera E. (2009). Delirium in advanced cancer leading to distress in patients and family caregivers. *J Palliat Care.* **25**:164–71.

Cole, M.G. (1999), Delirium: effectiveness of systematic interventions, *Dementia Ger Cogn Dis*, **10**, 406–11.

Cole, M.G., Primeau, F.J., Bailey, R.F., Bonnycastle, M.J.,Masciarelli, F., Engelsmann, F., Pepin, M.J., and Ducic, D. (1994). Systematic intervention for elderly inpatient with delirium: a randomized trial. *Can. Med. Assoc. J.* **151**, 965–70.

Cole, M.G., Primeau, F.J. and Elie, L.M. (1998), Delirium: prevention, treatment, and outcome studies, *J Geriatr Psychiatry Neurol*, **11** 126–37.

Cole, M.G., Primeau, F.J., Bailey, R.F., Bonnycastle, M.J., Masciarelli, F., Engelsmann, F., Pepin, M.J. and Ducic, D. (2002), Systematic intervention for elderly inpatient with delirium: a randomized trial. *Can Med Ass J*, **151**, 965–70.

Cook I.A. (2004). Guideline Watch: Practice Guideline for the Treatment of Patients with Delirium. *American Psychiatric Association.*

Copeland LA, Zeber JE, Pugh MJ, Mortensen EM, Restrepo MI, Lawrence VA. (2008). Postoperative complications in the seriously mentally ill: a systematic review of the literature. *Ann Surg.* **248**:31–38.

Corruble E, Chouinard VA, Letierce A, Gorwood PA, Chouinard G. (2009). Is DSM-IV bereavement exclusion for major depressive episode relevant to severity and pattern of symptoms? A case-control, cross-sectional study. *J Clin Psychiatry.* **70**(8):1091–97.

Cowan, J.D. and Walsh, D. (2001), Terminal sedation in palliative medicine - definition and review of the literature, *Supp Care Cancer*, **9**, 403–407.

Cox, J.M. and Pappagallo, M. (2001), Modafinil: a gift to portmanteau, *Am J Hosp Palliat Care*, **18** 408–10.

Coyle, N., Breitbart, W., Weaver, S. and Portenoy, R. (1994). Delirium as a contributing factor to "crescendo" pain: three case reports. *J Pain Symptom Manage*, **9**, 44–47.

Crammer, J. (2002). Subjective experience of a confusional state, *Br J Psychiatry*, **180**, 71–75.

Craven, J.L. (1991), Cyclosporine-associated organic mental disorders in liver trasplant recipients, *Psychosomatics*, **32**, 94–102.

Crum, R.M., Anthony, J.C., Basset, S.S. and Folstein, M.F. (1993), Population-based norms for the Mini-Mental State Examination by age and educational level, *JAMA*, **269**, 2386–91.

Curyto, K.J., Johnson, J., TenHave, T., Mossey, J., Knott, K. and Katz, I.R. (2001), Survival of hospitalized patients with delirium: a prospective study, *Am J Geriatr Psychiatry*, **9**, 141–47.

Daeninck, P.J. and Bruera, E. (1999), Opioid use in cancer pain. Is a more liberal approach enhancing toxicity, *Acta Anaesthesiol Scand*, **43**, 924–8.

Daeppen, J., Gache, P., Landry, U., Sekera, E., Schweizer, V., Gloor, S. and Yersin, B. (2002). Symptom-triggered vs fixed-schedule doses of benzodiazepine for alcohol withdrawal: a randomized treatment trial. *Arch Intern Med*. **27**, 1117–21.

Dalmau J, Gleichman AJ, Hughes EG, Rossi JE, Peng X, Lai M, Dessain SK, Rosenfeld MR, Balice-Gordon R, Lynch DR. (2008). Anti-NMDA-receptor encephalitis: case series and analysis of the effects of antibodies. *Lancet Neurol*. **7**:1091–8.

Dangler, L.A., O'Donnell, J., Gingrich, C. and Bope, E.T. (1996), What do family members expect from the family physician of a deceased loved one? *Fam Med* **28**, 694–97.

Daniels, R.J. (1998), Serotonin syndrome due to venlafaxine overdose. *J Accident Emerg Med* **15** 333–4.

Dasgupta M, Hillier LM (2010). Factors associated with prolonged delirium: a systematic review. *Int Psychogeriatr*. 1–22. [Epub ahead of print]

Davies, B., Reimer, J.C. and Martens, N. (1994). Family functioning and its implications for palliative care. *J Pall Care* **10**, 29–36.

Davis MP (2007). Does trazodone have a role in palliating symptoms? *Support Care Cancer* **15**: 221–4.

Davis, M.P. and Walsh, D. (2001), Clinical and ethical questions concerning delirium study on patienyts with advaced cancer, *Arch In*tern Med, **161**, 296–7.

De Angelis, L. (1989). Radiation-induced dementia inpatients cured of brain metastases, *Neurology*, **39**, 789–96.

DeCarolis DD, Rice KL, Ho L, Willenbring ML, Cassaro S (2007). Symptom-driven lorazepam protocol for treatment of severe alcohol withdrawal delirium in the intensive care unit. *Pharmacotherapy*. **27**:510–18.

de Carvalho WB, Fonseca MC (2008). Pediatric delirium: a new diagnostic challenge of which to be aware. *Crit Care Med* **36**:1986–7

De Conno, F., Caraceni, A., Martini, C., Spoldi, E., Salvetti, M. and Ventafridda, V. (1991a), Hyperalgesia and myoclonus with intrathecal infusion of high-dose morphine. *Pain* **47**, 337–9.

De Conno, F., Spoldi, E., Caraceni, A. and Ventafridda, V. (1991b), Does pharmacological treatment affect the sensation of breathlessness in terminal cancer patients. *Palliative Medicine* **5**, 237–43.

De Conno, F., Caraceni, A., Groff, L., Brunelli, C., Donati, I., Tamburini, M. and Ventafridda, V. (1996), Effect of home care on the place of death of advanced cancer patients, *Eur J Cancer*, **32A** 1142–7.

De Deyn, P.P., D'Hooge, R., Van Bogaert, P.P. and Marescau, B. (2001), Endogenous guanidino compounds as uremic neurotoxins. *Kydney International*, Suppl **78**, S77–83.

de Graeff A, Dean M. (2007). Palliative sedation therapy in the last weeks of life: a literature review and recommendations for standards. *J Palliat Med.* **10**:67–85.

de Haes H, Teunissen S. (2005). Communication in palliative care: a review of recent literature. *Curr Opin Oncol.* **17**:345–50.

Delmas G, Rothmann C, Flesch F. (2008). Acute overdose with controlled-release levodopa-carbidopa. *Clin Toxicol (Phila).* **46**(3):274–7.

Denikoff, K., Rubinow, D.R. and Papa, M.Z. (1987), Neuropsychiatric effects of treatment with interleuki-2 and lymphocyte-activated killer cells, *Ann Intern Med*, **107** 293–300.

de Paulis T. (2002). Perospirone (Sumitomo Pharmaceuticals). *Curr Opin Investig Drugs.* **3**:121–9.

Derogatis, L.R., Morrow, G.R., Fetting, J., Penman, D., Piasetsky, S. and Schmale, A.M. (1983), The prevalence of psychiatric disorders among cancer patients., *JAMA* **249**, 751–7.

de Rooij SE, van Munster BC, Korevaar JC, Levi MJ (2007). Cytokines and acute phase response in delirium. *Psychosom Res* **62**, 521–5.

de Stoutz, N.D., Tapper, M. and Faisinger, R.L. (1995), Reversible delirium in terminally ill patients. *J Pain Sympt Manage*, **10**, 249–53.

Deutsch, G. and Eisemberg, H.M. (1987), Frontal blood flow changes in recovery from coma, *J Cereb Blood Flow Metab*, **7**, 29–34.

Deutsche Lezak, M. (1995), *Neuropsychological assessment.*

Devlin JW, Roberts RJ, Fong JJ, Skrobik Y, Riker RR, Hill NS, Robbins T, Garpestad E. (2010). Efficacy and safety of quetiapine in critically ill patients with delirium: a prospective, multicenter, randomized, double-blind, placebo-controlled pilot study. *Crit Care Med.* **38**:419–27.

Dillen L, Fontaine JR, Verhofstadt-Denève L. (2008). Are normal and complicated grief different constructs? a confirmatory factor analytic test. *Clin Psychol Psychother.* **15**(6):386–95.

Dilling, H., Classification. In: M.G. Gelder, J.J.j. Lopez-Ibor and N. Andreasen (eds.) (200). New Oxford Textbook of Psychiatry, vol **1**. Oxford University Press, New York, pp. 109–33.

DiSalvo, T.G. and O'Gara, P.T. (1995), Torsade de Pointes caused by high dose intravenous haloperidol in cardiac patients. *Clin Cardiol*, **18** 285–90.

Dixon, D. and Craven, J. (1993), Continuous infusion of haloperidol. *Am J Psychiatry* **150**, 673.

Dolan, M.M., Hawkes, W.G., Zimmerman, S.I., Morrison, R.S., Gruber-Baldini, A.L., Hebel, J.R. and Magaziner, J. (2000), Delirium on hospital admission in aged hip fracture patients: prediction of mortality and 2-year functional outcomes. *J Gerontol* **55**, M527–534.

Driessen M, Lange W, Junghanns K, Wetterling T. (2005). Proposal of a comprehensive clinical typology of alcohol withdrawal—a cluster analysis approach. *Alcohol Alcohol.* **40**:308–313.

Dropcho, E. (2002), Remote neurologic manifestations of cancer. *Neurol Clin*, **20** 85–122.

Dubois, M.J., Bergeron, N., Dumont, M., Dial, S. and Skrobik, Y. (2001), Delirium in an intensive care unit: a study of risk factors. *Intensive Care Med* **27**, 1297–1304.

Duckett, S. and Scotto, M. (1992), An unusual case of sundown syndrome subsequent to a traumatic head injury. *Brain Injury* **6**, 189–91.

Dulfano, M.J. and Ishikawa, S. (1965), Hyercapnia: mental changes and extrapulmonary complications. *Ann Intern Med* **63**, 829–41.

Dumont I, Kissane D. (2009). Techniques for framing questions in conducting family meetings in palliative care. *Palliat Support Care.* **7**:163–70.

Dumont S, Turgeon J, Allard P, Gagnon P, Charbonneau C, Vézina L. (2006). Caring for a loved one with advanced cancer: determinants of psychological distress in family caregivers. *J Palliat Med.* **9**:912–21.

Dunlop, R.J. (1989). Is terminal restlessness sometimes drug induced. *Palliative Medicine* **3** 65–6.

Dunne, J.W., Leedman, P.J. and Edis, R.H. (1986), Inobvious stroke: a cause of delirium and dementia. *Aust Nz J Med* **16**, 771–8.

Duppils, G.S. and Wikblad, K. (2000), Acute confusional states in patients undergoing hip surgery. a prospective observation study. *Gerontology* **46**, 36–43.

Egbert, A.M., Parks, L.H., Short, L.M. and Burnett, M.L. (1990). Randomized trial of postoperative patient-controlled analgesia vs intramuscular narcotics in frail elderly men. *Arch Intern Med* **150**, 1897–1903.

Eidelman, L.A., Putterman, D., Putterman, C. and Sprung, C.L. (1996), The spectrum of septic encephalopathy. *JAMA* **275**, 470–3.

Eisendrath, S.J. and Ostroff, J.W. (1990), Ranitidine-associated delirium. *Psychosomatics* **31**, 98–100.

Elble, R.J. (2000). Diagnostic criteria for essential tremor and differential diagnosis. *Neurology* **54**, S2–S6.

Ely, E.W. (2001), Delirium in mechanically ventilated patients. Validity and reliability of the Confusion Assessment Method for the Intensive Care Unit (CAM-ICU). *JAMA* **286**, 2703–10.

Ely, E.W., Margolin, R., Francis, J., May, L., Truman, B., Dittus, R., Speroff, T., Gautam, S., Bernard, G.R. and Inouye, S.K. (2001), Evaluation of delirium in critically ill patients: validation of the Confusion Assessment Method for the Intensive Care Unit (CAM-ICU). *Crit Care Med* **29**, 1481–3.

Ely EW., Truman B, Manzi DJ, Sigl JC, Shintani A, Bernard GR. (2004). Consciousness monitoring in ventilated patients : bispectral EEG monitors arousal not delirium. *Intensive Care Med* **30**, 1537–43.

Emanuel, E.J., Fairclough, D.L., Slutsman, J., Alpert, H., Baldwin, D. and Emanuel, L.L. (1999), Assistance form family members, friends, paid care givers, and volunteers in the care of the terminally ill patients. *N Engl J Med* **341**, 956–63.

Engel, G.L. and Romano, J. (1959), Delirium a syndrome of cerebral insufficiency. *J Chronic Diseases* **9**, 260–77.

Enyert, G. and Burman, M.E. (1999). A qualitative study of self-transcendence in caregivers of terminally ill patients. *Am J Hosp Palliat Care* **16**, 455–62.

Eriksson, S. (1999). Social and environmental contributants to delirium in the elderly. *Dementia Ger Cogn Dis* **10**, 350–2.

Erkinjutti, T., Wikstrom, J., Palo, J. and Autio, K. (1986). Dementia among medical inpatients. Evaluation of 2000 consecutive admission. *Arch Intern Med* **146**, 1923–6.

Ernst E. (2003). Serious psychiatric and neurological adverse effects of herbal medicines—a systematic review. *Acta Psychiatr Scand.* **108**(2):83–91. Review.

Erwin, W.E., Williams, D.B. and Speir, W.A. (1998), Delirium tremens. *South Med J* **91**, 425–32.

Evans, A.J. (1994). Anticipatory grief: a theoretical challenge. *J Pall Med* **8**, 159–65.

Ewing G, Rogers M, Barclay S, McCabe J, Martin A, Campbell M, Todd C (2006). Palliative care in primary care: a study to determine whether patients and professionals agree on symptoms. *Br J Gen Pract.* **56**(522):27–34.

Ey, H., Bernard, P. and Brisset, C. (1989). Manuel de psychiatrie. *Masson, Paris.*

Factor, S.A., Molho, E.S. and Brown, D.L. (1998), Acute delirium after withdrawal of amantadine in Parkinson's disease. *Neurology* **50**, 1456–8.

Fadul N, Kaur G, Zhang T, Palmer JL, Bruera E. (2007). Evaluation of the memorial delirium assessment scale (MDAS) for the screening of delirium by means of simulated cases by palliative care health professionals. *Support Care Cancer.* **15**(11):1271–6.

Fahn, S., Marsden, C.D. and Van Woert, M.H. (1986), Definition and classification of myoclonus. In: S. Fahn, C.D. Marsden and M. Van Woert (eds), Advances in Neurology, vol. **43**. Myoclonus. Raven Press, New York, pp. 1–5.

Fainsinger, R. and Bruera, E. (1992), Treatment of delirium in a terminally ill patient. *J Pain Sympt Manage* **7**, 54–6.

Fainsinger, R., Miller, M.J., Bruera, E., Hanson, J. and MacEachern, T. (1991), Symptom control during the last week of life on a palliative care unit. *J Palliat Care* **7**, 5–11.

Fainsinger, R., Tapper, M. and Bruera, E. (1993), A perspective on the management of delirium in terminally ill patients on a palliative care unit. *J Palliat Care* **9**, 4–8.

Fainsinger, R., Landman, W., Hoskings, M. and Bruera, E. (1998), Sedation for uncontrolled symptoms in a South African Hospice. *J Pain Sympt Manage* **16**, 145–52.

Fainsinger, R., De Moissac, D., Mancini, I. and Oneschuk, D. (2000a), Sedation for delirium and other symptoms in terminally ill patients in Edmonton. *J Pall Care* **16**, 5–10.

Fainsinger, R., Waller, A., Bercovici, M., Bengston, K., Landman, W., Hosking, M., Nunez-Olarte, J.M. and deMoissac, D. (2000b), A multicentre international study of sedation for uncontrolled symptoms in terminally ill patients. *Pall Med* **14**, 257–65.

Fallowfield LJ, Jenkins VA, Beveridge HA. (2002). Truth may hurt but deceit hurts more: communication in palliative care. *Palliat Med.* **16**:297–303

Farber, I.J. (1959), Acute brain syndrome. (Clinical study of 122 patients). *Dis Nerv System* **20**, 296–99.

Farber, S.J., Egnew, T.R. and Herman-Bertsch, J.L. (1999), Issues in end-of-life care: family practice faculty perceptions. *J Fam Pract* **48**, 525–30.

Farberow, N.L., Schneiderman, E.S. and Leonard, C.V. (1963), Suicide among general medical and surgical hospital patients with malignant neoplasms, vol. **9**. US Veterans Administration, Washington.

Farrell, K.R. and Ganzini, L. (1995), Misdiagnosing delirium as depression in medically ill elderly patients. *Arch Intern Med* **155**, 2459–64.

Farrington, J., Stoudemire, A. and Tierney, J. (1995), The role of ciprofloxacin in a patient with delirium due to multiple etiologies. *Gen Hosp Psychiatry* **17**, 43–53.

Faulkner, A. and Maguire, P. (1994), Talking to cancer patients and their relatives, Oxford University Press, Oxford.

Fayers P, Hjermstad MJ, Ranhoff AH, Kaasa S, Skogstad L., Klepstad P, Loge JH. (2005). Which minimental state exam items can be used to screen for delirium and cognitive impairment? *J Pain Sympt Manage* **30** :41–50

Feldstein, M.A. and Buschman Gemma, P. (1995), Oncology nurses and chronic compounded grief, *Cancer Nurs* **18**, 228–36.

Fenelon, G., Marie, S. and Guillard, A. (1993), Hallucinose musicale: 7 cas. *Rev Neurol* **149**, 8–9.

Fennig, S. and Mauas, L. (1992), Ofloxaacin-induced delirium. *J Clin Psychiatry* **53**, 137–8.

Ferguson, J.A., Suelzer, C.J., Eckert, G.J., Zhou, X.H. and Dittus, R.S. (1996), Risk factors for delirium tremens development. *J Gen Intern Med* **11**, 10–414.

Fernandez, F., Levy, J.K. and Mansell, P.W. (1989), Management of delirium in terminally ill AIDS patients. *Int J Psychiatry Me*d **19**, 165–72.

Fernandez F, Ruiz P, (eds). (2006). Psychiatric Aspects of HIV/AIDS. 1st edn. Lippincott Williams and Wilkins, Philadelphia.

Ferrell, B.R. (1998). *The family.* In: D. Doyle, G.W.C. Hanks, and N. MacDonald (eds), Oxford Textbook of Palliative Medicine, 2nd edn, pp. 909–17. Oxford University Press, New York.

Ferro, J., Caeiro, L. and Verdelho, A. (2002). Delirium in acute stroke. *Curr Opin Neurol* **15**, 51–5.

Fink, M. (1993). Post-ECT delirium. *Convuls Ther* **9**, 326–30.

Fischer, P. (2001). Successful treatment of nonanticholinergic delirium with a cholinesterase inhibitor. *J Clin Psychopharmacol* **21**, 118.

Fitzgerald, R.G. and Parkes, C.M. (1998), Coping with loss: Blindness and loss of other sensory and cognitive functions. *BMJ* **316**, 1160–3.

Flacker, J.M. and Lipsitz, L.A. (1999a), Neural mechanisms of delirium: current hypotheses and evolving concepts. *J Gerontol Biol Sci* **54A** B239–46.

Flacker, J.M. and Lipsitz, L.A. (1999b), Serum anticholinergic activity changes with acute illness in elderly medical patients. *J Gerontol MS* **54A**, M12–16.

Flacker, J.M. and Wei, J.Y. (2001), Endogenous anticholinergic sustances may exist during acute illness in elderly medical patiens. *J Gerontol A* **56**, M353–5.

Folstein, M., Folstein, S. and McHugh, P. (1975), Mini-mental state. *J Psychiatr Res* **12**, 189–98.

Fong TG, Jones RN, Shi P, Marcantonio ER, Yap L, Rudolph JL, Yang FM, Kiely DK, Inouye SK (2009). Delirium accelerates cognitive decline in Alzheimer disease. *Neurology* **72**, 1570–5.

Formaglio, F. and Caraceni, A. (1998), Meningeal metastases clinical aspects and diagnosis. *Ital J Neurol Sci* **19**, 133–49.

Forsman, A. and Ohman, R. (1977). Applied pharmacokinetics of haloperidol in man, *Curr Ther Res*, **21** 396–411.

Forstmeier S, Maercker A. (2007). Comparison of two diagnostic systems for Complicated Grief. *J Affect Disord.* **99**(1-3):203–211.

Fountain, A. (2001), Visual hallucinations: a prevalence study among hospice inpatients. *Pall Med* **15** 19–25.

Francis, J. and Kapoor, W.N. (1992), Prognosis after hospital discharge of older medical patients with delirium. *J Am Geriatr Soc* **40** 601–6.

Francis, J., Martin, D. and Kapoor, W.N. (1990), A prospective study of delirium in hospitalized elderly. *JAMA* **263**, 1097–1101.

Francis, J.F. (1999). Three millenia of delirium research: moving beyond echoes of the past. *JAGS* **47**, 1382.

Franco, K., Litaker, D., Locala, J. and Bronson, D. (2001). The cost of delirium in surgical patients. *Psychosomatics* **42**, 68–73.

Frankl, V. (1984), Man's search for meaning, Simon and Shuster, New York.

Fredreriks, J.A.M. (2000), Inflammation of the mind. On the 300th anniversary off Gerard van Swieten. *J History Neurosci* **9** 307–10.

Frenk, H. (1983), Pro-and anticonvulsant actions of morphine and the endogenous opioids: involvement and interaction of multiple opiate and non-opiate systems. *Brain Res* **287**, 197–210.

Frenk, H., Watkins, L.R., Miller, J. and Mayer, D.J. (1984), Nonspecific convulsions are induced by morphine but not D-ala-methionine-enkephalinamide at cortical sites. *Brain Res* **299**, 51–9.

Freudenreich, O. and Menza, M. (2000), Zolpidem-related delirium: a case report. *J Clin Psychiatry* **61**, 449–50.

Frye, M.A., Coudreaut, M.F., Hakeman, S.M., Shah, B.G., Strouse, T.B. and Skotzko, C.E. (1995), Continuous droperidol infusion for management of agitated delirium in an intensive care unit. *Psychosomatics* **36**, 301–5.

Fukutani, Y., Katsukawa, K., Matsubara, R., Kobayashi, K., Nakamura, I. and Yamaguchi, N. (1993), Delirium associated with Joseph disease. *J Neurol Neurosurg Psychiatry* **56**, 1207–12.

Fuller BE, Loftis JM, Rodriguez VL, McQuesten MJ, (2009). HauserPsychiatric and substance use disorders comorbidities in veterans with hepatitis C virus and HIV coinfection. *Curr Opin Psychiatry* **22**:401–8.

Fulton, R. and Gottesman, D.J. (1989), Anticipatory grief: a psychosocial concept reconsidered. *Br J Psychiatry* **137**, 45–54.

Fulton, G., Madden, C. and Minichiello, V. (1996), The social construction of anticipatory grief. *Soc Sci Med* **43**, 1349–58.

Gagnon, B., Bielech, M., Watanabe, S., Walker, P., Hanson, J. and Bruera, E. (1999), The use of intermittent subcutaneous injections of oxycodone for opioid rotation in patients with cancer pain. *Support Care Cancer* **7**, 265–70.

Gagnon, P., Allard, P., Masse, B. and DeSerres, M. (2000), Delirium in terminal cancer: a prospective study using daily screening, early diagnosis and continuous monitoring. *J Pain Symptom Manage* **19**, 412–26.

Gagnon, B., Lawlor, P.G., Mancini, I.L., Pereira, J.L., Hanson, J. and Bruera, E. (2001), The impact of delirium on the circadian distribution of breakthrough analgesia in advanceed cancer patients. *J Pain Sympt Manage* **22**, 826–33.

Gagnon P, Charbonneau C, Allard P, Soulard C, Dumont S, Fillion L. (2002). Delirium in advanced cancer: a psychoeducational intervention for family caregivers. *J Palliat Care* **18**:253–61.

Gagnon B, Graeme L, Schreier G. (2005). Methylphenidate hydrochloride improves cognitive functions in patients with advanced cancer and hypoactive delirium: a prospective clinical study. *Rev Psychiatr Neurosci* **30**: 100–107

Galanakis, P., Bickel, H., Gradinger, R., Von Gumppenberg, S. and Forstl, H., Acute confusional state in the elderly following hip surgery: incidence, risk factors and complications., *Int J Geriatr Psychiatry*, **16** (2001) 349–55.

Galeno (1978), Galen on the affected parts. Karger, Basel.

Galinkin, J.L., Fazi, L.M., Cuy, R.M., Chiavacci, R.M., Kurth, C.D., Shah, U.K., Jacobs, I.N. and Watcha, M.F. (2000), Use of intranasal fentanyl in children undergoing myringotomy and tube placement during halothane and sevoflurane anesthesia. *Anesthesiology* **93**, 1378–83.

Gallagher, R. (1998). Nicotine withdrawal as an etiologic factor in delirium. *J Pain Sympt Manage* **16**, 76–77.

Galski, T., Williams, B. and Ehle, H.T. (2000), Effects of opioids on driving ability. *J Pain Sympt Manage* **19**, 200–8.

Galynker, I.I. and Tendler, D.S. (1997), Nizatidine-induced delirium. *J Clin Psychiatry* **58**, 327.

Gamberini M, Bolliger D, Lurati Buse GA, Burkhart CS, Grapow M, Gagneux A, Filipovic M, Seeberger MD, Pargger H, Siegemund M, Carrel T, Seiler WO, Berres M, Strebel SP, Monsch AU, Steiner LA. (2009). Rivastigmine for the prevention of postoperative delirium in elderly patientsundergoing elective cardiac surgery—a randomized controlled trial. *Crit Care Med.* **37**:1762–8.

Garges, H.P., Varia, I. and Doraiswamy, P.M. (1998), Cardiac complications and delirium associated with valerian root withdrawal. *JAMA* **280**, 1566–7.

Garza, M.B., Osterhoudt, K.C. and Rutstein, R. (2000). Central anticholinergic syndrome from orphenadrine in a 3 year old. *Ped Emergency Care* **16**(*2*), *97–8.*

Gaudreau JD, Gagnon P, Harel F, Roy MA, Tremblay A. (2005a). Psychoactive medications and risk of delirium in hospitalized cancer patients. *J Clin Oncol.* **23**(27):6712–8.

Gaudreau JD, Gagnon P, Harel F, Tremblay A, Roy MA. (2005b). Fast, systematic, and continuous delirium assessment in hospitalized patients: the nursing delirium screening scale. *J Pain Symptom Manage* **29**(4):368–75.

Gaudreau JD, Gagnon P, Roy MA, Harel F, Tremblay A (2005c). Association between psychoactive medications and delirium in hospitalized patients: a critical review *Psychosomatics* **46**, 302–16.

Gavazzi, C., Stacchiotti, S., Cavalletti, R. and Lodi, R. (2001), Confusion after antibiotics. *Lancet* **357** 1410.

Gelfand, S.B., Indelicato, J. and Benjamin, G. (1992), Using intravenous haloperidol to control delirium. *Psychopharmacology* **43**, 215.

Gemert van LA, Schuurmans MJ. (2007). The Neecham Confusion Scale and the Delirium Observation Screening Scale: capacity to discriminate and ease of use in clinical practice. *BMC Nurs.* **6**:3.

Gerlach AT, Murphy CV, Dasta JF. (2009). An updated focused review of dexmedetomidine in adults. *Ann Pharmacother* **43**:2064–74.

Gerritsen van der Hoop, R., De Angelis, L. and Posner, J. (1990), Neurotoxicity of combined radiation and chemotherapay. In: J. Hildebrand (ed.), Neurological adverse reaction to anticancer drugs. Springer Verlag, Berlin, pp. 45–53.

Geschwind, N. (1982), Disorders of attention: a frontier in neuropsychology. *Phil Trans R Soc Lond, B* **298**, 173–85.

Giacino, J.P. (1997), Disorders of consciousness: differential diagnosis and neuropathologic features. *Sem Neurol* **17**, 105–11.

Gibson, G.E., Blass, J.P., Huang, H. and Freeman, G.B. (1991), The cellular basis of delirium and its relevance to age-related disorders including Alzheimer disease. *Internatl Psychogeriatrics* **3**, 373–95.

Gijtenbeek, J.M.M., van den Bent, M.J. and Vecht, C.L. (1999), Cyclosporine neurotoxicity: a review. *J Neurol* 339–46.

Gil, R. (1989), Neurologie pour le practicien. Simep, Paris.

Gill, D. and Mayou, R. (2000). Delirium. In: M.G. Gelder, J.J.J. López-Ibor and N. Andreasen (eds), New Oxford Textbook of Psychiatry, vol **1**. Oxford University Press, New york, pp. 382–7.

Gill, M., LoVecchio, F. and Selden, B. (1999). Serotonin syndrome in a child after a single dose of fluvoxamine. *Ann Emerg Med* **33**, 457–9.

Gillman, P.K. (1995). Possible serotonin syndrome with moclobemide and pethidine. *Med J Australia* **162**, 554.

Gillman, P.K. (1998). Serotonin syndrome: history and risk. *Fundamental Clin Phamacol* **12**, 482–91.

Gillman, P.K. (1999). The serotonin syndrome and its treatment. *J Psychopharmacology* **13**, 100–9.

Givens JL, Jones RN, Inouye SK. (2009).The overlap syndrome of depression and delirium in older hospitalized patients. *J Am Geriatr Soc.***57**(8):1347–53.

Given, C.W., Stmmel, M., Given, B., Osuch, J., Kurtz, M.E. and Kurtz, J.C. (1993). The influence of cancer patients' symptoms and fucntional states on patients' depressiona and familiy caregivers' reaction and depression. *Health Psychol* **12**, 277–85.

Glare, P., Walsh, T.D. and Pippenger, C.E. (1990), Normorphine, aneurotoxic metabolite? *Lancet* **335**, 725–6.

Glaser R. (2005). Stress-associated immune dysregulation and its importance for human health: a personal history of psychoneuroimmunology. *Brain Behav Immun.* **19**:3–11.

Glassman, A. and Bigger, J.J. (2001). Antipsychotic drugs: prolonged QTc interval, torsade de pointes, and sudden death. *Am J Psychiatry* **158**, 1774–82.

Glavina, M.J. and Robertshaw, R. (1988). Myoclonic spasms following intrathecal morphine. *Anaesthesia* **43**, 389–90.

Glick, R.E., Sanders, K.M. and Stern, T.A. (1996), Failure to record delirium as a complication of intraaortic balloon pump treatment: a retrospective study. *J Geriatr Psychiatry Neurol* **9**, 97–9.

Godfrey A, Conway R, Leonard M, Meagher D, Olaighin G. (2009). A classification system for delirium subtyping with the use of a commercial mobility monitor. *Gait Posture* **30**:245–52.

Godfrey A, Conway R, Leonard M, Meagher D, Olaighin GM. (2010). Motion analysis in delirium: a discrete approach in determining physical activity for the purpose of delirium motoric subtyping. *Med Eng Phys.* **32**:101–10.

Goldstein, J.M., (2000) The new generation of antipsychotic drugs: how are atipycal are they? *Int'l Neuropsychopharmacol* **3**, 339–49.

Gordon, D. and Peruselli, C. (2001), Narrazione e fine della vita. Nuove possibilità per valutare qualità della vita e della morte. Franco Angeli, Milano.

Grace JB, Holmes J. (2006). The management of behavioural and psychiatric symptoms in delirium. *Expert Opin Pharmacother* **7**:555–61.

Graham, J., Ramirez, A.J., Cull, A., Finlay, I., Hoy, A. and Richards, M.A. (1996), Job stress and satisfaction among palliative physicians. *Pall Med* **10**, 185–94.

Grassi L. (2007). Bereavement in families with relatives dying of cancer. *Curr Opin Support Palliat Care* **1**(1):43–9.

Grassi L., Antonelli T. (2009). Psychotropic drugs. In Walsh D. (ed.) Palliative Medicine Textbook. Elsevier, New York, pp 759–67.

Grassi, L., Pavanati, M., Bedetti, A., Bicocchi, R. and AIDS Care, S.-S. (1995), Analysis of psychiatric consultations in patients with HIV infection and related syndromes. *AIDS Care* **7**, S73–7.

Grassi, L., Biancosino, B., Pavanati, M., Agostini, M. and Manfredini, R. (2001a), Depression or hypoactive delirium? A report of ciprofloxacin-induced mental disorder in a patient with chronic obstructive pulmonary disease. *Psychother Psychosom* **70**, 58–9.

Grassi, L., Caraceni, A., Beltrami, E., Zamorani, M., Maltoni, M., Monti, M., Luzzani, M., Mercadante, S. and De Conno, F. (2001b), Assessing delirium in cancer patients the Italian versions of the Delirium Rating Scale and the Memorial Delirium Assessment Scale. *J Pain Symptom Manage* **21**, 59–68.

Grbich, C., Parker, D. and Maddocks, I. (2001), The emotions and coping strategies of caregivers of family members with a terminal cancer. *J Palliat Care* **17**, 30–6.

Green B, Pettit T., Faith L, Seaton K. (2004). Focus on levomepromazine. *Curr Med Res Opin* **12**: 1877–81.

Gregory, D. (1994), The myth of control: suffering in palliative care. *J Pall Care* **10**, 18–22.

Gregory, R.E., Grossman, S. and Sheidler, V.R. (1992), Grand mal seizures associated with high-dose intravenous morphine: incidence and possible etiologies. *Pain* **51**, 255–8.

Greiner, F.C. (1817), Der traum und das fieberhafte Irreseyn. F.A. Brockhaus, Altenburg.

Greisinger, A.J., Lorimor, R.J., Aday, L.A., Winn, R.J. and Baile, W.F. (1997), Terminally ill cancer patients. Their most important concerns. *Cancer Pract* **5** 147–54.

Grobe, M.E., Ilstrup, D.M. and Ahman, D. (1981), Skills needed by family memmebrs to maintain the care of an advanced cancer patient. *Cancer Nurs* 371–5.

Groeneweg, M., Gyr, K., Amrein, R., Scollo-Lavizzari, G., Williams, R., Yoo, J.Y. and Schalm, S.W. (1996), Effect of flumazenil on the electroencephalogram of patients with portosystemic encephalopathy. Results of a double blind placebo-controlled multicenter trial. *Electroencephalogr Clin Neurophysiol* **98**, 29–34.

Groff, L. (1993), Risultati di un programma di assistenza domiciliare per pazienti oncologici in fase avanzata, Faculty of Medicine and Surgery, Oncology Specialty School. Universita' degli Studi di Mialno, Milan.

Grossman, S.A., Trump, D.L., Chen, D.C.P., Thomson, G. and Camargo, E.E. (1982), Cerebrospinal fluid abnormalities in patients with neoplastic meningitis. *Am J Med* **73**, 641–7.

Grover S, Malhotra S, Bharadwaj R, Bn S, Kumar S. (2009). Delirium in children and adolescents. *Int J Psychiatry Med* **39**:179–87.

Gueguen JA, Bylund CL, Brown RF, Levin TT, Kissane DW (2009). Conducting family meetings in palliative care: themes, techniques, and preliminary evaluation of a communication skills module. *Palliat Support Care* **7**:171–9.

Gupta N, de Jonghe J, Schieveld J, Leonard M, Meagher D. (2008). Delirium phenomenology: what can we learn from the symptoms of delirium? *J Psychosom Res*. **65**, 215–22.

Gupta, R.M., Parvizi, J., Hanssen, A.D. and Gay, P.C. (2001), obstructive sleep apnea syndrome Postoperative complications in patients with undergoing hip or knee replacement: a case-control study. *Mayo Clin Proc* **76**, 897–905.

Gustafson, Y., Brannstrom, B., Norberg, A., Bucht, G. and Winblad, B. (1991a), Underdiagnosis and poor documenttaion of acute confusional states in elderly hip fracture patients. *JAGS* **39**, 760–5.

Gustafson, Y., Olsson, T., Eriksson, S., Asplund, K. and Bucht, G. (1991b), Acute confusional state in stroke patients. *Cerebrovasc Dis* **1** 257–64.

Gyr, K., Meier, R., Haussler, J., Bouletreau, P., Fleig, W.E., Gatta, A., Holstege, A., Pomier-Layragues, G., Schalm, S.W., Groeneweg, M., Scollo-Lavizzari, G., Ventura, E., Zeneroli, M.L., Williams, R., Yoo, Y. and Amrein, R. (1996), Evaluation of the efficacy and safety of flumazenil in the treatment of portal systemic encephalopathy: a double blind, randomised, placebo controlled multicentre study. *Gut* **39**, 319–24.

Haddad, P. and Anderson, I. (2002), Antipsychotic-related QTc prolongation, torsade de pointes and sudden death. *Drugs* **62**, 1649–71.

Hagen, N. and Swanson, R. (1997), Strychnine-like multifocal myoclonus and seizures in extremely high-dose opioid administration: treatment strategies. *J Pain Symptom Manage* **14**, 51–8.

Hagstam, K.M. (1971), EEG frequency content related to chelical blood parameters in chronic uremia. *Scand J Urol Nephrol* Suppl 7.

Haines, J., Barclay, P. and Wauchob, T. (2001). Optimising management of delirium: Withdrawal of Droleptan (droperidol). *BMJ* **322**, 1603.

Hall, D.E., Kahan, B. and Snitzer, J. (1994). Delirium associated with hypophosphatemia in a patient with anorexia nervosa. *J Adolesc Health* **15**, 176–8.

Hall, W. and Zador, D. (1997). The alcohol withdrawal syndrome. *Lancet* **349**, 1897–1900.

Hamilton, S. and Malone, K. (2000), Serotonin syndrome during treatment with paroxetine and risperidone. *J Clin Psychopharmacol* **20**, 103–05.

Han CS, Kim YK. (2004). A double-blind trial of risperidone and haloperidol for the treatment of delirium. *Psychosomatics.* **45**(4):297–301.

Han, L., McCusker, J., Cole, M., Abrahamovicz, M., Primeau, F. and Elie, M. (2001). Use of medications with anticholinergic effect predicts clinical severity of delirium symptoms in older medical inpatients. *Arch Intern Med* **161** 1099–1105.

Hancock K, Clayton JM, Parker SM, Wal der S, Butow PN, Carrick S, Currow D, Ghersi D, Glare P, Hagerty R, Tattersall MH (2007). Truth-telling in discussing prognosis in advanced life-limiting illnesses: a systematic review. *Palliat Med* **21**:507–17.

Harrison, J., Haddad, P. and Maguire, P. (1995), The impact of cancer on key relatives: a comparison of relative and patient concerns. *Eur J Cancer* **31A**, 1736–40.

Hart, R., Best, A., Sessler, C. and Levenson, J.L. (1997), Abbreviated cognitive test for deliririum. *J Psychosom Res* **43**, 417–23.

Hart, R., Levenson, J., Sessler, C., Best, A., Schwartz, S. and Rutherford, L. (1996), Validation of a cognitive test for delirium in medical ICU patients. *Psychosomatics* **37**, 533–46.

Hatherill S, Flisher A. (2009). Delirium in children with HIV/AIDS. *J Child Neurol.* **24**:879–83.

Hattori H, Kamiya J, Shimada H, Akiyama H, Yasui A, Kuroiwa K, Oda K, Ando M, Kawamura T, Harada A, Kitagawa Y, Fukata S (2009). Assessment of the risk of postoperative delirium in elderly patients using E-PASS and the NEECHAM Confusion Scale. *Int J Geriatr* Psychiatry **24**:1304–10.

Hayakawa Y, Sekine A, Shimizu T (2004). Delirium induced by abrupt discontinuation of paroxetine. *J Neuropsychiatry Clin Neurosci.* **16**:119–20.

Hays, J.C., Kasl, S.V. and Jacobs, S.C. (1994), The course of psychological distress following threatened and actual conjugal bereavement. *Psychol Med* **24**, 411–21.

Heckmann, J.G., Birklein, F. and Neundorfer, B. (2000), Omeprazole-induced delirium. *J Neurol* **247**, 56–57.

Hendler, N., Cimini, C., Long, T. and Long, D. (1980), Comparison of cognitive impairment due to benzodiazepines and to narcotics. *Am J Psychiatry* **137**, 828–30.

Henon, H., Lebert, F., Durieu, I., Godefroy, O., Lucas, C., Pasquier, F. and Leys, D. (1999), Confusional state in stroke. Relation to preexisting dementia, patient characteristics and outcome. *Stroke* **30**, 773–9.

Heritch, A.J., Capwell, R. and Roy-Byrne, P.P.J.C.P. (1987). A case of psychosis and delirium following withdrawal from triazolam. *J Clin Psychiatry* **48**, 168–69.

Hermann, I., Denekens, J., Van den Eynden, B., Van Royen, P., Verrept, H. and Maes, R. (1999), General practitioners caring for terminally ill patients resident in a hospice. *Support Care Cancer* **7**, 437–8.

Hickey, M. (1990), What are the needs of families of critically ill patients? A review of the literature since 1976. *Heart Lung* **19**, 401–15.

Hillbom M, Pieninkeroinen I, Leone M. (2003). Seizures in alcohol-dependent patients: epidemiology, pathophysiology and management. *CNS Drugs* **17**:1013–30.

Hileman, J.W., Lackey, N.R. and Hassanein, R.S. (1992), Identifying the needs of home caregivers of patients with cancer. *Onc Nurs Forum* **19**, 771–7.

Hill, C.D., Risby, E. and Morgan, N. (1992), Cognitive deficits in deliririum: assessment over time. *Psychopharmacol Bull* **28**, 401–7.

Hinds, C. (1985), The needs of families who care for patients with cancer at home. Are we meeting them? *J Adv Nurs* **10**, 575–81.

Hinton, J. (1981), Sharing or withholding awareness of the dying between husband and wife. *J Psyhcosom Res* **25** 337–43.

Hinton, J. (1994), Can home maintain an acceptable quality of life for patients with terminal cancer and their relatives. *Pall Med* **8**, 183–96.

Hippocrates with an English traslation by WHS Jones, William Heinemann LTD, London, 1931.

Hjermstad M, Loge JH, Kaasa S (2004).Methods for assessment of cognitive failure and delirium in palliative care patients: implications for practice and research. *Palliat Med* **18**(6):494–506.

Holder, G., Brand, S., Hatzinger, M. and Holsboer-Trachsler, E. (2002), Reduction of daytime sleepiness in a depressive patient during adjunct treatment with modafinil. *J Psychiatry Res* **36** 49–52.

Honma, H., Kohsaka, M., Suzuki, I., Fukuda, N., Kobayashi, R., Sakakibara, S., Matubara, S. and Koyama, T. (1998), Motor activity rhythm in dementia with delirium. *Psychiatry Clin Neurosci* **52**, 196–8.

Hooten, W. and Pearlson, G. (1996), Delirium caused by tacrine and ibuprofen interaction [letter]. *Am J Psychiatry* **153** 842.

Horowitz, M.J., Bonanno, G.A. and Holen, A. (1993), Pathological grief: diagnosis and explanation, *Psychosom Med* **55**, 260–73.

Horowitz, M.J., Siegel, B., Holen, A., Bonanno, G.A., Milbrath, C. and Stinson, C. (1997), Diagnostic criteria for complicated grief disorder. *Am J Psychiatry* **154** 904–10.

Hottensen D. (2010). Anticipatory grief in patients with cancer. *Clin J Oncol Nurs* **14**(1):106–7.

Houts, P.S., Rusenas, I., Simmonds, M.A. and Hufford, D.L. (1991), Information needs of families of cancer patients: a literature review and recommendations. *J Cancer Educ* **6**, 255–61.

Huang, S.C., Tsai, S.J., Chan, C.H., Hwang, J.P. and Sim, C.B. (1998), Characteristics and outcome of delirium in psychiatric inpatients. *Psychiatry Clin Neurosci* **52**, 47–50.

Hudetz JA, Patterson KM, Iqbal Z, Gandhi SD, Byrne AJ, Hudetz AG, Warltier DC, Pagel PS (2009). Ketamine attenuates delirium after cardiac surgery with cardiopulmonary bypass. *J Cardiothorac Vasc Anesth.* **23**:651–7.

Hudson PL, Aranda S, Kristjanson LJ. (2004). Meeting the supportive needs of family caregivers in palliative care: challenges for health professionals. *J Palliat Med* **7**(1):19–25.

Hudson PL, Hayman-White K, Aranda S, Kristjanson LJ (2006a). Predicting family caregiver psychosocial functioning in palliative care. *J Palliat Care.* **22**:133–40.

Hudson PL, Kristjanson LJ, Ashby M, Kelly B, Schofield P, Hudson R, Aranda S, O'Connor M, Street A (2006b). Desire for hastened death in patients with advanced disease and the evidence base of clinical guidelines: a systematic review. *Palliat Med* **20**:693–701.

Hudson P, Quinn K, Kristjanson L, Thomas T, Braithwaite M, Fisher J, Cockayne M (2008). Evaluation of a psycho-educational group programme for family caregivers in home-based palliative care. *Palliat Med* **22**:270–80.

Huf G, Coutinho E, Adams C, for the TREC Collaborative Group. (2007). Rapid tranquillisation in psychiatric emergency settings in Brazil: pragmatic randomized controlled trial of intramuscular haloperidol versus intramuscular haloperidol plus promtheazine. *BMJ* **335**:869–72.

Hughes JR. (2009). Alcohol withdrawal seizures. *Epilepsy Behav* **15**:92–7.

Hughes, R.J. (1980), Correlations between EEG and chemical changes in uremia. *Electroencephalogr Clin Neurophysiol* **48**, 583–94.

Hui D, Bush SH, Gallo LE, Palmer JL, Yennurajalingam S, Bruera E (2010). Neuroleptic dose in the management of delirium in patients with advanced cancer. *J Pain Symptom Manage* **39** :186–96.

Hung, Y, Huang T (2006). Lorazepam and diazepam rapidly relieve the catatonic features in major depression. *Cliin Neuropharmacol* **29**, 144–47

Hurst SA, Mauron A (2006). The ethics of palliative care and euthanasia: exploring common values. *Palliat Med.* **20**:107–12.

Ildegarda di Bingen, Cause e cure delle infermità, Sellerio, Palermo, 1997

Immers HE, Schuurmans MJ, van de Bijl JJ. Recognition of delirium in ICU patients: a diagnostic study of the NEECHAM confusion scale in ICU patients. *BMC Nurs.* 2005 Dec 13;**4**:7. :7.

Inouye, S.K., Delirium in hospitalized older patients: recognition and risk factors, *J Geriatr Psychiatry Neurol*, **11** (1998) 118–25.

Inouye, S.K. and Charpentier, P.A., Precipitating factors for delirium in hospitalized elderly persons. Predictive model and interrelationship with baseline vulnerability, *JAMA*, **275** (1996) 852–57.

Inouye, S.K., van Dyck, C.H., Alessi, C.A., Balkin, S., Siegal, A.P. and Horwitz, R.I., Clarifying confusion: the confusion assessment method. A new method for detection of delirium, *Ann Intern Med*, **113** (1990) 941–48.

Inouye, S.K., Viscoli, C.M., Horwitz, R.I., Hurst, L.D. and Tinetti, M.E., A predictive model for delirium in hospitalized elderly medical patients based on admission characteristics, *Ann Intern Med*, **119** (1993) 474–81.

Inouye, S.K., Bogardus, S.T., Charpentier, P.A., Leo-Summers, L., Acampora, D., Holford, T.R. and Coeney, L.M., A multicomponent intervention to prevent delirium in hospitalized older patients, *N Engl J Med*, **340** (1999a) 669–76.

Inouye, S.K., Schlesinger, M.J. and Lyndon, T.J., Delirium: a symptom of how hospital care is failing older persons and a window to improve quality of hospital care, *Am J Med*, **106** (1999b) 565–73.

Inouye, S.K., Foreman, M.D., Mion, L.C., Katz, K.H. and Cooney, L.M.J., Nurses' recognition of delirium and its symptoms: comparison of nurse and researcher ratings, *Arch Intern Med*, **161** (2001) 2467–73.

Inouye SK, Bogardus ST Jr, Williams CS, Leo-Summers L, Agostini JV: The role of adherence on the effectiveness of nonpharmacologic interventions: evidence from the delirium prevention trial. *Arch Intern Med.* 2003; **163**:958–64.

Irwin MR, Miller AH. Depressive disorders and immunity: 20 years of progress and discovery. *Brain Behav Immun.* 2007;**21**:374–83.

Itil, T. and Fink, M., EEG and behavioral apects of the interaction of anticholinergic hallucinogens with centrally active compounds., *Prog Brain Res*, **28** (1968) 149–68.

Jackson, C.W., Markowitz, J.S. and Brewerton, T.D., Delirium associated with clozapine and benzodiazepine combination, *Ann Clin Psychiatry*, **7** (1995) 139–41.

Jackson, J.H., Selected writings, Hodder and Stoughton, London, 1932.

Jackson K, Lipman A. Drug therapy for delirium in terminally ill patients. *Cochrane database of systematic reviews* 2004; (2):CD004770.

Jackson, T., Ditmanson, L. and Phibbs, B., Torsade de pointes and low-dose oral haloperidol, *Arch Intern Med*, **157** (1997) 2013–5.

Jacobs, S., Hansen, F., Kaasl, S., Ostfield, A., Berkman, L. and Kim, K., Anxiety disorders during acute bereavement : risk and risk factors, *J Clin Psychiatry*, **51** (1990) 269–74.

Jacobs, S., Pathologic grief: maladaptation to loss, American Psychiatrc Press, Washington, 1993.

Jacobs, S., Mazure, C. and Prigerson, H., Diagnostic criteria for traumatic grief, *Death Stud*, **24** (2000) 185–99.

Jacobson, S. and Jerrier, H., EEG in delirium, *Sem Clin Neuropsychiatry*, **5** (2000) 86–92.

Jacobson, S. and Schreibman, B. (1997). Behavioral and pharmacologic treatment of delirium. *Am. Fam. Physician* **56**, 2005–12.

Jacobson, S.A., Leuchter, A.F. and Walter, D.O., Conventional and quantitative EEG in the diagnosis of delirium among the elderly. *J Neurol Neurosurg Psychiatry*, **56** (1993a) 153–58.

Jacobson, S.A., Leuchter, A.F., Walter, D.O. and Weiner, H., Serial quantitative EEG among elderly subjects with delirium, *Biol Psychiatry*, **34** (1993b) 135–40.

Jacobson SA, Dwyer PC, Machan JT, Carskadon MA. Quantitative analysis of rest-activity patterns in elderly postoperative patients with delirium: support for a theory of pathologic wakefulness. *J Clin Sleep Med.* 2008;4:137–42.

Jellema, J.G., Hallucinations during sustained-release morphine and methadone administration, *Lancet*, **i** (1987) 392.

Jenkins, B.G. and Kraft, E., Magnetic resonance spectroscopy in toxic encephalopathy and neurodegeneration, *Curr Opin Neurol*, **12** (1999) 753–60.

Jennings, M.T., Neurological complications of radiotherapy. In: R.G. Wiley (Ed.), Neurological complications of cancer, Mrcel Dekker Inc, New York, 1995, pp. 219–40.

Jo S, Brazil K, Lohfeld L, Willison K. Caregiving at the end of life: perspectives from spousal caregivers and care recipients. *Palliat Support Care.* 2007 Mar;5(1):11–7.

Johns, M.W., Daytime sleepiness, snoring, and obstructive sleep apnea. The Epworth sleepiness scale, *Chest*, **103** (1993) 30–36.

Johnson, J.C., Kerse, N.M., Gottlieb, G., Wanich, C., Sullivan, E. and Chen, K., Prospective versus retrospective methods of identifying patients with delirium, *J Am Geriatr Soc*, **40** (1992) 316–319.

Johnson JG, Zhang B, Prigerson HG. Investigation of a developmental model of risk for depression and suicidality following spousal bereavement. *Suicide Life Threat Behav.* 2008 Feb;38(1):1–12.

Johnson, L.C., Spinweber, C.L., Gomez, S.A. and Matteson, L.T., Daytime sleepiness, performance, mood, nocturnal sleep: the effect of benzodiazepine and caffeine and their relationship, *Sleep*, **13** (1990) 121–35.

Justice AC, McGinnis KA, Atkinson JH, Heaton RK, Young C, Sadek J, Madenwald T, Becker JT, Conigliaro J, Brown ST, Rimland D, Crystal S, Simberkoff M; Veterans Aging Cohort 5-Site Study Project Team Psychiatric and neurocognitive disorders among HIV-positive and negative veterans in care: Veterans Aging Cohort Five-Site Study. *AIDS*. 2004;**18** Suppl 1:S49–59.

Kagawa-Singer, M. and Blackhall, L.J., Negotiating cross-cultural issues at the end of life, *JAMA*, **286** (2001) 2993–3001.

Kales HC, Kamholz BA, Visnic SG, Blow FC. Recorded delirium in a national sample of elderly inpatients: potential implications for recognition. *J Geriatr Psychiatry Neurol*. 2003;**16**:32–38.

Kalisvaart KJ, de Jonghe JF, Bogaards MJ, Vreeswijk R, Egberts TC, Burger BJ, Eikelenboom P, van Gool WA. Haloperidol prophylaxis for elderly hip-surgery patients at risk for delirium: a randomized placebo-controlled study. *J Am Geriatr Soc*. 2005 **53**:1658–66

Kalivas, KK, Bourgeois JA Catatonia after liver and kidney transplantation (2009) *Gen Hosp Psychiatry* **31**, 196–98

Karam EG, Tabet CC, Alam D, Shamseddeen W, Chatila Y, Mneimneh Z, Salamoun MM, Hamalian M. Bereavement related and non-bereavement related depressions: a comparative field study. *J Affect Disord*. 2009;**112**(1-3):102–10.

Karena, M., Meehan, K.M., Wang, H., David, S.R., Nisivoccia, J., Jones, B., Beasley, J., Feldman, P.D., Mintzer, J., Beckett, L. and Breier, A., Comparison of Rapidly Acting Intramuscular Olanzapine, Lorazepam, and Placebo; A Double-blind, Randomized Study in Acutely Agitated Patients with Dementia, *Neuropsychopharmacology*, **26** (2002) 494–504.

Karki SD, Masood GR. Combination risperidone and SSRI-induced serotonin syndrome. *Ann Pharmacother*. 2003 Mar;**37**, 388–91.

Karnik NS, Joshi SV, Paterno C, Shaw R. Subtypes of pediatric delirium: a treatment algorithm. *Psychosomatics*. 2007;**48**:253–57.

Katirji, M.B., Visual hallucinations and cyclosporine, *Trasplantation*, **43** (1987) 768–69.

Katz, L. and Chochinov, H.M., The spectrum of grief in palliative care. In: P.R.K. Bruera E (Ed.), Topics in palliative care - Vol **2**., Oxford University Press, New York, 1998, pp. 295–310.

Kaufer, D., Catt, K., Lopez, O. and De, K.S., Dementia with Lewy bodies: response of delirium-like features to donepezil., *Neurology*, **51** (1998) p1512.

Kawashima T, Yamada S. Delirium caused by donepezil: a case study. *J Clin Psychiatry*. 2002;**63**:250-251

Kay, D.C., Eisenstein, R.B. and Jasinski, D., Morphine effects on human REM state, waking state and NREM sleep, *Psychopharmacologia*, **14** (1969) 404–416.

Kazmierski J, Kowman M, Banach M, Fendler W, Okonski P, Banys A, Jaszewski R, Sobow T, Kloszewska. Clinical utility and use of DSM-IV and ICD-10 Criteria and The Memorial Delirium Assessment Scale in establishing a diagnosis of delirium after cardiac surgery. *Psychosomatics*. 2008;**49**:73–76.

Kelly B, McClement S, Chochinov HM. Measurement of psychological distress in palliative care. *Palliat Med*. 2006;**20**:779–89.

Kemeny ME. Psychobiological responses to social threat: evolution of a psychological model in psychoneuroimmunology. *Brain Behav Immun*. 2009;**23**:1–9.

Kendler KS, Myers J, Zisook S. Does bereavement-related major depression differ from major depression associated with other stressful life events? *Am J Psychiatry*. 2008;**165**(11):1449–55.

Kesavan, S. and Sobala, G.M., Serotonin syndrome with fluoxetine plus tramadol, *J Royal Soc Med*, **92** (1999) 474–75.

Khan A, Levy P, DeHorn S, Miller W, Compton S. Predictors of mortality in patients with delirium tremens. *Acad Emerg Med* . 2008;**15**:788–90.

Khawaja, I.S., Marotta, R.F. and Lippmann, S., Herbal medicine as a factor in delirium, *Psychiatr Serv*, **50** (1999) 969–70.

Khouzam, H.R., Donnelly, N.J. and Ibrahim, N.F., Psychiatric morbidity in HIV patients, *Can J Psychiatry*, **43** (1998) 51–56.

Kiely DK, Jones RN, Bergmann MA, Marcantonio ER. Association between psychomotor activity delirium subtypes and mortality among newly admitted post-acute facility patients. *J Gerontol A Biol Sci Med Sci.* 2007;**62**:174–79.

Kiely DK, Jones RN, Bergmann MA, Murphy KM, Orav EJ, Marcantonio ER. Association between delirium resolution and functional recovery among newly admitted postacute facility patients. *J Gerontol A Biol Sci Med Sci.* 2006;**61**:204–208.

Kiely DK, Marcantonio ER, Inouye SK, Shaffer ML, Bergmann MA, Yang FM, Fearing MA, Jones RN. Persistent delirium predicts greater mortality. *J Am Geriatr Soc.* 2009;**57**:55–61.

Kim KY,McCartney JR, Kaye W, Boland RJ, and Niaura R. The effect of cimetidine and ranitidine on cognitive function in postoperative cardiac surgery. Int. *J. Psychiatry Med.* 1996;**26**, 295–307.

Kim KY, Bader GM, Kotlyar V, Gropper D. Treatment of delirium in older adults with quetiapine. *J Geriatr Psychiatry Neurol.* 2003;**16**:29–31.

Kinney, H.C., Korein, J., Panigrahy, A., Dikkes, P. and Goode, R., Neuropathological findings in the brain of Karen Ann Quinlan, *N Engl J Med*, **330** (1994) 1469–75.

Kissane, D.W. and Bloch, S., Family grief, *Br J Psychiatry*, **164** (1994) 720–40.

Kissane, D.W., Bloch, S., Burns, W.I., McKenzie, D. and Posterino, M., Psychological morbidity in the families of patients with cancer, *Psych-Oncology*, **3** (1994a) 47–56.

Kissane, D.W., Bloch, S., Burns, W.I., Patrick, J.D., Wallace, C.S. and McKenzie, D., Perceptions of famlily functioning and cancer, *Psych-Oncology*, **3** (1994b) 259–69.

Kissane, D.W., Bloch, S., Onghena, P., McKenzie, D.P., Snyder, R.D. and Dowe, D.L., The Melbourne Family Grief Study, II: Psychosocial morbidity and grief in bereaved families, *Am J Psychiatry*, **153** (1996) 659–66.

Kissane, D.W., Bloch, S., McKenzie, D., McDowall, A. and Nitzan, R. (1998), Family grief therapy: a preliminary acount of a new model to promote healthy family functioning during palliative care and bereavement, *Psych-Oncology*, **7** 14–25.

Kissane DW, McKenzie M, McKenzie DP, Forbes A, O'Neill I, Bloch S. Psychosocial morbidity associated with patterns of family functioning in palliative care: baseline data from the Family Focused Grief Therapy controlled trial. *Palliat Med.* 2003;**17**(6):527–37.

Kissane DW, McKenzie M, Bloch S, Moskowitz C, McKenzie DP, O'Neill I. Family focused grief therapy: a randomized, controlled trial in palliative care and bereavement. *Am J Psychiatry.* 2006;**163**(7):1208–18.

Klagsbrun, S.C., Patient, family, amd staff suffering, *J Pall Care*, **10** (1994) 14–17.

Kloke, M., Bingel, U. and Seeber, S., Complications of spinal opioid therapy: myoclonus, spastic musce tone and spinal jerking, *Support Care Cancer*, **2** (1994) 249–52.

Knapp CA. Research in pediatric palliative care: closing the gap between what is and is not known. *Am J Hosp Palliat Care.* 2009;**26**:392–98.

Kobayashi, K., Takeuchi, O., Suzuki, M. and Yamaguchi, N., A retrospective study on delirium type, *Jpn J Psychiatry Neurol*, **46** (1992) 911–917.

Koponen, H., Partanen, J., Paakkonen, A., Mattila E and Rikkinen, P.J., EEG spectral analysis in delirium., *J Neurol* Neurosurg Psychiatry, **52** (1989) 980–85.

Koponen, H.J. and Riekkinen, P.J., A prospective study of delirium in elderly patients admitted to a psychiatric hospital, *Psychol Med*, **23** (1993) 103–109.

Kornblith, A.B., Does palliative care palliate?, *J Clin Oncol*, **19** (2001) 2111–2113.

Korones DN. Pediatric palliative care. *Pediatr Rev.* 2007;**28**:46–56.

Kristjanson, L.J., The family as a unit of treatment. In: R.K. Portenoy and E. Bruera (Eds.), Topics in palliative care - Volume 1, Oxford University Press, New york, 1997, pp. 245–62.

Kristjanson LJ, Aoun S. Palliative care for families: remembering the hidden patients. *Can J Psychiatry.* 2004;**49**(6):359–65.

Kristjanson, L.J. and Ashercraft, T., The family's cancer journey: a literature review, *Cancer Nurs*, **17** (1994) 1–17.

Kristjanson, L.J., Dudgeon, D. and Adaskin, E., Family members' perceptions of palliative cancer care: predictors of family functioning and family members' health, *J Pall Care*, **12** (1996) 10–20.

Kroeger D, de Lecea L. The hypocretins and their role in narcolepsy. *CNS Neurol Disord Drug Targets.* 2009;**8**:271–80.

Kruszewski SP, Paczynski RP, Kahn DA. Gabapentin-induced delirium and dependence. *J Psychiatr Pract.* 2009;**15**:314–319

Kubler-Ross, E., On death and dying, Macmillan, New York, 1969.

Kumar CN, Andrade C, Murthy P. A randomized, double-blind comparison of lorazepam and chlordiazepoxide in patients with uncomplicated alcohol withdrawal. *J Stud Alcohol Drugs.* 2009;**70**:467–74.

Kupfer, A., Aeschlimann, C. and Cerny, T., Methylene blue and neurotoxic mechanism of ifosfamide encephalopathy, *Eur J Clin Pharmacol*, **50** (1996) 249–52.

Kurita GP, Lundorff L, Pimenta CA, Sjøgren P. (2009) The cognitive effects of opioids in cancer: a systematic review. *Support Care Cancer* **17**, 11–21.

Kurtz, M.E., Kurtz, J.C., Given, C.W. and Given, B., Relationship of caregiver reactions and depression to cancer patients' symptoms, functional states and depression. A longitudinal view., *Soc Sci Med*, **40** (1995) 837–46.

Kutner JS, Kilbourn KM. Bereavement: addressing challenges faced by advanced cancer patients, their caregivers, and their physicians. *Prim Care.* 2009 Dec;**36**(4):825–44.

Lacasse H, Perreault M, Williamson D. Systematic review of antipsychotics for the treatment of hospital-associated delirium in medically or surgically ill patients. *Ann Pharmacother.* 2006; **40**:1966–73.

Laccetti, M., Manes, G., Uomo, G., Lioniello, M., Rabitti, P.G. and Balzano, A., Flumazenil in the treatment of acute hepatic encephalopathy in cirrhotic patients: a double blind randomized placebo controlled study, *Dig Liver Dis*, **32** (2000) 335–38.

Lalonde, B., Uldall, K.K. and Berghuis, J.P., Delirium in AIDS patients: discrepancy between occurrence and health care provider identification., *AIDS Patient Care STDS*, **10** (1996) 282–87.

Langner R, Maercker A. Complicated grief as a stress response disorder: evaluating diagnostic criteria in a German sample. *J Psychosom Res.* 2005;**58**(3):235–42.

Lannen PK, Wolfe J, Prigerson HG, Onelov E, Kreicbergs UC. Unresolved grief in a national sample of bereaved parents: impaired mental and physical health 4 to 9 years later. *J Clin Oncol.* 2008;**26**(36):5870–76.

Langenbucher, J., Martin, C.S., Labouvie, E., Sanjuan, P.M., Bavly, L., Pollock, N.K. and 68:799-809, Toward the DSM-V: the Withdrawal-Gate Model versus the DSM-IV in the diagnosis of alcohol abuse and dependence., *J Consult Clin Psychol*, **68** (2000) 799–809.

Lapin, S.L., Auden, S.M., Goldsmith, L.J. and Reynolds, A.M., Effects of sevoflurane anaesthesia on recovery in children: a comparison with halothane, *Paediatr Anaesth*, **9** (1999) 283–86.

Lasagna, L. and DeKornfeld, T.J., Methotrimeprazine, a new phenothiazine derivative with analgesic properties., *Journal of the American Medical Association*, **178** (1961) 887–90.

Laurila JV, Pitkala KH, Strandberg TE, Tilvis RS.: Impact of Different Diagnostic Criteria on Prognosis of Delirium: A Prospective Study. *Dement Geriatr Cogn Disord.* **18** (2004) 240–44

Laurila JV, Pitkala KH, Strandberg TE, Tilvis RS.: The impact of different diagnostic criteria on prevalence rates for delirium. *Dement Geriat*r Cogn Disord. **16** (2003)156–62.

Lawlor, P., The panorama of opioid-related cognitive dysfunction in patients with cancer: a critical literature appraisal, *Cancer*, **94** (2002) 1836–53.

Lawlor, P., Gagnon, B., Mancini, I., Pereira, J. and Bruera, E., Phenomenology of delirium and its subtypes in advanced cancer patients: a prospective study, *J Palliat Care*, **14** (1998) 106.

Lawlor, P.G., Fainsinger, R.L. and Bruera, E.D., Delirium at the end of life. Critical issues in clinical practice and research, *JAMA*, **284** (2000a) 2427–29.

Lawlor, P.G., Gagnon, B., Mancini, I.L., Pereira, J.L., Hanson, J., Suarez-Almazor, M.E. and Bruera, E.D., Occurrence, causes and outcome of delirium in patients with advanced cancer, *Arch Intern Med*, **160** (2000b) 786–94.

Lawlor, P.G., Nekolaichuk, C., Gagnon, B., Mancini, I.L., Pereira, J.L. and Bruera, E.D., Clinical utility, factor analysis and further validation of the Memorial Delirium Assessment Scale (MDAS) in advanced cancer patients, *Cancer* (2000c).

Lawlor, P., Gagnon, B., Mancini, I.L., Pereira, J.L., Hanson, J., Suarez-Almazor, M.E. and Bruera, E., In reply to Davis et al., *Arch Intern Med*, **161** (2001) 297–99.

Lederberg, M., The family of the cancer patients. In: H. J. (Ed.), Psycho-Oncology, Oxford University Press, New York, 1998a, pp. 981–93.

Lederberg, M., Oncology staff stress and related interventions. In: J. Holland (Ed.), Psycho-Oncology, Oxford University Press, New York, 1998b, pp. 1035–48.

Lee, D.O. and Lee, C.D., Serotonin syndrome in a child associated with erytromycin and sertraline, *Pharmacotherapy*, **19** (1999) 894–96.

Lee JH, Jang MK, Lee JY, Kim SM, Kim KH, Park JY, Lee JH, Kim HY, Yoo JY. Clinical predictors for delirium tremens in alcohol dependence. *J Gastroenterol Hepatol.* 2005;**20**:1833–37.

Lee KU, Won WY, Lee HK, Kweon YS, Lee CT, Pae CU, Bahk WM. Amisulpride versus quetiapine for the treatment of delirium: a randomized, open prospective study. *Int Clin Psychopharmacol.* 2005;**20**:311–314.

Leentjens AF, Diefenbacher A. A survey of delirium guidelines in Europe. *J Psychoso*m Res. 2006;**61**:123–28

Leentjens AF, Schieveld JN, Leonard M, Lousberg R, Verhey FR, Meagher DJ. A comparison of the phenomenology of pediatric, adult, and geriatric delirium. *J Psychosom Res.* 2008;**64**:219–23.

Leinonen, E., Koponen, H.J. and Lepola, U., Delirium during fluoxetine treatment, *Ann Clin Psychiatry*, **5** (1993) 255–57.

Leipzig, R.M., Goodman, H., Gray, G., Erle, H. and Reidenberg, M.M., Reversible, narcotic-associated mental status impairment in patients with metastatic cancer, *Pharmacology*, **35** (1987) 47–54.

Leis, A.M., Kristjanson, L., Koop, P. and Laizner, A., Family health and the palliative care trajectory: a cancer research agenda, *Cancer Prevent Control*, **1** (1997) 352–60.

Lemkau, J.P., Mann, B., Little, D., Whitecar, P., Hershberger, P. and Schumm, J.A., A questionnaire survey of family practice physicians' perceptions of bereavement care, *Arch Fam Med*, **9** (2000) 822–29.

Lemperiere, T. and Feline, A., Psychiatrie de l'adulte, Masson, Paria, 1977.

Leo RJ, Baer D. Delirium associated with baclofen withdrawal: a review of common presentations and management strategies. *Psychosomatics.* 2005;**46**:503–507.

Leonard M, Raju B, Conroy M, Donnelly S, Trzepacz PT, Saunders J, Meagher D. (2008) Reversibility of delirium in terminally ill patients and predictors of mortality. *Palliat Med.* **22**, 848–54.

Leonard M, Spiller J, Keen J, MacLullich A, Kamholtz B, Meagher D. Symptoms of depression and delirium assessed serially in palliative-care inpatients *Psychosomatics.* 2009 Sep-Oct;**50**(5):506–14

Leso, L. and Schwartz, T.L., Ziprasidone treatment of delirium, *Psychosomatics*, 43 (2002) 61–62.

Leung JM, Sands LP, Rico M, Petersen KL, Rowbotham MC, Dahl JB, Ames C, Chou D, Weinstein P. Pilot clinical trial of gabapentin to decrease postoperative delirium in older patients. *Neurology.* 2006a 10;**67** :1251–3.

Leung JM, Sands LP, Vaurio LE, Wang Y. Nitrous oxide does not change the incidence of postoperative delirium or cognitive decline in elderly surgical patients. *Br J Anaesth.* 2006b;**96** :754–60.

Leung JM, Sands LP, Paul S, Joseph T, Kinjo S, Tsai T. 2009 Does postoperative delirium limit the use of patient-controlled analgesia in older surgical patients? *Anesthesiology.* **111**, 625–31.

Levenson, J.A., Should psychostimulants be used to treat delirious patients with depressed mood, *J CLin Psychiatry*, **53** (1992) 69.

Levenson, J.L., High-dose intravenous haloperidol for agitated delirium following lung transplantation, *Psychosomatics*, **36** (1995) 66–68.

Levin, T., Petrides, G., Weiner, J., Saravay, S., Multz, A.S. and Bailine, S., Intractable delirium associated with ziconotide successfully treated with electroconvulsive therapy, *Psychosomatics*, **43** (2002) 63–66.

Levine, P., Silberfarb, P. and Lipowski, Z., Mental disorders in cancer patients: A study of 100 psychiatric referrals., *Cancer*, **42** (1978) 1385–91.

Levkoff, S.E., Evans, D.A., Lipzin, B., Cleary, P.D., Lipsitz, L.A., Wetle, T.T., Reilly, C.H., Pilgrim, D.M., Schor, J. and Rowe, J., Delirium. The occurence and persistence of symptoms among elderly hospitalized patients, *Arch Intern Med*, **152** (1992) 334–40.

Levkoff, S.E., Lipzin, B., Cleary, P., Wetle, T., Evans, D., Rowe, J. and Lipsitz, L., Subsyndromal delirium, *Am J Geriatr Psychiatry*, **4** (1996) 320–29.

Lewis, F.M., Strengthening family support: cancer and the family, *Cancer*, **65** (1990) 752–59.

Liao S and Arnold RM. Caring for caregivers: The essence of palliative care. *J Pall Med.* 2006;**9**:1172–74.

Lichtenthal W.G., Cruess D.G., Prigerson H.G.: A case for establishing complicated grief as a distinct mental disorder in DSM-V. *Clinical Psy*chology Review, 2004; **24**: 637–62.

Lin CE, Mao WC. Mania complicated with delirium following cessation of long-term lithium therapy. *Gen Hosp Psychiatry.* 2010;**32**:102–104.

Lindenbaum, J., Healton, E., Savage, D., Brust, J., Garrett, T., Podell, E., Marcell, P., Stabler, S. and Allen, R., Neuropsychiatric disorders caused by cobalamin deficiency in the absence of anemia or macrocytosis., *N Engl J Med*, **318** (1988) 1720–28.

Lindesay, J., The concept of delirium, *Dement Geriatr Cogn Disord*, **10** (1999) 310–314.

Lipowski, Z.J. (1980). Delirium: acute brain failure in man. Charles C. Thomas, Springfield Ill.

Lipowski ZJ Differentiating delirium from dementia in the elderly. *Clin Gerontol* 1982; **1**:3.

Lipowski, Z.J. Etiology. In Delirium: acute confusional states, Oxford University Press, New York Oxford, 1990a, pp. 109–40.

Lipowski, Z.J., Delirium: acute confusional states, Oxford University Press, New York, 1990b, 490 pp.

Lipowski, Z.J., Update on delirium, *Psychiatric Clinics of North America*, **15** (1992) 335–45.

Lipsitt, D.R. and Lipsitt, M.P., Guidelines for working with familes in consultation. liaison psychiatry. In: F.K. Judd, G.D. Burrows and D.R. Lipsitt (Eds.), Handbook of studies on general hospital psychiatry, Elsevier, Amsterdam, 1991, pp. 179–94.

Liptzin, B., What criteria should be used for the diagnosis of delirium?, *Dementa Geriatr Cogn Disord*, **10** (1999) 364–67.

Liptzin, B. and Levkoff, S.E., An empyrical study of delirium subtypes, *Br J Psychiatry*, **161** (1992) 843–45.

Liptzin, B., Levkoff, S.E., Cleary, P.D., Pilgrim, D.M., Reilly, C.H., Albert, M. and Wetle, T.W., An empirical study of diagnostic criteria for delirium, *Am J Psychiatry*, **148** (1991) 454–57.

Liptzin B, Laki A, Garb JL, Fingeroth R, Krushell R. Donepezil in the prevention and treatment of post-surgical delirium. *Am J Geriatr Psychiatry.* 2005 **13**;1100–6.

Liston, E. and Sones, D., Postictal Hyperactive Delirium in ECT: Management with Midazolam, *Convuls Ther*, **6** (1990) 19–25.

Litaker, D., Locala, J., Franco, K., Bronson, D.L. and Tannous, Z.M.-A.-. Preoperative risk factors for postoperative delirium., *Gen Hosp Psychiatry*, **23** (2001) 84–69.

Ljubisavljevic V, Kelly B Risk factors for development of delirium among oncology patients. *Gen Hosp Psychiatry.* 2003 Sep-Oct;**25**(5):345–52.

Löf L, Berggren L, Ahlström G.: Severely ill ICU patients recall of factual events and unreal experiences of hospital admission and ICU stay—3 and 12 months after discharge. *Intensive Crit Care Nurs.* 2006 Jun;**22**(3):154–66.

Lonergan E, Britton AM, Luxenberg J, Wyller T. Antipsychotics for delirium. *Cochrane Database Syst Rev.* 2007 Apr **18**;(2):CD005594.

Lonergan E, Luxenberg J, Areosa Sastre A. Benzodiazepines for delirium. *Cochrane Database Syst Rev.* 2009 Oct 7;(4):CD006379.

Lotsch, J., Kobal, G., Stockman, A., Brune, K. and Geisslinger, G., Lack of analgesic activity of morphine-6-glucuronide after short-term intravenous administration in healthy volunteers, *Anestesiology*, **87** (1997) 1348–58.

Lowery DP, Wesnes K, Ballard CG. Subtle attentional deficits in the absence of dementia are associated with an increased risk of post-operative delirium. *Dement Geriatr Cogn Disord.* 2007;**23**:390–94.

Lowery DP, Wesnes K, Brewster N, Ballard C. Quantifying the association between computerised measures of attention and confusion assessment method defined delirium: a prospective study of older orthopaedic surgical patients, free of dementia. *Int J Geriatr Psychiatry.* 2008;**23**:1253–60.

Lowery DP, Wesnes K, Brewster N, Ballard C. Subtle deficits of attention after surgery: quantifying indicators of sub syndrome delirium. *Int J Geriatr Psychiatry.* 2010 Jan 6. [Epub ahead of print]

Luetz A, Heymann A, Radtke FM, Chenitir C, Neuhaus U, Nachtigall I, von Dossow V, Marz S, Eggers V, Heinz A, Wernecke KD, Spies CD. Different assessment tools for intensive care unit delirium: which score to use? *Crit Care Med.* 2010 Feb;**38**(2):409–18.

Lundorff LE, Jønsson BH, Sjøgren P. Modafinil for attentional and psychomotor dysfunction in advanced cancer: a double-blind, randomised, cross-over trial. *Palliat Med.* 2009;**23**:731–38.

Lundström M, Edlund A, Bucht G, Karlsson S, Gustafson Y. Dementia after delirium in patients with femoral neck fractures. *J Am Geriatr Soc.* 2003 Jul;**51**(7):1002–6.

Lynch, E.P., Lazor, M.A., Gellis, J.E., Orav, J., Goldman, L. and Marcantonio, E.R., The impact of postoperative pain on the development of postoperative delirium, *Anesth Analg,* **86** (1998) 781–85.

MacDonald, A.J.D., Can delirium be separated from dementia?, *Dement Geriatr Cogn Disord,* **10** (1999) 386–88.

Macdonald, G.A., Frey, K.A., Agranoff, B.W., Minoshima, S., Koeppe, R.A., Kuhl, D.E., Shulkin, B.L. and Lucey, M.R., Cerebral benzodiazepine receptor binding i vivo in patients with recurrent hepathic encephalopathy, *Hepatology,* **26** (1997) 277–82.

MacDonald, N., Der, L., Allan, S. and Champion, P., Opioid hyperexcitability: the application of alternate opioid therapy, *Pain,* **53** (1993) 353–55.

Mach, J.J., Kabat, V., Olson, D. and Kuskowski, M., Delirium and right-hemisphere dysfunction in cognitively impaired older persons., *Int Psychogeriatr,* **8** (1996) p373–82.

Maciejewski PK, Zhang B, Block SD, Prigerson HG. An empirical examination of the stage theory of grief. *JAMA.* 2007;**297**(7):716–23

Macleod, A.D. and Whitehead, L.E., Dysgraphia in terminal delirium, *Palliat Med,* **11** (1997) 127–32.

Maddocks, I., Somogyi, A., Abbott, F. and et al, Attenuation of morphin-induced delirium in palliative care by substitution with infusion of oxycodone, *J Pain Sympt Manage,* **12** (1996) 182–89.

Madi, S. and Langonnet, F., Postoperative agitation. A new cause (French), *Cahiers d' Anesthesiologie,* **36** (1988) 509–512.

Maes, M., Vanoolaeghe, E., Degroote, J., Altamura, C. and Roels, C., Linear CT-scan measurement in alcohol-dependent patients without delirium tremens., *Alcohol,* **20** (2000) 117–23.

Magoun, H.W., An ascending reticular activating system in the brainstem, *Arch Neurol Psychiatry,* **67** (1952) 145–54.

Maguire, P., Communication with terminally ill patients and their families. In: H.M. Chochinov and W. Breitbart (Eds.), Handbook of psychiatry in palliative medicine, Oxford University Press, New York, 2000, pp. 291–301.

Main, J., Improving management of bereavement in general practice based on a survey of recently bereaved subjects in a single general practice, *Br J Gen Pract,* **50** (2000) 863–66.

Makker, R. and Yanny, W., Postoperative delirium mimicking epilepsy, *Anaesthesia,* **55** (2000) 74–78.

Maldonado JR. Delirium in the acute care setting: characteristics, diagnosis and treatment. *Crit Care Clin.* 2008;**24**:657–722

Maldonado JR, Wysong A, van der Starre PJ, Block T, Miller C, Reitz BA. Dexmedetomidine and the reduction of postoperative delirium after cardiac surgery. *Psychosomatics.* 2009; **50**:206–217.

Maltoni, M., Nanni, O. and Pirovano, M., Successful validation of the palliative prognostic score in terminally ill cancer patients., *J Pain Symptom Manage*, **17** (1999) 240–47.

Maltoni M, Pittureri C, Scarpi E, Piccinini L, Martini F, Turci P, Montanari L, Nanni O, Amadori D. Palliative sedation therapy does not hasten death: results from a prospective multicenter study. *Annals of Oncology*. 2009; **20**: 1163–69.

Manepalli, J., Grossberg, G.T. and Mueller, C., Prevalence of delirium and urinary tract infections in a psychogeriatic unit, *J Geriatr Psychiatry Neurol*, **3** (1990) 198–202.

Manos, P. and Wu, R., The duration of delirium in medical and postoperative patients referred for psychiatric consultation, *Ann Clin Psychiatry*, **9** (1997) 219–26.

Marcantonio, E., Ta, T., Duthie, E. and Resnick, N., Delirium severity and psychomotor types: their relationship with outcomes after hip fracture repair, *J Am Geriatr Soc*, **50** (2002) 850–57.

Marcantonio, E.R., Goldman, L., Mangione, C.M., Ludwig, L.E., Muraca, B., Haslauer, C.M., Donaldson, M.C., Whittemore, A.D., Sugarbaker, D.J., Poss, R., Haas, S., Cook, E.F., Orav, E.J. and Lee, T.H., A clinical prediction rule for delirium after elective noncardiac surgery, *JAMA*, **271** (1994a) 134–39.

Marcantonio, E.R., Juarez, G., Goldman, L., Mangione, C.M., Ludwig, L.E., Lind, L., Katz, N., Cook, E.F., Orav, J. and Lee, T.H., The relationship of postoperative delirium with psychoactive medication, *JAMA*, **272** (1994b) 1518–22.

Marcantonio, E.R., Goldman, L., Orav, E.J., Cook, E.F. and Lee, T.H., The association of intraoperative factors with the development of postoperative delirium, *Am J Med*, **105** (1998) 380–84.

Marcantonio, E.R., Flacker, J.M., Michaels, M. and Resnick, N.M., Delirium is independently associated with poor functional recovery after hip fracture, *J Am Geriatr Soc*, **48** (2000) 618–24.

Marcantonio, E.R., Flacker, J.M., Wright, R.J. and Resnick, N.M., Reducing delirium after hip fracture: a randomized trial, *J Am Geriatr Soc*, **49** (2001) 678–79.

Marder, S.R.A., Antipsychotic mediciations. In: A.F. Schatzberg and C.B. Nemeroff (Eds.), Textbook of Psychopharmacology, American Psychiatric Press, Washington, 1998, pp. 309–21.

Margolese, H.C. and Chouinard, G., Serotonin syndrome from addition of low-dose trazodone to nefazodone, *Am J Psychiatry*, **157** (2000) 1022.

Marik PE. Propofol: therapeutic indications and side-effects. *Curr Pharm Des.* 2004;**10**:3639–49.

Marino J, Russo J, Kenny M, Herenstein R, Livote E, Chelly JE. Continuous lumbar plexus block for postoperative pain control after total hip arthroplasty. A randomized controlled trial. *J Bone Joint Surg Am.* 2009 **91** :29–37.

Mark, B.Z., Kunkel, E.J., Fabi, M.B. and Thompson, T.L.n., Pimozide is effective in delirium secondary to hypercalcemia when other neuroleptics fail, *Psychosomatics*, **34** (1993) 446–50.

Massie, M.J., Holland, J.C. and Glass, E., Delirium in terminally ill cancer patients., *American Journal of Psychiatry*, **140** (1983) 1048–50.

Matsuoka, Y., Miyake, Y., Arakaki, H., Tanaka, K., Saeki, T. and Yamawaki, S., Clinical utility and validation of the Japanese version of the Memorial Delirium Assessment Scale in a psychogeriatric inpatient setting, *Gen Hosp Psychiatry*, **23** (2001) 36–40.

Matsushima, E., Nakajima, K., Moriya, H., Matsuura, M., Motomiya, T. and Kojima, T., A psychophysiological study of the development of delirium in coronary care units, *Biol Psychiatry*, **41** (1997) 1211–1217.

Matsushita T, Matsushima E, Maruyama M. Early detection of postoperative delirium and confusion in a surgical ward using the NEECHAM confusion scale. *Gen Hosp Psychiatry*. 2004 Mar-Apr;**26**(2):158–63.

Mayer, S.A., Chong, J.Y., Ridgway, E., Min, K.C., Commichau, C. and Bernardini, G.L.N.A.-. Delirium from nicotine withdrawal in neuro-ICU patients., *Neurology*, **57** (2001) 551–53.

Mayo-Smith, M.F., Pharmacological management of alcohol withdrawal. A meta-analysis and evidence-based practice guideline. American Society of Addiction Medicine Working Group on Pharmacological Management of Alcohol Withdrawal., *JAMA*, **278** (1997) 144–51.

Mayo-Smith MF, Beecher L, Fischer T, Gorelick D, Guillaume J, Hill A, et al. Management of alcohol withdrawal delirium. An evidence-based practice guideline. *Arch Intern Med* 2004; **164**:1405–12.

McAllister-Williams, R. and Ferrier, I., Rapid tranquillisation: time for a reappraisal of options for parenteral therapy, *B J Psychiatry*, **180** (2002) 485–89.

McAvay GJ, Van Ness PH, Bogardus ST Jr, Zhang Y, Leslie DL, Leo-Summers LS, Inouye SK. Depressive symptoms and the risk of incident delirium in older hospitalized adults. *J Am Geriatr Soc*. 2007;**55**:684–91.

McClement S, Chochinov HM, Hack T, Hassard T, Kristjanson LJ, Harlos M. Dignity therapy: family member perspectives. *J Palliat Med*. 2007;**10**(5):1076–82.

McClement, S.E. and Woodgate, R.L., Research with families in palliative care: conceptual and methodological challenges, *Eur J Cancer Care*, **7** (1998) 247–54.

McCowan, C. and Marik, P., Refractory delirium tremens treated with propofol: a case, *Crit Care Med*, **28** (2000) 1781–84.

McCusker, J., Cole, M., Bellavance, F. and Primeau, F., Reliability and validity of a new measure of severity of delirium., *Int Psychogeriatr*, **10** (1998) p421–33.

McCusker, J., Cole, M., Abrahamowicz, M., Han, L., Podoba, J. and Ramman-Haddad, L., Environmental risk factors for delirium in hospitalized older people., *J Am Geriatr Soc*, **49** (2001a) 1327–34.

McCusker, J., Cole, M.G., Dendukuri, N., Belzile, E. and Primeau, F., Delirum in older medical inpatients and subsequent cognitive and functional status: a prospective study, *Can Med Ass J*, **165** (2001b) 575–83.

McCusker, J., Cole, M., Abrahamowicz, M., Primeau, F. and Belzile, E., Delirium predicts 12-month mortality., *Arch Intern Med*, **162** (2002) 457–63.

McCusker J, Cole MG, Dendukuri N, Belzile E. The delirium index, a measure of the severity of delirium: new findings on reliability, validity, and responsiveness. *J Am Geriatr Soc*. 2004;**52**:1744–9.

McDermott, J.L., Gideonse, N. and Campbel, J.W., Acute delirium associated with ciprofloxacin administration in a hospitalized elderly patient, *J Am Geriat Soc*, **39** (1991) 909–910.

McKeon A, Frye MA, Delanty N. The alcohol withdrawal syndrome. *J Neurol Neurosurg Psychiatry*. 2008;**79**:854–62.

McMillan SC. Interventions to facilitate family caregiving at the end of life. *J Palliat Med*. 2005;**8** Suppl 1:S132–139.

McMillan SC, Small BJ, Weitzner M, Schonwetter R, Tittle M, Moody L, Haley WE. Impact of coping skills intervention with family caregivers of hospice patients with cancer: a randomized clinical trial. *Cancer*. 2006;**106**(1):214–22.

McSherry M, Kehoe K, Carroll JM, Kang TI, Rourke MT. Psychosocial and spiritual needs of children living with a life-limiting illness. *Pediatr Clin North Am*. 2007;**54**:609–29.

McWilliams K, Keeley PW, Waterhouse ET. Propofol for terminal sedation in palliative care: a systematic review. *J Palliat Med.* 2010;**13**:73–76.

Meagher, D. and Trzepacz, P., Delirium phenomenology illuminates pathophysiology, management, and course., *J Geriatr Psychiatry Neurol*, **11** (1998) p150–6; discussion 157-8.

Meagher D., Trzepacz P.T.: Phenomenological distinctions needed in DSM-V: Delirium, Subsyndromal Delirium, and Dementias. *J Neuropsychiatry Clin Neurosci.* 2007; **19**:468–70.

Meagher, D., O'Hanlon, D., O'Mahony, E. and Casey, P., The use of environmental startegies and psychotropic medication in the management of delirium, *Br J Psychiatry*, **168** (1996) 512–515.

Meagher, D., O'Hanlon, D., O'Mahony, E., Casey, P. and Trzepacz, P., Relationship between etiology and phenomenologic profile in delirium., *J Geriatr Psychiatry Neurol*, **11** (1998) p146–9; discussion 157-8.

Meagher, D., O'Hanlon, D., O'Mahony, E., Casey, P. and Trzepacz, P., Relationship between symtpoms and motoric subtype of delirium, *J Neuropsychiatry Clin Neurosci*, **12** (2000) 51–56.

Meagher, D.J., Delirium: optimizing management, *Br Med J*, **322** (2001) 144–49.

Meagher DJ, Moran M, Raju B, Gibbons D, Donnelly S, Saunders J, Trzepacz PT Phenomenology of delirium. Assessment of 100 adult cases using standardised measures. *Br J Psychi*atry. 2007 Feb;**190**:135–41.

Meagher DJ, MacClullich AM, Laurila JV. Defining delirium for the International Classification of Diseases, 11th Revision. *J Psychosom Res.* 2008;**65**:207–214.

Meagher DJ, Moran M, Raju B, Gibbons D, Donnelly S, Saunders J, Trzepacz PT. Motor symptoms in 100 patients with delirium versus control subjects: comparison of subtyping methods. *Psychosomatics.* 2008; **49**:300–308.

Mellins CA, Havens JF, McDonnell C, Lichtenstein C, Uldall K, Chesney M, Santamaria EK, Bell J. Adherence to antiretroviral medications and medical care in HIV-infected adults diagnosed with mental and substance abuse disorders. *AIDS Care.* 2009;**21**:168–77.

Menza, M.A., Murray, G.B., Holmes, V.F. and Rafuls, W.A., Decreased extrapyramidal symptoms with intravenous haloperidol, *J Clin Psychiatry*, **48** (1987) 278–80.

Mercadante, S., Dantrolene treatment of opioid-induced myoclonus, *Anesth Analg*, **81** (1995) 1307–1308.

Mercadante, S., Alkalinization is troublesome in advanced cancer patients with dyspnea (letter), *J Pain Sympt* Manage, **13** (1997) 316–317.

Mercadante, S., Pilocarpine as an adjuvant to morphine therapy, *Lancet*, **351** (1998) 338–39.

Mercadante, S., De Conno, F. and Ripamonti, C., Propofol in terminal care, *J Pain Sympt Manage*, **10** (1995) 639–42.

Mermelstein, H., Clarithromycin-induced delirium in a general hospital., *Psychosomatics*, **39** (1998) p540–2.

Mesulam, M.M., Waxman, S.G., Geschwind, N. and Sabin, T.D., Acute confusional state with right cerebral artery infarction, *J Neurol Neurosurg Psychiatry*, **39** (1976) 84–89.

Mesulam, M.-M., Attention, confusional states, and neglect. In: M.-M. Mesulam (Ed.), Principles of behavioral neurology, Vol. **26**, F. Plum, J.R. Baringer and S. Gilman, F.A. Davis, Philadelphia, 1985, pp. 125–68.

Metitieri, T., Bianchetti, A. and Trabucchi, M., Delirium as a predictor of survival in older patients with cancer, *Arch Intern Med*, **160** (2000) 2866–68.

Meyer, H.P., Legemate, D.A., van den Brom, W. and Rothuizen, J., Improvement of chronic hepatic encephalopathy in dogs by the benzodiazepine receptor partial inverse agonist sarmazenil but not by the antagonist flumazenil, *Metabolic Brain Disease*, **13** (1998) 241–51.

Middleton, W., Burnett, P., Raphael, B. and Martinek, N., The bereavement response: a cluster analysis, *Br J Psychiatry*, **169** (1996) 167–71.

Mieda M, Sakurai T. Integrative physiology of orexins and orexin receptors. *CNS Neurol Disord Drug Targets*. 2009;8:281–95.

Milisen, K., Foreman, M.D., Abraham, I.L., De Geest, S., Godderis, J., Vandermeulen, E., Fischler, B., Delooz, H.H., Spiessens, B. and Broos, P.L., A nurse-lead interdisciplinary intervention program for delirium in elderly hip-fracture patients, *J Am Geriatr Soc*, **49** (2001) 523–32.

Milisen K, Steeman E, Foreman MD. Early detection and prevention of delirium in older patients with cancer. *Eur J Cancer Care*. 2004;**13**: 494–500

Milisen K, Lemiengre J, Braes T, Foreman MD. Multicomponent intervention strategies for managing delirium in hospitalized older people: systematic review. *J Adv Nurs*. 2005;**52**:79–90.

Miller MO. Evaluation and management of delirium in hospitalized older patients. *Am Fam Physician*. 2008;**78**:1265–70.

Minagawa, H., Yosuke, U., Yamawaki, S. and Ishitani, K., Psychiatric morbidity in terminally ill cancer patients, *Cancer*, **78** (1996) 1131–37.

Miotto, K., Darakjian, J., Basch, J., Murray, S., Zogg, J. and Rawson, R.-Gamma-hydroxybutyric acid: patterns of use, effects and withdrawal., *Am J Addict*, **10** (2001) 232–41.

Mitchell GK. How well do general practitioners deliver palliative care? A systematic review. *Palliat Med*. 2002 Nov;**16**(6):457–64.

Mittal D, Jimerson NA, Neely EP, Johnson WD, Kennedy RE, Torres RA, Nasrallah HA. Risperidone in the treatment of delirium: results from a prospective open-label trial. *J Clin Psychiatry*. 2004 May;**65**(5):662–7.

Monette, J., Galbaud du Fort, G., Fung, S.H., Massoud, F., Moride, Y., Arsenault, L. and Afilalo, M., Evaluation of the confusion assessment method (CAM) as a screening tool for delirium in the emergency room, *Gen Hosp Psychiatry*, **23** (2001) 20–25.

Monte R, Rabuñal R, Casariego E, Bal M, Pértega S. Risk factors for delirium tremens in patients with alcohol withdrawal syndrome in a hospital setting. *Eur J Intern Med*. 2009;**20**:690–94.

Morandi A, Pandharipande P, Trabucchi M, Rozzini R, Mistraletti G, Trompeo AC, Gregoretti C, Gattinoni L, Ranieri MV, Brochard L, Annane D, Putensen C, Guenther U, Fuentes P, Tobar E, Anzueto AR, Esteban A, Skrobik Y, Salluh JI, Soares M, Granja C, Stubhaug A, de Rooij SE, Ely EW. Understanding international differences in terminology for delirium and other types of acute brain dysfunction in critically ill patients. *Intensive Care Med*. **34** (2008) 1907–1915.

Morita, T., Tsunoda, J., Inoue, S. and Chihara, S., The palliative prognostic index: a scoring system for survival prediction of terminally ill cancer patients, *Support Care Cancer*, **7** (1999) 128–33.

Morita, T., Otani, H., Tsunoda, J., Inoue, S. and Chihara, S., Succesful palliation of hypoactive delirium due to multiorgan failure by oral methylphenidate, *Supp Care Cancer*, **8** (2000) 134–37.

Morita, T., Tsuneto, S. and Shima, Y., Proposed definitions for terminal sedation, *Lancet*, **358** (2001) 335–36.

Morita T, Tsunoda J, Inoue S, Chihara S, Oka K. Communication Capacity Scale and Agitation Distress Scale to measure the severity of delirium in terminally ill cancer patients: a validation study. *Palliat Med*. 2001 May;**15**(3):197–206.

Morita, T., Tei, Y., Tsunoda, J., Inoue, S. and Chihara, S., Increased plasma morphine metabolites in terminally ill cancer patients with delirium: an intra-individual comparison., *J Pain Symptom Manage*, **23** (2002) 107–113.

Morita T, Hirai K, Sakaguchi Y, Tsuneto S, Shima Y. (2004) Family-perceived distress from delirium-related symptoms of terminally ill cancer patients. *Psychosomatics* **45**, 2107-113.

Morita T, Takigawa C, Onishi H, Tajima T, Tani K, Matsubara T, Miyoshi I, Ikenaga M, Akechi T, Uchitomi Y; Japan Pain, Rehabilitation, Palliative Medicine, and Psycho-Oncology (PRPP) Study Group. Opioid rotation from morphine to fentanyl in delirious cancer patients: an open-label trial. *J Pain Symptom Manage*. 2005 Jul;**30**:96–103.

Morita T, Akechi T, Ikenaga M, Inoue S, Kohara H, Matsubara T, et al. (2007) Terminal delirium: recommendations from bereaved families. *J Pain Symp Manag*, **34** 579–89.

Morrison, R.S., Siu, A.L., Leipzig, R.M., Cassel, C.K. and Meier, D.E., The hard task of improving the quality of care at the end of life, *Arch Intern Med*, **160** (2000) 743–47.

Moruzzi, G. and Magoun, H.W., Brain stem reticular formation and activation of the EEG, *Electroenceph Clin Neurophysiol*, **1** (1949) 455–73.

Moss, J.H., Anileridine-induced delirium, *J Pain Sympt Manage*, **10** (1995) 318–20.

Muller, N., Klages, U. and Gunther, W., Hepatic encephalopathy presenting as delirium and mania. The possible role of bilirubin, *Gen Hosp Psychiatry*, **16** (1994) 138–40.

Mussi, C., Ferrari, R., Ascari, S. and Salvioli, G., Importance of serum anticholinerigic activity in the assessment of elderly patients with delirium, *J Geriatr Psychiatry Neurol*, **12** (1999).

Nakamura, J., Yoshimura, R., Okuno, T., Ueda, N., Yoshimura, R., Eto, S., Terao, T., Nakamura, J., Hachida, M., Yasumoto, K., Egami, H., Maeda, H., Nishi, M. and Aoyagi, S., Association of plasma free-3-methoxy-4-hydroxyphenyl (ethylene)glycol, natural killer cell activity and delirium in postoperative patients, *Int Clin Psychopharmacol*, **16** (2001) 339–43.

Namba M, Morita T, Imura C, Kiyohara E, Ishikawa S, Hirai K. Terminal delirium: families' experience. *Palliat Med*. 2007;**21**:587–94.

Neelon VJ, Champagne MT, Carlson JR, Funk SG: The NEECHAM Confusion Scale: construction, validation, and clinical testing. *Nursing Research*. 1996, **45**:324–30.

Neumarker, K.H.P.P.-. Karl Bonhoeffer and the concept of Symptomatic psychoses., *Hist Psychiatry*, **12** (2001) 213–26.

Newman, J.P., Terris, D.J. and Moore, M., Trends in the management of alcohol withdrawal syndrome, *Laryngoscope*, **105** (1995) 1–7.

Ni K, Cary M, Zarkowski P. Carisoprodol withdrawal induced delirium: A case study. *Neuropsychiatr Dis Treat*. 2007;**3**:679–82.

Nicholas, L.M. and Lindsey, B.A., Delirium presenting with symtoms of depression, *Psychosomatics*, **36** (1995) 471–79.

Nickell, P.V., Histamine-2 receptor blockers and delirium, *Ann Intern Med*, **115** (1991) 658.

Niedermeyer, E., Ribeiro, M. and Hertz, S., Mixed-type encephalopathies: preliminary considerations, *Clin Electroenceph*, **30** (1999) 12–15.

Nieves, A.V. and Lang, A.E., Treatment of excessive daytime sleepiness in patients with Parkinsn's disease with modafinil, *Clin Neuropharmacol*, **25** (2002) 111–114.

Nijboer, C., Tempelaar, R., Sanderman, R., Triemstra, M., Sprujit, R.J. and Van den Bos, G., Cancer and caregiving the impact on the caregiver's health, *Psycho-Oncology*, **7** (1998) 3–13.

Noimark D. Predicting the onset of delirium in the post-operative patient. *Age Ageing*. 2009;**38**:368–73.

Normann, C., Brandt, C., Berger, M. and Walden, J., Delirium and persistent dyskinesia induced by a lithium-neuroleptic interaction, *Pharmacopsychiatry*, **31** (1998) 201–204.

Northouse, L.L., Family issues in cancer care. In: R.J. Goldberg (Ed.), Psychiatric aspects of cancer, Karger, Basel, 1988, pp. 82–101.

Norton, J.W., Gabapentin withdrawal syndrome., *Clin Neuropharmacol.*, **24** (2001) 245–46.

Nyatanga B. Culture, palliative care and multiculturalism. *Int J Palliat Nurs.* 2002;8:240–46.

O'Connor MF. Bereavement and the brain: invitation to a conversation between bereavement researchers and neuroscientists. *Death Stud.* 2005;**29**:905–22.

O'Dowd, M.A. and McKegney, F.P., AIDS patients compared with others seen in psychiatric consultation., *Gen Hosp Psychiatry*, **12** (1990) 50–55.

Okamoto Y, Matsuoka Y et al, Trazodone in the treatment of delirium. *J Clin Psychopharmacol* 1999; **19**(3): 280–82

O'Keeffe, S.T., Rating the severity of delirium: the delirium assessment scale, *Int J Geriatr Psychiatry*, **9** (1994) 551–56.

O'Keeffe, S.T., Clinical subtypes of delirium in the elderly, *Dement Geriatr Cogn Disord*, **10** (1999) 380–85.

O'Keeffe, S.T. and Chonchubhair, A., Postoperative delirium in the elderly, *Br J Anaesth*, **73** (1995) 673–87.

O'Keeffe, S.T. and Devlin, J.G., Delirium and dexamethasone suppression test in the elderly, *Neuropsych*obiology, **30** (1994) 153–56.

O'Keeffe, S.T., Tormey, W.P., Glasgow, R. and Lavan, J.N., Thiamine deficiency in hospitalized elderly patients, *Gronyology*, **40** (1994) 18–24.

Okon TR. Spiritual, religious, and existential aspects of palliative care. *J Palliat Med.* 2005;8:392–41.

Okon TR, George ML. Fentanyl-induced neurotoxicity and paradoxic pain. *J Pain Symptom Manage.* 2008 Mar;**35**(3):327–33.

Okugawa G, Kato M, Wakeno M, Koh J, Morikawa M, Matsumoto N, Shinosaki K, Yoneda H, Kishimoto T, Kinoshita T. Randomized clinical comparison of perospirone and risperidone in patients with schizophrenia: Kansai Psychiatric Multicenter Study. *Psychiatry Clin Neurosci.* 2009;**63**:322–28.

Olmedo R, Hoffman RS. Withdrawal syndromes. *Emerg Med Clin North Am.* 2000;**18**:273–88.

Olofson, S.M., Weitzener, M.A., Valentine, A.D., Baile, W.F. and Meyers, C.A., A retrospective study of the psychiatric management and outcome of delirium in the cancer patient, *Supp Care Cancer*, **4** (1996) 351–57.

Onrust, S.V., McClellan K. Perospirone. *CNS Drugs.* 2001;**15**(4):329–37.

Osmon, D.C., Luria-Nebraska neuropsychological battery case study: a mild drug related confusional state, *Int J Clin Neuropsychology*, **6** (1984).

Osse, B.H., Vernooij-Dassen, M.J., de Vree, B.P., Schade, E. and Grol, R.P., Assessment of the need for palliative care as perceived by individual cancer patients and their families: a review of instruments for improving patient participation in palliative care, *Cancer*, **88** (2000) 900–911.

Ouimet S, Riker R, Bergeron N, Cossette M, Kavanagh B, Skrobik Y Subsyndromal delirium in the ICU: evidence for a disease spectrum. *Intensive Care Med.* 2007;**33**:1007–1013.

Overshott R, Karim S, Burns A. Cholinesterase inhibitors for delirium. *Cochrane Database Syst Rev.* 2008 Jan **23**;(1):CD005317.

Owens, M.J. and Riscj, S.C., Atypical antipsychotics. In: A.F. Schatzberg and C.B. Nemeroff (Eds.), Textbook of Psychopharmacology, American Psychiatric Press, Washington, 1998, pp. 323–48.

Pae CU, Lee SJ, Lee CU, Lee C, Paik IH. A pilot trial of quetiapine for the treatment of patients with delirium. *Hum Psychopharmacol.* 2004;**19**:125–27.

Page CB, Duffull SB, Whyte IM, Isbister GK. Promethazine overdose: clinical effects, predicting delirium and the effect of charcoal. *QJM*. 2009 Feb;**102**(2):123–31. Epub 2008 Nov 28. PubMed PMID: 19042969.

Palmstierna, T., A model for predicting alcohol withdrawal delirium, *Psychiatr Serv*, **52** (2001) 820–23.

Pandharipande P, Shintani A, Peterson J, Pun BT, Wilkinson GR, Dittus RS, Bernard GR, Ely EW. Lorazepam is an independent risk factor for transitioning to delirium in intensive care unit patients. *Anesthesiology*. 2006;**104** :21–6.

Pandharipande P, Pun B, Herr D, Girard T, Miller R, Shintani A, et al. Effect of sedation with dexmedetomidine vs lorazepam on acute brain dysfunction in mechanically ventilated patients. *JAMA*. 2008; **298**:2644–53.

Papersack, T., Garbusinski, J., Robberecht, J., Beyer, I., Willems, D. and Fuss, M., Clinical relevance of thiamine status amongst hospitalized elderly patients, *Gerontology*, **45** (1999) 96–101.

Parellada E, Baeza I, de Pablo J, Martínez G. Risperidone in the treatment of patients with delirium. *J Clin Psychiatry*. 2004 Mar;**65**(3):348–53.

Parker SM, Clayton JM, Hancock K, Walder S, Butow PN, Carrick S, Currow D, Ghersi D, Glare P, Hagerty R, Tattersall MH. A systematic review of prognostic/end-of-life communication with adults in the advanced stages of a life-limiting illness: patient/caregiver preferences for the content, style, and timing of information. *J Pain Symptom Manage*. 2007;**34**:81–93.

Parkes, C.M., Bereavement. In: D. Doyle, G.W.C. Hanks and N. MacDonald (Eds.), Oxford Textbook of palliative medicine. 2nd Ed, Oxford University Press, New York, 1998a, pp. 995–1010.

Parkes, C.M., Bereavement: studies of grief in adult life. 3rd ed, Pelican, Harmondsworth, 1998b.

Parkes, C.M., Coping with loss - Bereavement in adult life, *BMJ*, **316** (1998c) 856–59.

Parkh, S.S. and Chung, F., Postoperative delirium in the elderly, *Anesth Analg*, **80** (1995) 1223–32.

Passik, S.D. and Cooper, M., Complicated delirium in a cancer patient successfully treated with olanzapine, *J Pain Symptom Manage*, **17** (1999) 219–23.

Patten, S.B., Williams, J.V., Haynes, L., Mc Cruden, J. and Arboleda-Flórez, J., The incidence of delirium in psychiatric inpatients units., *Can J Psychiatry*, **42** (1997) 858–63.

Payne, S. and Relf, M., The assessment of need for bereavement follow-up in palliative and hospice care, *Pall Med*, **8** (1990) 291–7.

Pearson A, de Vries A, Middleton SD, Gillies F, White TO, Armstrong IR, Andrew R, Seckl JR, Maclullich AM. Cerebrospinal fluid cortisol levels are higher in patients with delirium versus controls. *BMC Res Notes*. 2010 **3**:33.

Peritogiannis V, Stefanou E, Lixouriotis C, Gkogkos C, Rizos DV. Atypical antipsychotics in the treatment of delirium. *Psychiatry Clin Neurosci*. 2009;**63**(5):623–31.

Perry, E., Walker, M., Grace, J. and Perry, R., Acetylcholine in mind: a neurotrasmitter correlate of consciousness, *Trends Neurosci*, **22** (1999) 273–80.

Perry, N.K., Venlafaxine-induced serotonin syndrome with relapse following amytriptiline, *Postgrad Med J*, **76** (2000) 254–56.

Peruselli, C., Paci, E., Franceschi, P. and et al, Outcome evaluation in a home palliative care service, *J Pain Sympt Manage*, **13** (1997) 158–67.

Petterson, K. and Rottemberg, D.A., Radiation damage to the brain. In: C.J. Vecht (Ed.), Handbook of clinical neurology vol **23**, Elsevier, Amsterdam, 1997, pp. 325–51.

Pintor L, Fuente E, Bailles E, Matrai S. Study on the efficacy and tolerability of amisulpride in medical/surgical inpatients with delirium admitted to a general hospital. *Eur Psychiatry.* 2009;**24**:450–55.

Pirovano, M., Maltoni, M., Nanni, O., Marinari, M., Indelli, M., Zaninetta, G., Petrella, V., Barni, S., Zecca, E., Scarpi, E., Labianca, R., Amadori, D. and Luporini, G., A new palliative prognostic score: a first step fo rthe staging of terminally ill cancer patients, *J Pain Symptom Manage*, **17** (1999) 231–39.

Pisani MA, Kong SY, Kasl SV, Murphy TE, Araujo KL, Van Ness PH. Days of delirium are associated with 1-year mortality in an older intensive care unit population. *Am J Respir Crit Care Med.* 2009;**180**:1092–97.

Pittenger C, Desan PH. Gabapentin abuse, and delirium tremens upon gabapentin withdrawal. *J Clin Psychiatry.* 2007;**68**:483–84.

Plaschke K, Thomas C, Engelhardt R, Teschendorf P, Hestermann U, Weigand MA, Martin E, Kopitz J. (2007a). Significant correlation between plasma and CSF anticholinergic activity in presurgical patients. *Neurosci Lett.* **417**, 16–20.

Plaschke K, Hill H, Engelhardt R, Thomas C, von Haken R, Scholz M, Kopitz J, Bardenheuer HJ, Weisbrod M, Weigand MA (2007b). EEG changes and serum anticholinergic activity measured in patients with delirium in the intensive care unit. *Anaesthesia.* **62**, 1217–23.

Plaschke K, von Haken R, Scholz M, Engelhardt R, Brobeil A, Martin E, Weigand MA. Comparison of the confusion assessment method for the intensive care unit (CAM-ICU) with the Intensive Care Delirium Screening Checklist (ICDSC) for delirium in critical care patients gives high agreement rate(s). *Intensive Care Med.* 2008;**34**(3):431–6.

Platt, M.M., Breitbart, W., Smith, M., Marotta, R., Weisman, H. and Jacobsen, P.B., Efficacy of neuroleptics in hypoactive delirium, *J Neuropsychiatry Clin Neurosci*, **6** (1994) 66–65.

Plum, F. and Posner, J. Psychogenic unresponsiveness, The diagnosis of stupour and coma, F.A. Davis, Philadelphia, 1980a, pp. 305–312.

Plum, F. and Posner, J.B. The diagnosis of stupor and coma, Vol. **19**, F.A. Davis, Philadelphia, 1980b.

Pompei, P., Foreman, M., Rudberg, M.A., Inouye, S.K., Braund, V. and Cassel, C.K., Delirium in hospitalized older persons: outcomes and predictors, *J Am Geriatr Soc*, **42** (1994) 809–815.

Pompei, P., Foreman, M., Cassel, C., Alessi, C. and Cox, D., Detecting delirium among hospitalized older patients, *Arch Intern Med*, **155** (1995) 301–307.

Portenoy RK, Foley KM, Inturrisi CE. The nature of opioid responsiveness and its implications for neuropathic pain: new hypotheses derived from studies of opioid infusions. *Pain.* 1990;**43**(3):273–86.

Posner, J. and Plum, F., Spinal-fluid pH and neurologic symtoms in systemic acidosis, *New Engl J Med*, **277** (1967) 605–615.

Posner, J., Swanson, A.G. and Plum, F., Acid-base balance in cerebrospinal fluid, *Arch Neurol*, **12** (1965) 479–96.

Posner J, Saper CB, Schiff ND. Plum and Posner's diagnosis of stupor and coma. Oxford: Oxford University Press; 2007.

Posner, J.B., Neurologic complications of cancer, Vol. **45**, F.A. Davis, Philadelphia, 1995.

Potter, J.M., Reid, D.B., Shaw, R.P., Hackett, P. and Hickman, P.E., Myoclonus associated with treatment with high doses of morphine: the role of supplemental drugs, *Br Med J*, **299** (1989) 150–53.

Pourcher, E., Filteau, M., Bouchard, R.H. and Baruch, P., Efficacy of the combination of buspirone and carbamazepine in early post-traumatic delirium, *Am J psychiatry*, **151** (1994) 150–51.

Prigerson HG, Maciejewski PK. Grief and acceptance as opposite sides of the same coin: setting a research agenda to study peaceful acceptance of loss. *Br J Psychiatry.* 2008;**193**(6):435–7.

Prigerson, H., Frank, E., Kasl, S., Reynolds, C.r., Anderson, B., Zubenko, G., Houck, P., George, C., and Kupfer, D. (1995). Complicated grief and bereavement-related depression as distinct disorders: preliminary empirical validation in elderly bereaved spouses. *Am. J. Psychiatry* **152**, 22–30.

Prigerson, H.G., Bierhals, A.J., Kasl, S.V., Reynolds, C.F.r., Shear, M.K., Newsom, J.T., and Jacobs, S. (1996). Complicated grief as a disorder distinct from bereavement-related depression and anxiety: a replication study. *Am. J. Psychiatry* **153**, 1484–6.

Prigerson, H.G., Bierhals, A.J., Kasl, S.V., Reynolds, C.F.r., Shear, M.K., Day, N., Beery, L.C., Newsom, J.T. and Jacobs, S., Traumatic grief as a risk factor for mental and physical morbidity, *Am J Psychiatry*, **154** (1997) 616–23.

Prigerson, H.G., Shear, M.K., Jacobs, S.C., Reynolds, C.F.r., Maciejewski, P.K., Davidson, J.R., Rosenheck, R., Pilkonis, P.A., Wortman, C.B., Williams, J.B., Widiger, T.A., Frank, E., Kupfer, D.J. and Zisook, S., Consensus criteria for traumatic grief. A preliminary empirical test, *Br J Psychiatry*, **174** (1999) 67–73.

Prigerson HG, Vanderwerker LC, Maciejewski PK. Prolonged grief disorder: a case for inclusion in DSM–V. In Handbook of Bereavement Research and Practice: 21st Century Perspectives (eds M Stroebe, R Hansson, H Schut, W Stroebe): 165–86. American Psychological Association Press, 2008.

Prigerson HG, Horowitz MJ, Jacobs SC, Parkes CM, Aslan M, Goodkin K, Raphael B, Marwit SJ, Wortman C, Neimeyer RA, Bonanno G, Block SD, Kissane D, Boelen P, Maercker A, Litz BT, Johnson JG, First MB, Maciejewski PK. Prolonged grief disorder: Psychometric validation of criteria proposed for DSM-V and ICD-11. *PLoS Med.* 2009 Aug;**6**(8):917–928.

Quill, T.E., Byock, I.R. and for-the-ACP-ASIM-end-of-life-consensus-panel, Responding to intractable terminal suffering. the role of terminal sedation and voluntary refusal of food and fluids, *Ann Intern Med*, **132** (2000) 408–414.

Rabins, P.V. Psychosocial and management aspects of delirium., *Int'l Psychogeriatrics*, **3** (1991) 319–24.

Rahakonen, T., Luukkainen-Markkulla, R., Paanila, S., Sivenius, S. and Sulkava, R., Delirium episode as a sign of undetected dementia among community dwelling elderly subjects: a 2 year follow-up study, *J Neurol Neurosurg Psychiatry*, **69** (2000) 519–21.

Ramirez, A., Addington-Hall, J. and Richards, M., ABC of palliative care: The carers., *BMJ*, **316** (1998) 208–211.

Rammonah, K.W., Rosenberg, J., Lynn, D.J., Blumenfeld, A.M. and Pollak Nagaraja, H.N., Efficacy and safety of modafinil (Provigil) for the treatment of fatigue in multple sclerosis: a two centre phase 2 study, *J Neurol Neurosurg Psychiat*, **72** (2002) 179–83.

Rando, T.A. Anticipatory grief: the term is a misnomer but the phenomenon exists, *J Palliat Care*, **4** (1988) 70–73.

Rao, V. and Lyketsos, C., The benefits and risks of ECT for patients with primary dementia who also suffer from depression, *Int J Geriatr Psychiatry.*, **15** (2000) 729–35.

Ravona-Springer, R., Dolberg, O.T., Hirschmann, S. and Grunhaus, L., Delirium in elderly patients treated with risperidone: a report of three cases, *J Clin Psycopharmacol*, **18** (1998) 171–72.

Rea RS, Battistone S, Fong JJ, Devlin JW. Atypical antipsychotics versus haloperidol for treatment of delirium in acutely ill patients. *Pharmacotherapy.* 2007 Apr;**27**(4):588–94.

Reade MC, O'Sullivan K, Bates S, Goldsmith D, Ainslie WR, Bellomo R. Dexmedetomidine vs. haloperidol in delirious, agitated, intubated patients: a randomised open-label trial. *Crit Care.* 2009;**13**(3):R75. Epub 2009 May 19.

Reeves RR, Burke RS. Carisoprodol: Abuse Potential and Withdrawal Syndrome. *Curr Drug Abuse Rev.* 2010 Jan 21. [Epub ahead of print]

Reeves RR, Hammer JS, Pendarvis RO. Is the frequency of carisoprodol withdrawal syndrome increasing? *Pharmacotherapy.* 2007;**27**:1462–66.

Reischies FM, Neuhaus AH, Hansen ML, Mientus S, Mulert C, Gallinat J. (2005) Electrophysiological and neuropsychological analysis of a delirious state: the role of the anterior cingulate gyrus. *Psychiatry Res.* Feb 28;**138**(2):171–81.

Resnick, M. and Burton, B.T., Droperidol vs haloperidol in the initial management of acutely agitated patients, *J Clin Psychiatry*, **45** (1984) 298–99.

Richtie, J., Steiner, W. and Abramowicz, M., Incidence and risk factors for delirium among psychiatric inpatients, *Psychiatr Serv*, **47** (1996) 727–30.

Riker, R.R., Fraser, G.L. and Cox, P.M., Continuous infusion of haloperidol controls agitation in critically ill patients, *Crit Care Med*, **22** (1994) 433–40.

Riker RR, Shehabi Y, Bokesch PM, Ceraso D, Wisemandle W, Koura F, Whitten P, Margolis BD, Byrne DW, Ely EW, Rocha MG; SEDCOM (Safety and Efficacy of Dexmedetomidine Compared With Midazolam) Study Group. Dexmedetomidine vs midazolam for sedation of critically ill patients: a randomized trial. *JAMA.* 2009 4;**301**(5):489–99.

Rinck, G.C., van den Bos, A.M., Kleijnen, J., de Haes, H.J.C.J.M., Schade, E. and Veenhof, C.H.N., Methodologic issues in effectiveness research on palliative cancer care: a systematic review, *J Clin Oncol*, **15** (1997) 1697–1707.

Robbins, T.W. and Everitt, B.J., Arousal systems and attention. In: M. Gazzaniga (Ed.), The cognitive neuroscience, MIT Press, Cambridge (MA), 1995, pp. 703–20.

Robertsson, B. Assessment scales in delirium, *Dementia Ger Cognit Dis*, **10** (1999) 368–79.

Robertsson, B., Karlsson, I., Styrud, E. and Gottfries, C., Confusional State Evaluation (CSE): an instrument for measuring severity of delirium in the elderly., *Br J Psychiatry*, **170** (1997) 565–70.

Robertsson, B., Blennow, K., Gottfries, C. and Wallin, A., Delirium in dementia, *Int J Geriatr Psychiatry*, **13** (1998) 49–56.

Robertsson, B., Olsson, L. and Wallin, A., Occurrence of delirium in different regional brain syndromes, *Dement Geriatr Cogn Disord*, **10** (1999) 278–83.

Robertsson, B., Blennow, K., Brane, G., Edman, A., Karlsson, I., Wallin, A. and Gottfries, C., Hyperactivity of the hypothalamic-pituitary-adrenal axis in demented patients with delirium, *Int J Clin Psychopharmacol*, **16** (2001) 39–47.

Robinson, L. and Stacy, R., Palliative care in the community: setting practice guidelines for primary care teams, *Br J Gen Pract*, **44** (1994) 461–64.

Robinson, L.A., Nuamh, I.F., Lev, E. and McCorkle, R., A prospective longitudinal investigation of spousal bereavement examining Parkes and Weiss' Bereavement Risk Index, *J Pall Care*, **11** (1995) 5–13.

Robson A, Scrutton F, Wilkinson L, Macleod F. The risk of suicide in cancer patients: a review of the literature. *Psychooncology.* 2010 Mar 9. [Epub ahead of print]

Rockwood, K., Educational interventions in delirium., *Dementia Ger Cogn Dis*, **10** (1999) 426–29.

Rockwood, K., Cosway, S., Stolee, P., Kydd, D., Carver, D., Jarret, P. and O'Brien, B., Increasing recognition of delirium in elderly patients, *J Am Geriat Soc*, **42** (1994) 252–56.

Rockwood, K., Gooodman, J., Flynn, M. and Stolee, P., Cross-validation of the delirium rating scale in older patients, *J Am Geriatr Soc*, **44** (1996) 839–42.

Rogawski MA. Update on the neurobiology of alcohol withdrawal seizures. *Epilepsy Curr.* 2005;5:225–30.

Rolfson, D.B., McElhaney, J.E., Rockwood, K., Finnegan, B.A., Entwistle, L.M., Wong, J.F. and Suarez-Almazor, M.E., Incidence and risk factors for delirium and other adverse outcomes in older adults after coronary artery bypass graft surgery, *Can J Cardiol*, **15** (1999) 771–76.

Rolland, J.S., Families, illness, and disability. An integrative model, Basic Books, New York, 1994.

Rosebush, P.I., Margetts, P. and Mazurek, M.F., Serotonin syndrome as a result of clomipramine monotherapy, *J Clin Pharmacol*, **19** (1999) 285–87.

Rosen, J., Sweet, R., Mulsant, B., Rifai, A.H., Pasternak, R. and Zubenko, G., The delirium rating scale in psychogeriatric inpatient setting, *J Neuropsychiatry Clin Neurosci*, **6** (1994) 30–35.

Rosenbraugh, C.J., Flockart, D.A., Yasuda, S.U. and Woosley, R.L., Visual hallucination and tremor induced by sertraline and oxycodone in a bone marrow trasplant recipient, *J Clin Pharmacol*, **41** (2001) 224–27.

Rosenfeld, M. and Dalmau, J., The clinical spectrum and pathogenesis of paraneoplastic disorders of the central nervous system., *Hematol Oncol Clin North Am*, **15** (2001) 1109–28.

Ross, C.A., Etiological models and their phenomenological variants. CNS arousal systems: possible role in delirium., *International Psychogeriatrics*, **3** (1991) 353–71.

Ross, C.A., Peyser, C.E., Shapiro, I. and Folstein, M.F., Delirium: phenomenologic and etiologic subtypes, *International Psychogeriatrics*, **3** (1991) 135–47.

Roth-Romer, S., Fann, J. and Syrjala, K., The importance of rcognizing and measuring delirium, *J Pain Sympt Manage*, **13** (1997) 125–27.

Rothschild, A.J., Delirium an SSRI-benztropine adverse effect?, *J Clin Psychiatry*, **56** (1995) 492–95.

Royal College of Physicians: The prevention, diagnosis and management of delirium in older people—national guidelines, 2006.

Royal College of Psychiatrists: Guidelines for the prevention, diagnosis and management of delirium in older people in hospital. 2006.

Rudolph JL, Babikian VL, Birjiniuk V, Crittenden MD, Treanor PR, Pochay VE, Khuri SF, Marcantonio ER. Atherosclerosis is associated with delirium after coronary artery bypass graft surgery. *J Am Geriatr Soc.* 2005;**53**:462–466.

Rudolph JL, Jones RN, Grande LJ, Milberg WP, King EG, Lipsitz LA, Levkoff SE, Marcantonio ER. mpaired executive function is associated with delirium after coronary artery bypass graft surgery. *J Am Geriatr Soc.* 2006 Jun;**54**(6):937–41.

Rudolph JL, Jones RN, Rasmussen LS, Silverstein JH, Inouye SK, Marcantonio ER. (2007). Independent vascular and cognitive risk factors for postoperative delirium. *Am J Med.* **120**:807–13.

Rudolph JL, Marcantonio ER, Culley DJ, Silverstein JH, Rasmussen LS, Crosby GJ, Inouye SK. (2008a) Delirium is associated with early postoperative cognitive dysfunction. *Anaesthesia.* Sep;**63**(9):941–7. Epub 2008 Jun 10.

Rudolph JL, Ramlawi B, Kuchel GA, McElhaney JE, Xie D, Sellke FW, Khabbaz K., Levkoff SE, Marcantonio ER. Chemokines are associated with delirium after cardiac surgery. *J Gerontol,* 2008b; **63A**: 184–89.

Rudolph JL, Jones RN, Levkoff SE, Rockett C, Inouye SK, Sellke FW, Khuri SF, Lipsitz LA, Ramlawi B, Levitsky S, Marcantonio ER. (2009). Derivation and validation of a preoperative prediction rule for delirium after cardiac surgery. *Circulation.* **119**, 229–36.

Ruokonen E, Parviainen I, Jakob SM, Nunes S, Kaukonen M, Shepherd ST, Sarapohja T, Bratty JR, Takala J; "Dexmedetomidine for Continuous Sedation" Investigators. Dexmedetomidine versus propofol/midazolam for long-term sedation during mechanical ventilation. *Intensive Care Med.* 2009;**35**:282–90.

Ryan K, Leonard M, Guerin S, Donnelly S, Conroy M, Meagher D. Validation of the confusion assessment method in the palliative care setting. *Palliat Med.* 2009;**23**:40–45.

Sachdev P, Andrews G, Hobbs MJ, Sunderland M, Anderson TM. Neurocognitive disorders: cluster 1 of the proposed meta-structure for DSM-V and ICD-11. *Psychol Med.* **39** (2009) 2001–2012.

Sales, E., Shulz, R. and Biegel, D., Predictors of strain in families of cancer patients: a review of the literature, *J Psychosoc Oncol,* **10** (1992) 1–26.

Salkind, A.R. Acute delirium induced by intravenous trimethprim-sulfamethoxazole therapy in a patient with acquired immunodeficiency syndrome, *Human Experimen Tox,* **19** (2000) 149–51.

Sandberg, O., Gustafson, Y., Brannstrom, B. and Bucht, G., Clinical profile of delirium in older patients, *J Am Geriatr Soc,* **47** (1999) 315–318.

Sandberg, O., Franklin, K., Bucht, G. and Y., G., Sleep apnea, delirium, depressed mood, cognition, and ADL ability after stroke, *J Am Geriatr Soc,* **49** (2001) 391–97.

Santamauro, J.T., Stover, D.E., Jules, E.K. and Maurer, J.R., Lung transplantation for chemotherapy-induced pulmonary fibrosis, *Chest,* **105** (1994) 310–2.

Sasajima, Y., Sasajima, T., Uchida, H., Kawai, S., Haga, M., Akasaka, N., Kusakabe, M., Inaba, M., Goh, K. and Yamamoto, H., Postoperative delirium in patients with lower limb ischemia: what are the specific markers, *Eur J Vasc Endovasc Surg,* **20** (2000) 132–37.

Sasaki Y, Matsuyama T, Inoue S, Sunami T, Inoue T, Denda K, Koyama T. A prospective, open-label, flexible-dose study of quetiapine in the treatment of delirium. *J Clin Psychiatry.* 2003;**64**:1316–21.

Sato S, Mizukami K, Moro K, Tanaka Y, Asada T. Efficacy of perospirone in the management of aggressive behavior associated with dementia. *Prog Neuropsychopharmacol Biol Psychiatry.* 2006;**30**:679–83.

Saunders C. Watch with me. *Nursing Times.* 1965; **61**:48–50.

Saunderson, E.M. and Ridsdale, L., General practitioners' beliefs and attitudes about how to respond to death and bereavement: a qualitative study, *BMJ,* **319** (1999) 293–96.

Scammell, T.E., Estabrooke, I.V., McCarthy, M.T., Chemelli, R.M., Yanagishawa, M., Miller, M.S. and Saper, C.B., Hypthalamic arousal regions are activaated during modafinil induced wakefulness, *J Neurosci,* **20** (2000) 8620–28.

Schachter, S.R. and Coyle, N., Palliative home care. Impact on families. In: H. J (Ed.), Psycho-Oncology, Oxford University Press, New York, 1998, pp. 1004–1015.

Schaefer, C., Queensbury, C.P. and Wi, S., Mortality following conjugal bereavement and the effects of shared environment, *Am J Epidemiol*, **141** (1995) 1142–51.

Schieveld JN, Leentjens AF. Delirium in severely ill young children in the pediatric intensive care unit (PICU). *J Am Acad Child Adolesc Psychiatr*, 2005; **44**:392–94.

Schieveld JN, Leroy PL, van Os J, Nicolai J, Vos GD, Leentjens AF. Pediatric delirium in critical illness: phenomenology, clinical correlates and treatment response in 40 cases in the pediatric intensive care unit. *Intensive Care Med.* 2007;**33**(6):1033–40.

Schieveld JN, Lousberg R, Berghmans E, Smeets I, Leroy PL, Vos GD, Nicolai J, Leentjens AF, van Os J. Pediatric illness severity measures predict delirium in a pediatric intensive care unit. *Crit Care Med.* 2008;**36**(6):1933–6.

Schieveld J.N.M., van der Valk J.A., Smeets I., Berghmans E., Wassenberg R., Leroy P.L.M.N., Vos G.D., van Os J.: Diagnostic considerations regarding pediatric delirium: a review and a proposal for an algorithm for pediatric intensive care units. *Intensive Care Med*, 2009; **35**:1843–49.

Schor, J.D., Levkoff, S.E., Lipsitz, L.A., Reilly, C.H., Cleary, P.D., Rowe, J.W. and Evans, D.A., Risk factors for delirium in hospitalized elderly, *JAMA*, **267** (1992) 827–31.

Schumacher, L., Pruitt, J.N. and Phillips, M.,Identifying patients "at risk" for alcohol withdrawal syndrome: a treatment protocol., *J. Neurosci Nurs*, 2000; **32**(3) 158–63.

Schuurmans MJ, Deschamps PI, Markham SW, Shortridge-Baggett LM, Duursma SA. The measurement of delirium: review of scales. *Res Theory Nurs Pract.* 2003 **17**:207–24.

Schwab, R.A. and Bachhuber, B.H., Delirium and lactic acidosis caused by ethanol and niacin coingestion, *Am J Emerg Med*, **9** (1991) 363–65.

Schwartz, T.L. and Masand, P., Treatment of delirium with quetiapine, *J Clin Psychiatry Primary Care Companion*, **2** (2000) 10–12.

Scott, J.C. and Stanski, D.R., Decreased fentanyl and alfentanil dose requirements with age. A simultaneous pharmacokinetic and pharmacodynamic evaluation., *J Pharmacol Clin Ther*, **240** (1987) 159–66.

Scott, J.C., Cooke, J.E. and Stanski, D.R., Electroencephalographic quantitation of opioid effect: comparative pharmacodyna, mics of fentanyl and sufentanil, *Anesthesiology*, **74** (1991) 34–42.

Seitz DP, Gill SS, van Zyl LT. Antipsychotics in the treatment of delirium: a systematic review. *J Clin Psychiatry.* 2007 Jan;**68**(1):11–21.

Sellal, F. and Collard, M., Sindrome confusionale, Encycl Méd Chir, Vol. **17**-044-C-30, Edition Scientifique et Médicales Elsevier SAS, 2001.

Seltzer, B. and Mesulam, M., Confusional states and delirium as a disorder of attention. In: F. Boller and J. Grafman (Eds.), Handbook of neuropsychology, Vol. **1**, Elsevier, Amsterdam, 1990, pp. 165–74.

Serdaru, M., Hausser-Hauw, C., Laplane, D., Buge, A., Castaigne, P., Goulon, M., Lhermitte, F. and Hauw, J., The clinical spectrum of alcoholic pellagra encephalopathy: A retrospective analysis of 22 cases studied pathologically., *Brain*, **111** (1988) 829–42.

Serio RN. Acute delirium associated with combined diphenhydramine and linezolid use. *Ann Pharmacother.* 2004 Jan;**38**(1):62–5.

Settle, E.C. and Ayd, F.J., Haloperidol: a quarter century of experience, *J Clin Psychiatry*, **44** (1983) 440–48.

Shapiro, B.A., Warren, J., Egol, A.B., Greenbaum, D.M., Jacobi, J., Nasraway, S.A., Schein, R.M., Spevetz, A. and Stone, J.R., Practice parameters for intravenous analgesia and sedation for adult patients in the intensive care unit: an executive summary. Society of Critical Care Medicine [see comments], *Crit Care Med*, **23** (1995) 1596–600.

Sharma, N.D., Rosman, H.S., Padhi, I.D. and Tisdale, J.E., Torsades de Pointes associated with intravenous haloperidol in critically ill patients, *Am J Cardiol*, **81** (1998) 238–40.

Shehabi Y, Grant P, Wolfenden H, Hammond N, Bass F, Campbell M, Chen J. Prevalence of delirium with dexmedetomidine compared with morphine based therapy after cardiac surgery: a randomized controlled trial (DEXmedetomidine COmpared to Morphine-DEXCOM Study). *Anesthesiology*. 2009;**111**:1075–84.

Sheldon, F. ABC of palliative care: Bereavement., *BMJ*, **316** (1998) 456–58.

Shelly, M.P., Sultan, M.A., Bodenham, A. and Park, G.R., Midazolam infusions in critically ill patients, *Eur J Anaesthesiol*, **8** (1991) 21–7.

Shibasaki Warabi Y, Idezuka J, Yamazaki M, Onishi Y. Triphasic waves detected during recovery from lithium intoxication. *Intern Med*. 2003 Sep;**42**(9):908–9.

Shinjo T, Morita T, Hirai K, Miyashita M, Sato K, Tsuneto S, Shima Y. Care for imminently dying cancer patients: family members' experiences and recommendations. *J Clin Oncol*. 2010;**28**:142–48.

Siddiqi N, Stockdale R, Britton AM, Holmes J. Interventions for preventing delirium in hospitalised patients. *Cochrane Database Syst Rev*. 2007; **18**;(2):CD005563.

Sidhu KS, Balon R, Ajluni V, Boutros N Standard EEG and the difficult-to-assess mental status. *Ann Clin Psychiatry*. 2009;**21**:103-108.

Siegel JM. The neurobiology of sleep. *Semin Neurol*. 2009;**29**:277–96.

Siegel, K., Ravis, V.H., Houts and Mor, V. Caregiver burden and unmet patient needs, *Cancer*, **68** (1991) 1131–40.

Silber, M.H. and Rye, D.B., Solving the mistery of nacolepsy. The hypocretin story., *Neurology*, **56** (2001) 1616–1618.

Silverman, G.K., Jacobs, S.C., Kasl, S.V., Shear, M.K., Maciejewski, P.K., Noaghiul, F.S. and Prigerson, H.G., Quality of life impairments associated with diagnostic criteria for traumatic grief, *Psychol Med*, **30** (2000) 857–62.

Simon, L., Jewell, N. and Brokel, Management of acute delirium in hospitalised elderly: a process of improvement project., *J Geriatr Nurs*, **18** (1997) 150–54.

Sinclair S, Pereira J, Raffin S. A thematic review of the spirituality literature within palliative care. *J Palliat Med*. 2006;**9**:464–79.

Sipahimalani, A. and Masand, P., Use of risperidone in delirium: case reports, *Ann Clin Psychiatry*, **9** (1997) 105–7.

Sipahimalani, A. and Masand, P., Olanzapine in the treatment of delirium., *Psychosomatics*, **39** (1998) 422–30.

Sivilotti, M.L., Burns, M.J., Aaron, C.K. and Greenberg, M.J. Pentobarbital for severe gamma-butyrolactone withdrawal. *Ann Emerg Med*, **38** (2001) 660–65.

Sjogren, P. and Banning, A., Pain, sedation and reaction time during long-term treatment of cancer patients with oral and epidural opioids, *Pain*, **39** (1989) 5–11.

Sjogren, P., Dragsted, L. and Christensen, C.B., Myoclonic spasms during treatment with high doses of intravenous morphine in renal failure, *Acta Anaes*thesiol Scand, **37** (1993a) 780–2.

Sjogren, P., Jonsson, T., Jensen, N.H., Drenck, N.E. and Jensen, T.S., Hyperalgesia and myoclonus in terminal cancer patients treated with continuous intravenous morphine, *Pain*, **55** (1993b) 93–7.

Sjogren, P., Jensen, N.-H. and Jensen, T.S., Disappearance of morphine induced hyperalgesia after discontinuining or substituting morphine with other opioid agonists, *Pain*, **59** (1994) 313–316.

Sjogren, P., Thunedborg, L.P., Christrup, L., Hansen, S.H. and Franks, J., Is development of hyperalgesia, allodynia and myoclonus related to morphine metabolism during long-term administration, *Acta Anaesthesio Scand*, **42** (1998) 1070–75.

Sjogren, P., Olsen, A.K., Thomsen, A.B. and Dalberg, J., Neuropsychological performance in cancer patients: the role of oral opioids, pain and performance status, *Pain*, **86** (2000) 237–45.

Skinner Cook, A. and Dworkin, D.S., Helping the bereaved. Therapeutic interventions for children, adolescents, and adults, Basic Books, New York, 1992.

Skrobik YK, Bergeron N, Dumont M, Gottfried SB. Olanzapine vs haloperidol: treating delirium in a critical care setting. *Intensive Care Med.* 2004;**30**:444–49.

Slatkin, N.E., Rhiner, M. and Bolton, T.M., Donezepil in the treatment of opiate induced sedation, *J Pain Sympt Manage*, **21** (2001) 425–38.

Smit O, van der Steen MS, van Houten M, Rahkonen T, Sulkava R, Laurila JV, Strandberg TE, Tulen JH, Zwang L, Macdonald AJ, Treloar A, Sijbrands EJ, Zwinderman AH, Korevaar JC. The association of the dopamine transporter gene and the dopamine receptor 2 gene with delirium, a meta-analysis. *Am J Med Genet B Neuropsychiatr Genet.* 2010 **153B**, 648–55.

Smith, D.L. and Wenegrat, B.G., A case report of serotonin syndrome associated with combined nefazodone and fluoxetine, *J Clin Psychiatry*, **61** (2000) 146.

Smith HA, Fuchs DC, Pandharipande PP, Barr FE, Ely EW. Delirium: an emerging frontier in the management of critically ill children. *Crit Care Clin.* 2009;**25**:593–614.

Smith, M.J., Breitbart, W.S. and Platt, M.M., A critique of instruments and methods to detect, diagnose, and rate delirium, *J Pain Symptom Manage*, **10** (1995) 35–77.

Snyder, S., Reyner, A., Schmeidler, J., Bogursky, E., Gomez, H. and Strain, J.J., Prevalence of mental disorders in newly admitted medical inpatients with AIDS, *Psychosomatics*, **33** (1992) 166–70.

Spunberg, J.J., Chang, C.H., goldman, M., Auricchio, E. and Bell, J.J., Quality of long-term survival following irradiation for intracranial tumors iinchildren under the age of two, *Int J Rad Onol Biol Phys*, **7** (1981) 727–36.

Stagno D, Gibson C, Breitbart W. The delirium subtypes: a review of prevalence, phenomenology, pathophysiology, and treatment response. *Palliat Support Care.* 2004;**2**:171–79.

Stahl, S.M., Essentials Psychopharmacology., Cambridge University Press, Cambridge, 2000.

Stanford, B.J. and Stanford, S.C., Postoperative delirium indicating an adverse drug interaction involving the selective serotonin reuptake inhibitor, paroxetine?, *J Psychopharmacology*, **13** (1999) 313–317.

Stanilla, J.K., de Leon, J. and Simpson, G.M., Clozapine withdrawal resulting in delirium with psychosis: a report of three cases, *J Clin Psychiatry*, **58** (1997) 252–55.

Starzl, T. E., Taylor, C. A. & Magoun, H. W. (1951). Collateral afferent excitation of reticular formation of brain stem. *J. Neurophysiol.* **14**, 479–96.

Stefano, G.B., Bilfinger, T.V. and Fricchione, G.L., The immune neuro-link and the macrophage: postcardiotomy delirium, HIV associate dementia and psychiatry, *Prog Neurobiol*, **42** (1994) 475–88.

Steg, R.E. and Garcia, E.G., Complex visual hallucinations and cyclosporine neurotoxicity, *Neurology*, **41** (1991) 1156.

Steinberg, R.B., Gilman, D.E. and Johnson, F.I., Acute toxic delirium in a patient using transdermal fentanyl, *Anesth Analg*, **75** (1992) 1014–1016.

Steinmetz, D., Walsh, M., Gabel, L.L. and Williams, P.T., Family physicians' involvement with dying patients and thier families. Attitudes, difficulties and strategies, *Arch Fam Med*, **2** (1993) 753–61.

Sternbach, H. The serotonin syndrome, *Am J Psychiatry*, **148** (1991) 705–713.

Stiefel, F. and Bruera, E., Psychostimulants for hypoactive-hypoalert delirium?, *J Palliat Care*, **7** (1991) 25–6.

Stiefel, F. and Morant, R., Morphine intoxication during acute reversible renal insufficiency, *J Palliat Care*, **7** (1991) 45–7.

Stiefel, F.C., Breitbart, W.S. and Holland, J.C., Corticosteroids in cancer: neuropsychiatric complications, *Cancer Invest*, **7** (1989) 479–91.

Stiefel, F., Fainsinger, R. and Bruera, E., Acute confusional states in patients with advanced cancer, *J Pain Symptom Manage*, **7** (1992) 94–8.

Stoudemine, A., Anfinson, T. and Edwards, J., Corticosteroid-induced delirium and dependency, *Gen Hosp Psychiatry*, **18** (1996) 196–202.

Strain JJ. Psychiatric diagnostic dilemmas in the medical setting. *Aust N Z J Psychiatry*. 2005;**39**:764–71.

Straker D.A., Shapiro P.A., Muskin P.R.: Aripiprazole in the Treatment of Delirium. *Psychosomatics* 2006; **47**:385–91.

Stroebe, M.S. and Stroebe, W., The mortality of bereavement. In: M.S. Stroebe, W. Stroebe and R.O. Hansson (Eds.), Handbook of bereavement: Theory, research, and intervention, Cambridge University Press, New York, 1993, pp. 175–95.

Stroebe, M.S., van Son, M., Stroebe, W., Kleber, R., Schut, H. and van den Bout, J., On the classification and diagnosis of pathological grief, *Clin Psychol Rev*, **20** (2000) 57–75.

Strouse, T.B., El-Saden, S., Bonds, C., Ayars, N. and Busuttil, W., Immunosuppressant neurotoxicity in liver trasplant recipients, *Psychosomatics*, **39** (1998) 124–33.

Suc, E., Kalifa, C., Brauner, R., Hambrand, J.L., Terrier-Lacombe, M.J., Vassal, G. and Lemerle, J., Brain tumors under the age of three the price of survival. A retrospective study of 20 long-term survivors, *Acta Neurochir*, **106** (1990) 93–98.

Susan B. The impact on the family of terminal restlessness and its management. *Palliat Med*. 2003; **17**:454–60.

Swart, E.L., van Schijndel, R.J., Strack, R.J.M., van Loenen, A. and Thijs, L.G., Continuous infusion of lorazepam versus midazolam in patients in the intensive care unit: sedation with lorazepam is easier to manage and is more cost-effective, *Crit Care Med*, **27** (1999) 1461–65.

Sweeting, H.N. and Gilhooly, M.L., Anticipatory grief: a review, *Soc Sci Med*, **30** (1990) 1073–80.

Swore Fletcher BA, Dodd MJ, Schumacher KL, Miaskowski C. Symptom experience of family caregivers of patients with cancer. *Oncol Nurs Forum*. 2008 Mar;**35**(2):E23–44.

Szeto, H.H., Inturrisi, C.E., Houde, R., Saal, R., Cheigh, J. and Reidengerg, M.M., Accumulation of normeperidine an active metabolite of meperidine, in patients with renal failure or cancer., *Ann Intern Med*, **86** (1977) 738–4l.

Szymanski, S., Jody, D., Leipzig, R., Masiar, S. and Lieberman, J., Anticholinergic delirium caused by retreatment with clozapine, *Am J Psychiatry*, **148** (1991) 1752.

Takanashi J. Two newly proposed infectious encephalitis/encephalopathy syndromes. *Brain Dev*. 2009 **31** 521–8.

Takeuchi T, Furuta K, Hirasawa T, Masaki H, Yukizane T, Atsuta H, Nishikawa T. Perospirone in the treatment of patients with delirium. *Psychiatry Clin Neurosci*. 2007;**61**:67–70.

Tamura Y, Chiba S, Takasaki H, Tabata K, Ishimaru Y, Ishimoto T. (2006) Biperiden-induced delirium model in rats: a behavioral and electroencephalographic study. *Brain Res.* 2006 **1115**, 194–9.

Tavcar, R. and Dernovsek, M.Z., Risperidone-induced delirium, *Can J Psychiatry*, **43** (1998) 194.

Taylor MA, Fink M. Catatonia in a psychiatric classification. (2003) *A home of its own Am J Psych* **160**, 1233–41.

Tei M, Ikeda M, Haraguchi N, Takemasa I, Mizushima T, Ishii H, Yamamoto H, Sekimoto M, Doki Y, Mori Risk factors for postoperative delirium in elderly patients with colorectal cancer. Surg Endosc. 2010 Feb 23. [Epub ahead of print]

Tejera, C.A., Saravay, S.M., Goldman, E. and Gluck, L., Diphenydramine-induced delirium on elderly hospitalized patients with mild dementia, *Psychosomatics*, **35** (1994) 399–402.

Teseo, P.J., Thaler, H.T., Lapin, J., Inturrisi, C.E., Portenoy, R.K. and Foley, K.M., Morphine-6-glucuronide concentratios and opioid-related side effects: a survey in cancer patients, *Pain*, **61** (1995) 46–54.

Thomas C, Hestermann U, Kopitz J, Plaschke K, Oster P, Driessen M, Mundt C, Weisbrod M. Serum anticholinergic activity and cerebral cholinergic dysfunction: an EEG study in frail elderly with and without delirium. *BMC Neurosci.* 2008.

Thomas, H., Schwartz, E. and Petrilli, R. Droperidol versus haloperidol for chemical restraint of agitated and combative patients, *Ann Emerg Med*, **21** (1992) 407–413.

Torres, R., Mittal, D. and Kennedy, R., Use of quetiapine in delirium. Case reports., *Psychosomatics*, **42** (2001) 347–49.

Towne, A., Waterhouse, E., Boggs, J., Garnett, L., Brown, A., Smith, J. and DeLorenzo, R., Prevelence of nonconvulsive status epilepticus in comatose patients., *Neurology*, **54** (2000a) 340–45.

Towne, A.R., Waterhouse, E.J., Boggs, J.G., Garnett, L.K., Brown, A.J., Smith, J.R.j. and De Lorenzo, R.J., Prevalence of non-convulsive status epilepticus in comatose patients, *Neurology*, **54** (2000b) 340–45.

Trachman, S.B., Begun, D.L. and Kirch, D.G., Delirium in a patient with carcinomatosis, *Psychosomatics*, **32** (1991) 455–57.

Treloar, A. and Macdonald, A., Outcome of delirium: Part 1. Outcome of delirium diagnosed by DSM-III-R, ICD-10 and CAMDEX and derivation of the Reversible Cognitive Dysfunction Scale among acute geriatric inpatients., *Int J Geriatr Psychiatry*, **12** (1997a) 609–13.

Treloar, A. and Macdonald, A., Outcome of delirium: part 2. Clinical features of reversible cognitive dysfunction—are they the same as accepted definitions of delirium?, *Int J Geriatr Psychiatry*, **12** (1997b) 614–618.

Trzepacz, P. and Dew, M.A., Further analysys of the delirium rating scale, *Gen Hosp Psychiatry*, **17** (1995) 75–79.

Trzepacz, P., Ho, V. and Mallavarapu, H., Cholinergic delirium and neurotoxicity associated with tacrine for Alzheimer's dementia, *Psychosomatics*, **37** (1996) 299–301.

Trzepacz, P., Mulsant, B., Amanda, D.M., Pasternak, R., Sweet, R. and Zubenko, G., Is delirium different when it occurs in dementia? A study using the delirium rating scale., *J Neuropsychiatry Clin Neurosci*, **10** (1998) 199–204.

Trzepacz, P.T., The neuropathogenesis of delirium. A need to focus our research, *Psychosomatics*, **35** (1994a) 374–91.

Trzepacz, P.T. A review of delirium assessment instruments, *Gen Hosp Psychiatry*, **16** (1994b) 397–495.

Trzepacz, P.T. Update on the neuropathogenesis of delirium, *Dement Geriatr Cogn Disord*, **10** (1999) 330–34.

Trzepacz PT, Meagher DJ: *Delirium, in The American Psychiatric Publishing Textbook of Psychosomatic Medicine*. Edited by Levenson JL. Washington, DC, American Psychiatric Publishing, 2005, pp 91–130.

Trzepacz, P.T., Teague, G.B., Lipowski, Z.J. (1985). Delirium and other organic mental disorders in a general hospital. *Gen. Hosp. Psychiatry* **7**, 101.

Trzepacz, P.T., Baker, R.W. and Greenhouse, J., A symptom rating scale for delirium, *Psychiatry Res*, **23** (1988a) 89–97.

Trzepacz, P.T., Brenner, R.P., Coffman, G.C. and van Thiel, D.H., Delirium in liver transplantation candidates: discriminant analysis of multiple test variables, *Biol Psychiatry*, **24** (1988b) 3–15.

Trzepacz, P.T., Brenner, R. and Van Thiel, D.H., A psychiatric study of 247 liver trasplantation candidates, *Psychosomatics*, **30** (1989a) 147–53.

Trzepacz, P.T., Sclabassi, R.J. and Van Thiel, D.H., Delirium a subcortical phenomenon?, *J Neuropsychiatry*, **1** (1989b) 283–90.

Trzepacz, P.T. and DiMartini, A., Survival of 247 liver trasplant candidates. Relationaship to pretrasplant psychiatric variables and presence of delirium, *Gen Hosp Psychiatry*, **14** (1992) 380–86.

Trzepacz, P.T., DiMartini, A. and Tringall, R.D., Psychofarmacologic issues in organ transplantation, *Psychosomatics*, **34** (1993) 290–98.

Trzepacz, P.T., Mittal, D., Torres, R., Kanary, K., Norton, J. and Jimerson, N., Validation of the delirium rating scale-revised-98: comparison with the delirium rating scale and the cognitive test for delirium, *J Neurosychiatry Clin Neurosci*, **13** (2001) 229–42.

Trzepacz, P.T., Tarter, R., Shah, A., Tringali, R., Faett, D.G., and Van Thiel, D.H. SPECT scan and cognitive findings in subclinical hepatic encephalopathy, *J Neuropsychiatry Clin Neurosci*, **6** (1994) 170–75.

Tsao YY, Gugger JJ. Delirium in a patient with toxic flecainide plasmaconcentrations: the role of a pharmacokinetic drug interaction with paroxetine. *Ann Pharmacother*. 2009 **43**:1366–9.

Tucker, G.J. The diagnosis of delirium and DSM-IV, *Dement Geriatr Cogn Disord*, **10** (1999) 359–63.

Tulsky JA. Interventions to enhance communication among patients, providers, and families. *J Palliat Med*. 2005;**8** Suppl 1:S95–102.

Tuma, R. and DeAngelis, L.M., Altered mental status in patients with cancer, *Arch Neurol*, **57** (2000) 1727–31.

Tune, L., Carr, S., Hoag, E. and Cooper, T., Anticholinergic effects of drugs commonly prescribed for the elderly: potential means for assessing risk of delirium, *Am J Psychiatry*, **149** (1992) 1393–94.

Tune, L., Carr, S., Cooper, T., Klug, B. and Golinger, R.C., Association of anticholinergic activity of prescribed medications with postoperative delirium, *J Neuropsychiatry Clin Neurosci*, **5** (1993) 208–210.

Turkel SB, Trzepacz PT, Tavaré CJ. Comparing symptoms of delirium in adults and children. *Psychosomatics*. 2006;**47**:320–324.

Twycross, R. Corticosteroids in advanced cancer [editorial; comment], *Bmj*, **305** (1992) 969–70.

Twycross, R. and Lichter, I., The terminal phase. In: D. Doyle, G.W.C. Hanks and N. MacDonald (Eds.), Oxford Textbook of palliative medicine. 2nd Ed, Oxford University Press, New York, 1998, pp. 977–92.

Tyler, H.R. Neurologic disorders in renal failure, *Am J Med*, **44** (1968) 734–48.

Uchiyama, M., Tanaka, K., K., I. and Toru, M., Efficacy of mianserin for symtoms of delirium in the aged: an open trial study, *Prog Neuropsychopharmacol Biol Psychiatry*, **20** (1996) 651–56.

Uldall, K.K. and Berghuis, J.P., Delirium in AIDS patients: recognition and medication factors., *AIDS Patient Care STDS*, **11** (1997) 435–41.

Uldall, K.K., Harris, V.L. and Lalonde, B., Outcomes associated with delirium in acutely hospitalized acquired immune deficiency syndrome patients, *Comprehensive psychiatry*, **41** (2000a) 88–91.

Uldall, K.K., Ryan, R., Berghuis, J.P. and Harris, V.L., Association between delirium and death in AIDS patients, *AIDS patients care & STDS*, **14** (2000b) 95–100.

Unseld, E., Ziegle, G., Gemeinhardt, A., Janssen, V. and Klotz, U., Possible interaction of fluoquinolones with the benzodiazepine-GABA-receptor complex, *Br J Clin Pharmacol*, **30** (1990) 63–70.

Vachon, M.L.S. (1998). The emotional problems of the patient. In Oxford textbook of palliative medicine, 2nd edn (ed. D. Doyle, G.W.C. Hanks, and N. MacDonald), pp. 883–907. Oxford University Press, New York.

van der Mast, R.C. Postoperative Delirium, *Dement Geriatric Cogn. Disord.*, **10** (1999) 401–405.

van der Mast, R.C. and Fekkes, D., Serotonin and aminoacids: partners in delirium, *Sem Clin Neuropsychiatry*, **5** (2000) 125–31.

van der Mast, R.C. and Roest, F.H.J., Delirium after cardiac surgery: a review of the literature, *J Psychosom Res*, **41** (1996) 109–113.

van der Mast, R.C., Fekkes, D., Moleman, P. and Pepplinkhizen, L., Is postoperative delirium related to reduced plasma tryptophan?, *Lancet*, **338** (1991) 851–52.

van der Mast, R.C., van den Broek, W.W., Fekkes, D., Pepplinkhuizen, L. and Habbema, J.D.F., Incidence of and preoperative predictors for delirium after cardiac surgery, *J Psycosomatics Res*, **46** (1999) 479–83.

van der Mast, R.C., van den Broek, W.W., Fekkes, D., Pepplinkhuizen, L. and Habbema, J.D., Is delirium after cardiac surgery related to plasma amino-acids and physical conditions, *J Neuropsychiatry Clin Neurosci*, **12** (2000) 57–63.

van der Molen-Eijgenraam, M., Blanken-Meijs, J.T., Heeringa, M. and van Grootheest, A.C., Delirium due to increase in clozapine level during an inflammatory reaction (in Dutch), *Nederlands Tijdschrift voor Geneeskunde*, **145** (2001) 427–30.

Van Deurzen E, Aenild-Baker C.: Existential perspectives on human issues. Palgrave McMillan, New York, 2005.

van Gool WA, van de Beek D, Eikelenboom P. Systemic infection and delirium: when cytokines and acetylcholine collide. *Lancet*. 2010 27;**375**:773–5.

van Hemert, A.M., van der Mast, R.C., Hengeveld, M.W. and Vorstenbosch, M., Excess mortality in general hospital patients with delirium: a 5-year follow-up of 519 patients seen in psychiatric consultation, *J Psychosomatic Res*, **38** (1994) 339–46.

van Leeuwen, A., Molders, J., Sterkmans, P., Mielants, P., Martens, C., Toussaint, C., Hovent, A., Desseilles, M., Koch, H., Devroye, A. and Parent, M., Droperidol in acutely agitated patients. A double-blind placebo-controlled study, *J Ner Ment Dis*, **164** (1977) 280–83.

van Munster BC, de Rooij SE, Yazdanpanah M, Tienari PJ, Pitkälä KH, Osse RJ, Adamis D. Genetic polymorphisms related to delirium tremens: a systematic review. *Alcohol Clin Exp Res*. 2007a Feb;**31**(2):177–84.

van Munster BC, Korevaar JC, de Rooij SE, Levi M, Zwinderman AH. The association between delirium and the apolipoprotein E epsilon4 allele in the elderly. *Psychiatr Genet*. 2007b;**17**:261–66.

van Munster BC, Korevaar JC, Zwinderman AH, Levi M, Wiersinga WJ, De Rooij SE. Time-course of cytokines during delirium in elderly patients with hip fractures *J Am Geriatr Soc*. 2008;**56**,1704–9.

van Munster BC, de Rooij SE, Korevaar JC. (2009a) The role of genetics in delirium in the elderly patient. *Dement Geriatr Cogn Disord*. **28**, 187–95.

van Munster BC, Korevaar JC, Zwinderman AH, Leeflang MM, de Rooij SE. The association between delirium and the apolipoprotein E epsilon 4 allele: new study results and a meta-analysis. *Am J Geriatr Psychiatry*. 2009b;**17**:856–62.

van Munster BC, Yazdanpanah M, Tanck MW, de Rooij SE, van de Giessen E, Sijbrands EJ, Zwinderman AH, Korevaar JC. Genetic polymorphisms in the DRD2, DRD3, and SLC6A3 gene in elderly patients with delirium. *Am J Med Genet B Neuropsychiatr Genet*. 2010a;**153B**:38–44

van Munster BC, de Rooij SE, Yazdanpanah M, Tienari PJ, Pitkälä KH, Osse RJ, Adamis D, Smit O, van der Steen MS, van Houten M, Rahkonen T, Sulkava R, Laurila JV, Strandberg TE, Tulen JH, Zwang L, MacDonald AJ, Treloar A, Sijbrands EJ, Zwinderman AH, Korevaar JC. The association of the dopamine transporter gene and the dopamine receptor 2 gene with delirium, a meta-analysis. *Am J Med Genet B Neuropsychiatr Genet*. 2010b;**153B**:648–655.

Van Praag, H., Falcon, M., Guendelman, D. and Frenk, H., The development of analgesic, pro- and anticonvulsant opiate effect in the rat, *Annali dell'Istituto Superiore di Sanita'*, **29** (1993) 419–29.

Van Rompaey B, Schuurmans MJ, Shortridge-Baggett LM, Truijen S, Elseviers M, Bossaert L.A. comparison of the CAM-ICU and the NEECHAM Confusion Scale in intensive care delirium assessment: an observational study in non-intubated patients. *Crit Care*. 2008;**12**(1):R16.

Van Rompaey B, Elseviers MM, Schuurmans MJ, Shortridge-Baggett LM, Truijen S, Bossaert L. Risk factors for delirium in intensive care patients: a prospective cohort study. *Crit Care*. 2009;**13**(3):R77.

van Steijn, J., Nieboer, P., Hospers, G., de Vries, E. and Mulder, N., Delirium after interleukin-2 and alpha-interferon therapy for renal cell carcinoma., *Anticancer Res*, **21** (2001) 3699–3700.

Vasconcelos, M., Silva, K., Vidal, G., Silva, A., Domingues, R. and Berditchevsky, C., Early diagnosis of pediatric Wernicke's encephalopathy., *Ped Neurol*, **20** (1999) 289–94.

Vaurio LE, Sands LP, Wang Y, Mullen EA, Leung JM. (2006). Postoperative delirium: the importance of pain and pain management **102**:1267–73.

Ventafridda, V., Ripamonti, C., De Conno, F., Tamburini, M. and Cassileth, B.R., Symptom prevalence and control during cancer patients' last days of life, *Journal of Palliative Care*, **6** (1990a) 7–11.

Ventafridda, V., Spoldi, E. and De, C.F., Control of dyspnea in advanced cancer patients [letter], *Chest*, **98** (1990b) 1544–5.

Venturini, I., Corsi, L., Avallone, R., Farina, F., Bedogni, G., Baraldi, C., Baraldi, M. and Zeneroli, M.L., Ammonia and endogenous benzodiazepine-like compounds in the pathogenesis of hepatic encephalopathy, *Scand J Gastroenterol*, **36** (2001) 423–35.

Verkerk M, van Wijlick E, Legemaate J, de Graeff A. (2007) A national guideline for palliative sedation in the Netherlands. *J Pain Symptom Manage.* **4** :666–70.

Vidal, S., Andrianjatovo, J.J., Dubau, B., Winnok, S. and Maurette, P., Encephalopathies postoperatoires: la carence en thiamine, une etiologie a ne pas meconnaitre, *Ann Fr Anesth Reanim*, **20** (2000).

Vidán MT, Sánchez E, Alonso M, Montero B, Ortiz J, Serra JA. An intervention integrated into daily clinical practice reduces the incidence of delirium during hospitalization in elderly patients. *J Am Geriatr Soc.* 2009;**57**:2029–36.

Viganò, A., Dorgan, M., Buckingham, J., Bruera, E. and Suarez-Almazor, M.E., Survival prediction in terminal cancer patients: a systematic review of the literature, *Pall Med*, **14** (2001) 363–74.

Vitiello, M.V., Bliwise, D.L. and Prinz, P.N., Sleep in Alzheimer's disease and the sundown syndrome, *Neurology*, **46** (1992) 83–93.

Vlajkovic GP, Sindjelic RP. Emergence delirium in children: many questions, few answers. *Anesth Analg.* 2007;**104**:84–91.

Voepel-Lewis T., Malviya S., Tait A.R.: A prospective cohort study of emergence agitation in the pediatric postanesthesia care unit. *Anesth Anal* **96** (2003), pp. 1625–30.

Voltz, R., Gultekin, H., Rosenfeld, M.R., Gerstner, E., Eichen, J., Posner, J. and Dalmau, J., A serologic marker of paraneoplastic limbic and brain-stem encephalitis in patients with testicular cancer, *N Engl J Med*, **340** (1999) 1788–95.

Wada, Y. and Yamaguchi, N., Delirium in the elderly: relationship of clinical symptoms to outcome, *Dementia*, **4** (1993) 113–116.

Wakefield JC, Schmitz MF, First MB, Horwitz AV. Extending the bereavement exclusion for major depression to other losses: evidence from the National Comorbidity Survey. *Arch Gen Psychiatry.* 2007;**64**(4):433–40.

Wallesch, C.W. and Hundsaltz, A., Language function in delirium: a comparison of single word processing in acute confusional state and probable Alzheimer's disease, *Brain & Language*, **46** (1994) 592–606.

Wasserstrom, W.R., Glass, J.P. and Posner, J.B., Diagnosis and treatment of leptomeningeal metastasis from solid tumors: Experience with 90 patients., *Cancer*, **49** (1982) 759–72.

Wasteson E, Brenne E, Higginson IJ, Hotopf M, Lloyd-Williams M, Kaasa S, Loge JH; European Palliative Care Research Collaborative (EPCRC). Depression assessment and classification in palliative cancer patients: a systematic literature review. *Palliat Med.* 2009;**23**:739–745.

Weaver MR, Conover CJ, Proescholdbell RJ, Arno PS, Ang A, Ettner SL; Cost Subcommittee of the HIV/AIDS Treatment Adherence, Health Outcomes, and Cost Study Group. Utilization of mental health and substance abuse care for people living with HIV/AIDS, chronic mental illness, and substance abuse disorders. *J Acquir Immune Defic Syndr.* 2008;**47**:449–58.

Webster, R. and Holroyd, S., Prevalence of psychotic symptoms in delirium, *Psychosomatics*, **41** (2000) 519–22.

Weed, H.G., Lutman, C.V., Young, D.C. and Schuller, D.E., Preoperative identification of patients at risk for delirium after major head and neck cancer surgery, *Laryngoscope*, **105** (1995) 1066–68.

Wei LA, Fearing MA, Sternberg EJ, Inouye SK. The Confusion Assessment Method: a systematic review of current usage. *J Am Geriatr Soc.* 2008;**56**(5):823–30.

Weiner, A.L. Meperidine as a potential cause of serotonin syndrome in the emergency department, *Academic Emerg Med*, **6** (1999) 156–58.

Weiner JS, Roth J. Avoiding iatrogenic harm to patient and family while discussing goals of care near the end of life. *J Palliat Med.* 2006;**9**:451–63.

Weitzener, M.A., Olofson, S.M. and Forman, A.D., Patients with malignant meningitis presenting with neuropsychiatric manifestations, *Cancer*, **76** (1995) 1804–1808.

Welborn, L.G., Hannallah, R.S., Norden, J.M., Ruttimann, U.E. and Callan, C.M., Comparison of emergence and recovery characteristics of sevoflurane, desflurane, and halothane in pediatric ambulatory patients, *Anesth Analg*, **83** (1996) 917–20.

Welch-McCaffery, D. (1988). Family issues in cancer care: current dilemmas and future directions. *J. Psychosoc. Oncol.* **6**, 199–211.

Wellisch, D.K., Family issues in palliative care. In: H.M. Chochinov and W. Breitbart (Eds.), Handbook of psychiatry in palliative medicine, Oxford University Press, New York, 2000, pp. 275–89.

Wellisch, D.K., Wolcott, D.L., Pasnau, R.O., Fawzy, F.I. and Landsverk, J., An evaluation of the psychosocial problems of the homebound cancer patient: relationship of patient adjustment to family problems, *J Psychosoc Oncol*, **7** (1989) 55–76.

Wengel, S., Roccaforte, W. and Burke, W., Donepezil improves symptoms of delirium in dementia: implications for future research., *J Geriatr Psychiatry Neurol*, **11** (1998) 159–61.

Wengs, W.J., Talwar, D. and Bernard, J., Ifosfamide-induced nonconvulsive status epilepticus, *Arch Neurol*, **50** (1993) 1104–1105.

Werz, M.A. and MacDonald, R.L., Opiate alkaloids antagonize postsynaptic glycine and GABA responses: correlation with convulsant action, *Bra Res*, **236** (1982) 107–119.

Whyte, J., Neurologic disorder of attention and arousal: assessment and treatment, *Arch Phys Med Rehabil* (1992) 1094–1103.

Wilkins-Ho, M. and Hollander, Y., Toxic delirium with low-dose clozapine, *Can J Psychiatry*, **42** (1997) 429–30.

Wilkinson A, Gavine A, Black K. Lithium toxicity presenting as delirium in an older patient. Practitioner. 2009 May;**253**(1718):28–30. PubMed PMID: 19517683.

Williams, J.B.W., Psychiatric classification. In: R.E. Hales, S.C. Yudofsky and J.A. Talbott (Eds.), Textbook of psychiatry, American Psychiatric Press, Washington, 1999, pp. 227–52.

Williams-Russo, P., Urquhart, B.L., Sharrock, N.E. and Charlson, M.E., Postoperative delirium: predictors and prognosis in elderly orhopedics patients, *J Am Geriatr Soc*, **40** (1992) 759–67.

Wilt, J.L., Minnema, A.M., Johnson, R.F. and Rosenblum, A.M., Torsade de pointes associated with the use of intravenous haloperidol, *Ann Intern Med*, **119** (1993) 391–4.

Winawer, N. Postoperative delirium., *Med Clin North Am*, **85** (2001) 1229–39.

Wise, M.G. and Trzepacz, P.T., Delirium (Confusional States). In: J.R. Rundell and M.G. Wise (Eds.), Textbook of Consultation-Liaison Psychiatry, American Psychiatric Press, Washington, 1996, pp. 259–74.

Wise, M.G., Gray, K.F. and Seltzer, B., Delirium, dementia and amnestic disorders. In: R.E. Hales, S.C. Yudorfsky and J.A. Talbott (Eds.), *Textbook of psychiatry*, American Psychiatric Press, Washington, 1999, pp. 317–62.

Wojnar, M., Bizon, Z. and Wasilewski, D., The role of somatic disorders and physical injury in the development and course of alcohol withdrawal delirium., *Alcohol Clin Exp Res*, **23** (1999) 209–213.

Wolf, H.G. and Curran, D., Nature of delirium and allied states. The disergastic reaction, *Arch Neurol Psychiatry*, **33** (1935) 1175–1215.

Wong CP, Chiu PK, Chu LW. Zopiclone withdrawal: an unusual cause of delirium in the elderly. *Age Ageing*. 2005;**34**:526–27.

Woof, W.R. and Carter, Y.H., The grieving adult and the general practitioner: a literature review in two parts (part 1), *Br J Gen Pract*, **47** (1997a) 443–48.

Woof, W.R. and Carter, Y.H., The grieving adult and the general practitioner: a literature review in two parts (part 2), *Br J Gen Pract*, **47** (1997b) 509–514.

Worden, J.W., Grief counseling and grief therapy. A handbook of the mental health pratctitioner, Springer, New York, 1991.

Worden JW.: Grief Counseling and Grief Therapy: A Handbook for the Mental Health Practitioner. Fourth Edition. Springer, New York, 2009.

World Health Organization, The ICD-10 Classification of Mental and Behavioral Disorders: Clinical Descriptions and Diagnostic Guidelines, WHO Publications, Geneva, 1992.

World Health Organization, The ICD-10 Classification of Mental and Behavioral Disorders: Diagnostic criteria for research, World Health Organization, Geneva, 1993.

World Health Organization, Diagnostic and managementg guidelines for mental disorders in primary care ICD 10 chapter V primary care version, Hogrefe and Huber, Gottingen, 1996.

World Health Organization, International classification of functioning and disability (ICDH-2) Full draft version, World Health Organization, Geneve, 2001.

World Health Organization: International Statistical Classification of Diseases and Related Health Problems 10th Revision -Version for 2007 (http://www.who.int/classifications/icd/icd10updates/en/)

Yaksh, T.L., Harty, G.J. and Onofrio, B.M., High doses of spinal morphine produce a nonopiate receptor mediated hyperesthesia: clinical and theoretic impliacations, Anesthesiology, **64** (1986) 590–97.

Yancik, R. Coping with hospice work stress, J Psychosoc Oncol, **2** (1984a) 19–35.

Yancik, R. Source of work stress for hospice staff., J Psychosoc Oncol, **2** (1984b) 21–31.

Yang FM, Marcantonio ER, Inouye SK, Kiely DK, Rudolph JL, Fearing MA, Jones RN. Phenomenological subtypes of delirium in older persons: patterns, prevalence, and prognosis. Psychosomatics. 2009;**50**:248–54.

Young CC, Lujan E. Intravenous ziprasidone for treatment of delirium in the intensive care unit. Anesthesiology. 2004;**101**:794–95.

Young, G.B., Major syndromes of impaired consciousness. In: G.B. Young, A.H. Ropper and C.F. Bolton (Eds.), Coma and impaired consciousness. A clinical perspective, McGraw-Hill, New York, 1998, pp. 39–78.

Young, G.B., Leung, L.S., Campbell, V., DeMelo, J., Schieven, J. and Tilsworth, R., The electroencephalogram in metabolic/toxic coma, *Am J EEG Technol*, **32** (1992) 243–59.

Young, G.B., McLachlan, R.S., Kreeft, J.H. and DeMelo, J., An electroencephalographic classification system for coma, *Can J Neurol Sci*, **24** (1997) 329–25.

Young J, Leentjens AF, George J, Olofsson B, Gustafson Y. Systematic approaches to the prevention and management of patients with delirium. *J Psychosom* Res. 2008;**65**:267–72.

Yue, M., Faisinger, R.L. and Bruera, E., Cognitive impairment in a patient with a normal mini-mental state examination (MMSE), *J Pain Symptom Manage*, **9** (1994) 51–53.

Zacny, J.P. A review of the effects of opioids on psychomotor and cognitive functioning in humans, *Exp Clin Psychopharmacol*, **3** (1995) 432–66.

Zacny JP, Gutierrez S. 2009 Within-subject comparison of the psychopharmacological profiles of oral hydrocodone and oxycodone combination products in non-drug-abusing volunteers. *Drug Alcohol Depende* **101**(1-2):107–14.

Zaider T, Kissane D. The assessment and management of family distress during palliative care. *Curr Opin Support Palliat Care*. 2009;**3**:67–71.

Zalsman, G., Hermesh, H. and Munitz, H., Alprazolam withdrawal delirium: a case report, *Clin Neuropharmacol*, **21** (1998) 201–202.

Zarate, C.A., Baldessarini, R.J., Siegel, A.J., Nakamura, A., McDonald, J., Muir-Hutchinson, L.A., Cherkerzian, T. and Tohen, M., Risperidone in the elderly: a pharmacoepidemiologic study, *J Clin Psychiatry*, **58** (1997) 311–317.

Zeimer, H. Paraneoplastic limbic encephalitis should not be overlooked as a possible cause of delirium in cancer patients, *Arch Intern Med*, **160** (2000) 2866.

Zeitlin, S.V. Grief and bereavement., *J Pall Care*, **28** (2001) 415–25.

Zeman, A. Consciousness, *Brain*, **124** (2001) 1263–89.

Zhang B, El-Jawahri A, Prigerson HG. Update on bereavement research: evidence-based guidelines for the diagnosis and treatment of complicated bereavement. *J Palliat Med*. 2006;**9**:1188–1203.

Ziske, C.G., Schottker, B., Gorschuler, M., Mey, U., Kleinschmidt, R., Schlegel, U., Sauerbruck, T. and Scmidt-Wolf, G.H., Acute transient encephalopathy after paclitaxel infusion. report of three cases, *Ann Oncol.*, **13** (2002) 629–31.

Zisook, S., Understanding and managing bereavement in palliative care. In: H.M. Chochinov and W. Breitbart (Eds.), Handbook of psychiatry in palliative medicine, Oxford University Press, New York, 2000.

Zou, Y., Cole, M., Primeau, F., McCusker, J., Bellavance, F. and Laplante, J., Detection and diagnosis of delirium in the elderly: psychiatrist diagnosis, confusion assessment method, or consensus diagnosis? *Int Psychogeriatr*, **10** (1998) 303–8.

Appendix 1

The Confusion Assessment Method (CAM) Instrument

This CAM instrument is reprinted from Inouye et al. (1990) with permission.

The CAM Instrument

Acute onset

1. Is there evidence of an acute change in mental status from the patient's baseline?

Inattention

The questions listed under this topic were repeated for each topic where applicable.

2. A. Did the patient have difficulty focusing attention, for example, being easily distractible, or have difficulty keeping track of what was being said?
      Not present any time during interview.
      Present at some time during interview, but in mild form.
      Present at some time during interview, in marked form.
      Uncertain.

   B. (If present of abnormal) Did this behaviour fluctuate during the interview, that is, tend to come and go or increase and decrease in severity?
      Yes.
      No.
      Uncertain.
      Not applicable.

   C. (If present of abnormal) Please describe this behaviour.

Disorganized thinking

3. Was the patient's thinking disorganized or incoherent, such as rambling or irrelevant conversation, unclear or illogical flow of ideas, or unpredictable switching from subject to subject?

Altered level of consciousness

4. Overall, how would you rate this patient's level of consciousness?
   Alert (normal).
   Vigilant (hyperalert, overly sensitive to environmental stimuli, started very easily).

Lethargic (drowsy, easily aroused).
Stupor (difficult to arouse).
Coma (unarousable).
Uncertain.

Disorientation

5. Was the patient disoriented at any time during the interview, such as thinking that he or she was somewhere other than the hospital, using the wrong bed, or misjudging the time of day?

Memory impairment

6. Did the patient demonstrate any memory problems during the interview, such as inability to remember events in the hospital, or have difficulty remembering instructions?

Perceptual disturbances

7. Did the patient have any evidence of perceptual disturbances, for example, hallucinations, illusions, or misinterpretations (such as thinking something was moving when it was not)?

Psychomotor agitation

8. (Part 1) At any time during the interview, did the patient have an unusually increased level of motor activity, such as restlessness, picking at bedclothes, tapping finger, or making frequent sudden changes of position?

Psychomotor retardation

8. (Part 2) At any time during the interview, did the patient have an unusually decreased level of motor activity, such as sluggishness, staring into space, staying in one position for a long time, or moving very slowly?

Altered sleep–wake cycle

9. Did the patient have evidence of disturbance of the sleep–wake cycle, such as excessive daytime sleepiness with insomnia at night?

The CAM Diagnostic Algorithm

This diagnosis of delirium by CAM requires the presence of Features 1 and 2 and either Feature 3 or 4.

Feature 1. Acute Onset and Fluctuating Course

This feature is usually obtained from a family member or nurse and is shown by positive responses to the following questions: Is there evidence of an acute change in mental status from the patient's baseline? Did the (abnormal) behaviour fluctuate during the day, that is, tend to come and go or increase and decrease in severity?

Feature 2. Inattention

This feature is shown by a positive response to the following question: Did the patient have difficulty focusing attention, for example, being easily distractible, or have difficulty keeping track of what was being said?

Feature 3. Disorganized thinking

This feature is shown by a positive response to the following question: Was the patient's thinking disorganized or incoherent, such as rambling or irrelevant conversation, unclear or illogical flow of ideas, or unpredictable switching from subject to subject?

Feature 4. Altered level of consciousness

This feature is shown by any answer other than 'alert' to the following question: Overall, how would you rate this patient's level of consciousness? Alert (normal), vigilant (hyperalert), lethargic (drowsy, easily aroused), stupor (difficult to arouse), or coma (unarousable).

Appendix 2

The Delirium Rating Scale (DRS)

Item 1: Temporal onset of symptoms

This item addresses the time course over which symptoms appear; the maximum rating is for the most abrupt onset of symptoms—a common pattern of delirium. Dementia is usually more gradual in onset (Lipowski 1982). Other psychiatric disorders, such as affective disorders, might be scored with 1 or 2 points on this item. Sometimes delirium can be chronic (e.g. in geriatric nursing home patients), and unfortunately only 1 or 2 points would be assessed in that situation.

0 Gradual onset change from longstanding behaviour, essentially a chronic or chronic-recurrent disorder

1 Gradual onset of symptoms, occurring within a 6-month period

2 Acute change in behaviour or personally occurring over a month

3 Abrupt change in behaviour, usually occurring over a 1- to 3-day period

Item 2: Perceptual disturbances

This item rates most highly the extreme inability to perceive differences between internal and external reality, while intermittent misperceptions such as illusions are given 2 points. Depersonalization and derealization can be seen in other organic mental disorder and thus are given only 1 point.

0 None evident by history or observation

1 Feelings of depersonalization or derealization

2 Visual illusions or misperceptions including macropsia, micropsia; e.g. may urinate in wastebasket or mistake bedclothes for something else

3 Evidence that the patient is markedly confused about external reality; e.g. not discriminating between dreams and reality

Item 3: Hallucination type

The presence of any type of hallucination is rated. Auditory hallucinations alone are rated with less weight because of their common occurrence in primary psychiatric disorders. Visual hallucinations are generally associated with organic mental syndromes, although not exclusively, and are given 2 points. Tactile hallucinations are classically described in delirium, particularly due to anticholinergic toxicity, and are given the most points.

0 Hallucination not present

1 Auditory hallucination only

2 Visual hallucinations present by patient's history or inferred by observation, with or without auditory hallucinations

3 Tactile, olfactory, or gustatory hallucinations present with or without auditory hallucinations

Item 4: Delusions

Delusions can be present in many different psychiatric disorders, but tend to be better organized and more fixed in non-delirious disorders and thus are given less weight. Chronic fixed delusions are probably most prevalent in schizophrenic disorders. New delusions may indicate affective and schizophrenic disorders, dementia, or substance intoxication but should also alert the clinician to possible delirium and are given 2 points. Poorly formed delusions, often of a paranoid nature, are typical of delirium (Lipowski 1980).

0 Not present

1 Delusions are systematized, i.e. well organized and persistent

2 Delusions are new and not part of a pre-existing primary psychiatric disorders

3 Delusions are not well circumscribed; are transient, poorly organized, and mostly in response to misperceived environmental cues; e.g. are paranoid and involve persons who are in reality caregivers, loved ones, hospital staff, etc.

Item 5: Psychomotor behaviour

This item describes degrees of severity of altered psychomotor behaviour. Maximum points can be given for severe agitation or severe withdrawal to reflect either the hyperactive or hypoactive variant of delirium (Lipowski 1980).

0 Not present

1 Mild restlessness, tremolousness, or anxiety evident by observation and a change from patient's usual behaviour

2 Moderate agitation with pacing, removing IVs, etc.

3 Severe agitation; patient needs to be restrained, may be combative, or has significant withdrawal from the environment, but not due to major depression or schizophrenic catatonia

Item 6: Cognitive status during formal testing

Information from the cognitive portion of a routine mental status examination is needed to rate this item. The maximum rating of 4 points is given for severe cognitive deficits while only 1 point is given for mild inattention, which could be attributed to pain and fatigue seen in medically ill persons. Two points are given for a relatively isolated cognitive deficit, such as memory impairment, which could be during dementia or organic amnestic syndrome as well as due to early delirium.

0 No cognitive deficits, or deficits that can be alternatively explained by lack of education or mental retardation

1 Very mild cognitive deficits that might be attributed to inattention due to acute pain, fatigue, depression, or anxiety associated with having a medical illness

2 Cognitive deficit largely in one major area tested, e.g. memory, but otherwise intact

3 Significant cognitive deficits that are diffuse, i.e. affecting many different areas tested. They must include periods of disorientation to time or place at least once each 24-h period; registration and/or recall are abnormal; concentration is reduced

4 Severe cognitive deficits, including motor or verbal perseverations, confabulations, disorientation to person, remote and recent memory deficits, and inability to cooperate with formal mental tests

Item 7: Physical disorder

Maximum points are given when a specific lesion or physiological disturbance can be temporally associated with the altered behaviour. Dementias are often not found to have a specific underlying medical cause, while delirium usually has at least one identifiable physical cause (Trzepacz et al. 1985).

0 None present or active

1 Presence of any physical disorder that might affect mental state

2 Specific drug, infection, metabolic, central nervous system lesion, or other medical problem that can be temporally implicated in causing the altered behaviour or mental status

Item 8: Sleep–wake cycle disturbance

Disruption of the sleep–wake cycle is typical in delirium, with demented person generally having significant sleep disturbance much later in their course (Lipowski 1982). Severe delirium is on a continuum with stupor and coma, and person with a resolving coma are likely to be delirious temporally.

0 Not present; awake and alert during the day, and sleep without significant disruption at night

1 Occasional drowsiness during the day and mild sleep continuity disturbance at night; may have nightmares but can readily distinguish from reality

2 Frequent napping and unable to sleep at night, constituting a significant disruption of or a reversal of the usual sleep–wake cycle

3 Drowsiness prominent, difficulty staying alert during the interview, loss of self-control over alertness and somnolence

4 Drifts into stuporous or comatose periods

Item 9: Lability of mood

Rapid shifts in mood can occur in various organic mental syndromes, perhaps due to a disinhibition of one's normal control. The patient may be aware of this lack of emotional control and may behave inappropriately relative to the situation or to his/her thinking state, e.g. crying for no apparent reason. Delirious patient may score points on any of these items depending upon the severity of the delirium and upon how their underlying psychological state 'colours' their delirious presentation. Patients with borderline personality disorder might score 1 or 2 points on this item.

0 Not present; mood stable

1 Affect/mood somewhat altered and changes over the course of hours; patient states that mood changes are not under self-control

2 Significant mood changes that are inappropriate to situation, including fear, anger, or tearfulness; rapid shifts of emotion, even over several minutes

3 Severe disinhibition of emotions, including temper outbursts, uncontrolled inappropriate laughter, or crying

Item 10: Variability of symptom

The hallmark of delirium is waxing and waning of symptoms, which is given 4 points on this item. Demented as well as delirious patients, who become more confused at night when environmental cues are decreased, could score 2 points.

0 Symptom stable and mostly present during daytime

1 Symptom worse at night

2 Fluctuating intensity of symptoms, such that they wax and wane during 24-h period

Total score _____

Reprinted from Trzepacz et al. (1988a) with permission from Elsevier.

The Delirium Rating Scale-Revised-98 (DRS-R-98)

Reprinted from Trzepacz et al. (2001) with permission.

This is a revision of the Delirium Rating Scale (Trzepacz et al. 1998). It is used for initial assessment and repeated measurements of delirium symptom severity. The sum of the 13 item scores provides a severity score. In all available ratings of delirium severity, reasonable time frames should be chosen between ratings to document meaningful changes because delirium symptom severity can fluctuate without interventions.

The DRS-R-98 Severity Scale

1. Sleep–wake cycle disturbance

Rate the sleep–wake pattern using all sources of information, including from family, caregivers, nurses' report, and patient. Try to distinguish sleep from resting with eyes closed.

0. Not present
1. Mild sleep continuity disturbance at night or occasional drowsiness during the day
2. Moderate disorganization of sleep–wake cycle (e.g. falling asleep during conversations, napping during the day, or several brief awakenings during the night with confusion/behavioural changes or very little night-time sleep)
3. Severe disruption of sleep–wake cycle (e.g. day–night reversal of sleep–wake cycle or several circadian fragmentation with multiple periods of sleep and wakefulness or severe sleeplessness)

2. Perceptual disturbances and hallucinations

Illusions and hallucinations can be of any sensory modality. Misperceptions are 'simple' if they are uncomplicated, such as a sound, noise, colour, spot, or flashes, and 'complex' if they are multidimensional, such a voices, music, people, animals, or scenes. Rate if reported by patient or caregiver, or inferred by observation.

0 Not present
1 Mild perceptual disturbances (e.g. feelings of derealization or depersonalization; or patient may not be able to discriminate dreams from reality)
2 Illusions present
3 Hallucinations present

3. Delusions

Delusions can be of any type, but are most often persecutory. Rate if reported by patient, family, or caregivers. Rate as delusional if ideas are unlikely to be true, yet are believed by the patient who cannot be dissuaded by logic. Delusional ideas cannot be explained, otherwise, by the patient's usual cultural or religious background.

0 Not present

1 Mildly suspicious, hypervigilant, or preoccupied

2 Unusual or overvalued ideation that does not reach delusional proportions or could be plausible

3 Delusional

4. Lability of affect

Rate the patient's affect as the outward presentation of emotion and not as a description of what the patient feels.

0 Not present

1 Affect somewhat altered or incongruent to situation; changes over the course of hours; emotion are mostly under self-control

2 Affect is often inappropriate or incongruent to situation; changes over the course of minutes; emotion are not consistently under self-control, thought they respond to redirection by others

3 Severe and consistent disinhibition of emotions; affect changes rapidly, is inappropriate to context, and does not respond to redirection by others

5. Language

Rate abnormalities of spoken, written, or sign language that cannot be attributed to dialect or stuttering. Assess fluency, grammar, comprehension, semantic content, and naming. Test comprehension and naming nonverbally if necessary by having patient follow commands or point.

0 Normal language

1 Mild impairment including word-finding or problems with naming or fluency

2 Moderate impairment including comprehension difficulties or deficit in meaningful communication (semantic content)

3 Severe impairment including nonsensical semantic content, word salad, muteness, or severely reduced comprehension

6. Thought process abnormalities

Rate abnormalities of thinking processes based on verbal or written output. If a patient does not speak or write, do not rate this item.

0 Normal thought process

1 Tangential or circumstantial

2 Associations loosely connected occasionally, but largely comprehensible

3 Associations loosely connected most of the time

7. Motor agitation

Rate by observation, including from other sources of observation, such as visitors, family, and clinical staff. Do not include dyskinesia, tics, or chorea.

0 No restlessness or agitation

1 Mild restlessness of gross motor movements or mild fidgetiness

2 Moderate motor agitation including dramatic movements of the extremities, pacing, fidgeting, removing IVs, etc.

3 Severe motor agitation, such as combativeness or a need for restraints or seclusion

8. Motor retardation

Rate movements by direct observation or from other sources of observation, such as family, visitors, and clinical staff. Do not rate components of retardation caused by Parkinsonian symptoms. Do not rate drowsiness or sleep.

0 No slowness of voluntary movements

1 Mildly reduced frequency, spontaneity, or speed of motor movements, to the degree that may interfere somewhat with the assessment

2 Moderately reduced frequency, spontaneity, or speed of motor movements, to the degree that it interferes with participation in activities of self-care

3 Severe motor retardation with few spontaneous movements

9. Orientation

Patients who cannot speak can be a visual or auditory presentation of multiple-choice answers. Allow patient to be wrong by up to 7 days instead of 2 days for patients hospitalized more than 3 weeks. Disorientation to person means not recognizing familiar persons and may be intact even if the person has naming difficulty but recognizes the person. Disorientation to person is most severe when one doesn't know one's own identity and is rare. Disorientation to person usually occurs after disorientation to time and/or place.

0 Oriented to person, place, and time.

1 Disoriented to time (e.g. by more 2 days or wrong month or wrong year) or to place (e.g. mane of building, city, state), but not both

2 Disoriented to time and place

3 Disoriented to person

10. Attention

Patients with sensory deficits or who are intubated or whose hand movements are constrained should be tested using an alternate modality besides writing. Attention can be assessed during the interview (e.g. verbal perseverations, distractibility, and diffi-culty with set shifting) and/or through use of specific tests, e.g. digit span.

0 Alert and attentive

1 Mildly distractible or mild difficulty sustaining attention, but able to refocus with cueing. On formal testing makes only minor errors and is not significantly slow in responses

2 Moderate inattention with difficulty focusing and sustaining attention. On formal test-ing, makes numerous errors and either requires prodding to focus or finish the task.

3 Severe difficulty focusing and/or sustaining attention with many incorrect or incomplete responses or inability to follow instructions. Distractible by other noises or events in the environment.

11. Short-term memory

Defined as recall of information (e.g. 3 items presented either verbally or visually) after a delay of about 2 to 3 minutes. When formally tested, information must be reg-istered adequately before recall is tested. The number of trials to register as well as effect of cueing can be noted on scoresheet. Patient should not be allowed to rehearse during the delay period and should be distracted during the time. Patient may speak or nonverbally communicate to the examiner the identity of the correct items. Short-term deficits noticed during the course of the interview can be used also.

0 Short-term memory intact

1 Recalls 2/3 items; may be able to recall third item after category cueing

2 Recalls 1/3 items; may be able to recall other item after category cueing

3 Recalls 0/3 items

12. Long-term memory

Can be assessed formally through interviewing for recall of past personal (e.g. past medical history or experiences that can be corroborated from another source) or gen-eral information that is culturally relevant. When formally tested, use a verbal and/or visual modality for 3 items that are adequately registered and recalled after at least 5 minutes. The patient should be not be allowed to rehearse during the delay period during formal testing. Make allowances for patients with less than 8 years of education or who are mentally retarded regarding general information question. Rating of the severity of deficits may involve a judgment about all the ways long-term memory is assessed, including recent and/or remote long-term memory ability informally tested during the interview as well as any formal testing of recent long-term memory using 3 items.

0 No significant long-term memory deficits

1 Recalls 2/3 items and/or has minor difficulty recalling details of other long-term information

2 Recalls 1/3 items and/or has moderate difficulty recalling other long-term information

3 Recalls 0/3 items and/or has severe difficulty recalling other long-term information

13. Visuospatial ability

Assess informally and formally. Consider patient's difficulty navigating one's way around living areas or environment (e.g. getting lost). Test formally by drawing or copying a design, by arranging puzzle pieces, or by drawing a map and identifying major cities, etc. Take into account any visual impairments that may affect performance.

0 No impairment

1 Mild impairment such that overall design and most details or pieces are correct; and/or little difficulty navigating in his/her surroundings

2 Moderate impairment with distorted appreciation of overall design and/or several errors of details or pieces, and/or needing repeated redirection to keep from getting lost in a newer environment; trouble locating familiar object in immediate environment

3 Severe impairment on formal testing; and/or repeated or getting lost in environment

DRS-R-98 Optional Diagnostic Items

These three items can be used to assist in the differentiation of delirium from other disorders for diagnostic and research purposes. They are added to the severity score for the total scale score, but are *not* included in the severity score.

14. Temporal onset symptoms

Rate the acuteness of onset of the initial symptoms of the disorder or episode being currently assessed, not their duration. Distinguish the onset of symptoms attributable to delirium when it occurs currently with a different pre-existing psychiatric disorder. For example, if a patient with major depression is rated during a delirium episode due to an overdose, then rate the onset of the delirium symptoms.

0 No significant change from usual or longstanding baseline behaviour

1 Gradual onset of symptoms, occurring over a period of several week to a month

2 Acute change in behaviour or personality occurring over days to a week

3 Abrupt change in behaviour occurring over a period of several hours to a day

15. Fluctuation of symptoms severity

Rate the waxing and waning of an individual or cluster of symptom(s) over the time frame being rated. Usually applies to cognition, affect, intensity of hallucinations, thought disorder, and language disturbance. Take into consideration that perceptual disturbance usually occur intermittently, but might cluster in period of greater intensity when other symptoms fluctuate in severity.

0 No symptom fluctuation

1 Symptoms intensity fluctuates in severity over hours

2 Symptoms intensity fluctuates in severity over minutes

16. Physical disorders

Rate the degree to which a psychological, medical, or pharmacological problem can be specifically attributed to have caused the symptom being assessed. Many patients have such a problem but they may or may not have a causal relationship to the symptoms being rated.

0 None present or active

1 Presence of any physical disorder that might affect mental state

2 Drug, infection, metabolic disorder, CSN lesion, or other medical problem that specifically can be implicated in causing the altered behaviour or mental state.

DRS-R-98 SCORESHEET

Name of patient: _____ Date: ___/___/___ Time: _____

Name of Rater: _____

SEVERITY SCORE: [ ] TOTAL SCORE: [ ]

Severity Item	Item Score				Optional Information
Sleep-wake cycle	0	1	2	3	Naps Nocturnal disturbance only Day-night reversal
Perceptual disturbances	0	1	2	3	Sensory type of illusion or hallucination: Auditory visual olfactory tactile Format of illusion or hallucination: simple complex
Delusions	0	1	2	3	Type of delusion: persecutory Nature: poorly formed systematized
Lability of affect	0	1	2	3	Type: angry anxious dysphoric Elated irritable
Language	0	1	2	3	Check here intubated, mute, etc.
Thought process	0	1	2	3	Check here intubated, mute, etc.
Motor agitation	0	1	2	3	Check here if restrained Type of restraints:
Motor retardation	0	1	2	3	Check here if restrained Type of restraints:
Orientation	0	1	2	3	Date: Place: Person:
Attention	0	1	2	3	
Shot-term memory	0	1	2	3	Record # of trials for registration of items: Check here if category cueing helped
Long-term memory	0	1	2	3	Check here if category cueing helped
Visuospatial ability	0	1	2	3	Check here if unable to use hands
Diagnostic Item	Item Score				
Temporal onset of symptom	0	1	2	3	Check here if symptoms appeared on a background of other psychopathology
Fluctuation of symptom severity	0	1	2		Check here if symptoms only appeared during the night

Fig. A5.1 The DRS-R-98 scoresheet.

Appendix 4

The Memorial Delirium Assessment Scale (MDAS)

The following is reprinted from Breitbart etal. (1997) with permission from Elsevier.

Instructions: Rate the severity of the following symptoms of delirium based on current interaction with subject or assessment of his/her behaviour or experience over past several hours (as indicated in each time).

Item 1—Reduced level of consciousness (awareness)

Rate the patient's current awareness of and interaction with the environment (interviewer, other people/object in the room; for example, ask patients to describe their surrounding).

☐	0	None	(Patient spontaneously fully aware of environment and interacts appropriately)
☐	1	Mild	(Patient is unaware of some elements in the environment, or not spontaneously interacting appropriately with the interviewer; becomes fully aware and appropriately interactive when prodded strongly; interview is prolonged but not seriously disrupted)
☐	2	Moderate	(Patient is unaware of some or all elements in the environment, or not spontaneously interacting appropriately with the interviewer; becomes incompletely aware and appropriately interactive when prodded strongly; interview is prolonged but not seriously disrupted)
☐	3	Severe	(Patient is unaware of all elements in the environment with no spontaneous interaction or awareness of the interviewer; so that the interview is difficult-to-impossible, even with maximal prodding)

Item 2—Disorientation

Rate current state by asking the following 10 orientation items: date, month, day, year, season, floor, name of hospital, city state, and country.

☐	0	None	(Patient knows 9-10 items)
☐	1	Mild	(Patient knows 7-8 items)
☐	2	Moderate	(Patient knows 5-6 items)
☐	3	Severe	(Patient knows no more than 4 items)

Item 3—Short-term memory impairment

Rate current state by using repetition and delayed recall of 3 words. Patient must immediately repeat and recall words 5 minutes later after an intervening task. Use alternate sets of 3 words for successive evaluations (e.g. apple, table, tomorrow; sky, cigar, justice).

☐   0   None   (All 3 words repeated and recalled)

☐   1   Mild   (All 3 words repeated, patient fails to recall 1)

☐   2   Moderate (All 3 words repeated, patient fails to recall 2-3)

☐   3   Severe   (Patient fails to repeat 1 or more words)

Item 4—Impaired digit span

Rate current performance by asking subjects to repeat first 3, 4, then 5 digits forward and then 3, then 4 backwards; continue to the next step only if patient succeeds at the previous one.

☐   0   None   (Patient can do at least 5 numbers forward and 4 backward)

☐   1   Mild   (Patient can do at least 5 numbers forward and 3 backward)

☐   2   Moderate (Patient can do 4-5 numbers forward, cannot do 3 backward)

☐   3   Severe   (Patient can do no more than 3 numbers forward)

Item 5—Reduced ability to maintain and shift attention

As indicated during the interview by questions needing to be rephrased and/or repeated because patient's attention wanders, patient loses track, patient is distracted by outside stimuli or over-absorbed in a task.

☐   0   None   (None of the above, patient maintains and shifts attention normally)

☐   1   Mild   (Above attentional problems occur once or twice without prolonging the interview)

☐   2   Moderate (Above attentional problems occur often, prolonging the interview without seriously disrupting it)

☐   3   Severe   (Above attentional problems occur constantly, disrupting and making the interview difficult-to-impossible)

Item 6—Disorganized thinking

As indicated during the interview by rambling, irrelevant, or incoherent speech, or by tangential, circumstantial, or faulty reasoning. Ask patient a somewhat complex question (e.g. 'Describe your current medical condition.').

☐   0   None   (Patient's speech is coherent and goal-directed)

☐   1   Mild   (Patient's speech is slightly difficult to follow; responses to questions are slightly off target but not so much as to prolong the interview)

☐   2   Moderate (Disorganized thought or speech are clearly present, such that interview is prolonged but not disrupted)

☐   3   Severe   (Examination is very difficult or impossible due to disorganized thinking or speech)

Item 7—Perceptual disturbance

Misperceptions, illusions, and hallucinations inferred from inappropriate behaviour during the interview or admitted by subject, as well as those elicited from nurse/family/chart accounts of the past several hours or of the time since last examination:

☐	0	None	(No misperceptions, illusions, hallucinations)
☐	1	Mild	(Misperceptions, or illusions related to sleep, fleeting hallucinations on 1-2 occasions without inappropriate behaviour)
☐	2	Moderate	(Hallucinations or frequent illusions on several occasions with minimal inappropriate behaviour that does not disrupt the interview)
☐	3	Severe	(Frequent or intense illusions or hallucinations with persistent inappropriate behaviour that disrupts the interview or seriously interferes with medical care)

Item 8—Delusions

Rate delusions inferred from inappropriate behaviour during the interview or admitted by patient, as well as delusions elicited from nurse/family/chart accounts of the past several hours or of the time since the previous examination

☐	0	None	(No evidence of misinterpretations or delusion)
☐	1	Mild	(Misperceptions, or suspiciousness without clear delusional ideas or inappropriate behaviour)
☐	2	Moderate	(Delusions admitted by the patient or evidenced by his/her behaviour that do not or only marginally disrupt the interview or interfere with medical care)
☐	3	Severe	(Persistent and/or intense delusions resulting in inappropriate behaviour, disrupting the interview or seriously interfering with medical care)

Item 9—Decreased or increased psychomotor activity

Rate activity over past several hours, as well as activity during the interview, by circling (a) hypoactive, (b) hyperactive, or (c) elements of both present

☐	0	None	(Normal psychomotor activity)
☐	1 a b c	Mild	(Hypoactivity is barely noticeable, expressed as slightly slowing of movement. Hyperactivity is barely noticeable or appears as simple restlessness)
☐	2 a b c	Moderate	(Hypoactivity is undeniable, with marked reduction in the number of movements or marked slowness of movement; subject rarely spontaneously moves or speaks. Hyperactivity is undeniable, subject moves almost constantly; in both cases, exam is prolonged as a consequence)
☐	3 a b c	Severe	(Hypoactivity is severe, patient does not move or speak without prodding; is catatonic. Hyperactivity is severe; patient is constantly moving, overreacts to stimuli, and requires surveillance and or restraint; getting through the exam is difficult or impossible)

Item 10—Sleep–wake cycle disturbance (disorder of arousal)

Rate patient's ability to either sleep or stay awake at the appropriate times. Utilize direct observation during the interview, as well as reports from nurses, family, patient, or charts describing sleep–wake cycle disturbance over the past several hours or since last examination. Use observations of the previous night for morning evaluations only.

☐	0	None	(At night sleep well; during the day, has no trouble staving awake)
☐	1	Mild	(Mild deviation from appropriate sleepfulness and wakefulness states: at night, difficulty falling asleep or transient night awakening; need medication to sleep well; during the day, reports periods of drowsiness or, during the interview, is drowsy but can easily awaken him/herself)
☐	2	Moderate	(Moderate deviations from appropriate sleepfulness and wakefulness states: at night, sleeplessness; during the day, patient spends most of the time sleeping or, during the interview, can only be roused to complete wakefulness by strong stimuli)
☐	3	Severe	(Severe deviations from appropriate sleepfulness and wakefulness states: at night, repeated and prolonged night awakening; during the day, reports of frequent and prolonged napping or, during the interview, cannot be roused to full wakefulness by any stimuli)

Appendix 5

The Nursing Delirium Screening Scale (Nu-DESC)

Features Description	Symptoms Rating (0-2)		
Time period	Midnight–8 AM	8 AM–4 PM	4 PM–Midnight
Symptom			
I. Disorientation			
Verbal or behavioural manifestation of not being oriented to time or place or misperceiving persons in the environment			
II. Inappropriate behaviour			
Behaviour inappropriate to place and/or for the person; e.g. pulling at tubes or dressings, attempting to get out of bed when that is contraindicated, and the like.			
III. Inappropriate communication			
Communication inappropriate to place and/or for the person; e.g. incoherence, noncommunicativeness, nonsensical or unintelligible speech			
IV. Illusions/hallucinations			
Seeing or hearing things that are not there; distortions of visual objects			
V. Psychomotor retardation			
Delayed responsiveness, few or no spontaneous actions/words; e.g. when the patient is prodded, reaction is deferred and/or the patient is unarousable			
Total score			

Symptoms are rated from 0 to 2 based on the presence and intensity of each symptom and individual ratings are added to obtain a total score per shift. The first four items of the Nu-DESC are included in the CRS.
Reproduced from Gaudreau et al. (2005b) with permission from Elsevier.

Index

Page numbers in *italic* indicate figures and tables.